RACIAL AND ETHNIC
DIFFERENCES IN DISEASE

RACIAL AND ETHNIC DIFFERENCES IN DISEASE

ANTHONY P. POLEDNAK, Ph.D.

Department of Community and Preventive Medicine
State University of New York at Stony Brook

New York   Oxford
OXFORD UNIVERSITY PRESS
1989

Oxford University Press

Oxford   New York   Toronto
Delhi   Bombay   Calcutta   Madras   Karachi
Petaling Jaya   Singapore   Hong Kong   Tokyo
Nairobi   Dar es Salaam   Cape Town
Melbourne   Auckland

and associated companies in
Berlin   Ibadan

Copyright © 1989 by Oxford University Press, Inc.

Published by Oxford University Press, Inc.,
200 Madison Avenue, New York, New York 10016

Oxford is a registered trademark of Oxford University Press

Library of Congress Cataloging-in-Publication Data
Polednak, Anthony P.
Racial and ethnic differences in disease / Anthony P. Polednak.
p.   cm.   Bibliography: p.   Includes index.   ISBN 0-19-505970-0
1. Medical anthropology.   2. Health and race.
3. Ethnic groups—Diseases.   I. Title.
GN296.P65   1989   616.07′1—dc 19   89-3121   CIP

9 8 7 6 5 4 3 2 1
Printed in the United States of America

To the memory of
Albert Damon, M.D., Ph.D. (1918–1973)

Preface

This book is intended for students and researchers in anthropology, public health, and medicine. A subdiscipline, called biomedical anthropology, has emerged within physical anthropology mainly during the past 15–20 years. Unique aspects of physical anthropology include the consideration of human populations as biocultural groups in an evolutionary perspective, continually subject to natural selection via differential mortality and fertility, and the focus of human variation and adaptation based on genetic and environmental influences. The main distinction of *biomedical* anthropology is its orientation toward the study of disease in modern populations. This contrasts with other applications of physical anthropology—for example, in archaeology, population genetics, paleopathology, forensic sciences, and human engineering. The present volume deals with some aspects of biomedical anthropology—that is, with biological and cultural variation by racial and ethnic group in relation to disease susceptibility, and prognosis or outcome after disease has been diagnosed.

This volume has been designed so that it can be used as a textbook for courses in biomedical anthropology at both advanced undergraduate and graduate levels. It could be supplemented by a basic textbook in medical statistics or biostatistics in an upper-level undergraduate course. Alternatively, in a graduate-level course in biomedical anthropology, such biostatistical training could be offered separately or obtained at a school of public health. Students in public health may also be interested in a course in biomedical anthropology, whether offered in a graduate school anthropology program or at a school of public health.

The book is organized by broad disease categories. Clinical applications of knowledge of racial and ethnic differences in disease are made apparent in this text, so that it should be of interest to clinicians who deal with patients of various racial and ethnic backgrounds. In dealing with such a broad range of diseases it is difficult to provide coverage of similar depth for specific disorders. The separate chapters on single-gene disorders, infectious and parasitic diseases, cardiovascular diseases, and cancers reflect the availability of more information on population differences in frequency but also to some extent the author's interests. In contrast, Chapter 9 covers a wide range of chronic diseases and other disorders, in less depth. The extensive bibliography should aid those readers interested in exploring these areas in more detail. Many individual studies are briefly summarized and critically appraised. It is hoped that the authors of these reports will understand that extensive discussion of each study was not feasible and that generalizations and interpretations may differ among scientists.

The idea for a book on this subject emerged some years ago from discussions with the late Dr. Albert Damon, who had a keen interest in certain areas of applied physical anthropology. Hopefully some measure of the original goal of increasing awareness of this area of applied physical anthropology can be achieved. The present volume is an expansion of a chapter in the author's *Host Factors in Disease* (Charles C. Thomas, publisher, 1987).

The author wishes to acknowledge the support of the Department of Community and Preventive Medicine at the School of Medicine of the State University of New York at Stony Brook, including access to word-processing equipment, during much of the writing of this book.

Stony Brook, N.Y.   A. P. P.
November 1988

Contents

RACIAL AND ETHNIC
DIFFERENCES IN DISEASE

1
Introduction: Concepts of Racial/Ethnic Group in Epidemiology

DEFINITIONS

Races are not artificial assemblages of "types" but natural units or populations that undergo evolutionary change. These groups differ slightly in gene frequencies and share some more or less distinct biological characteristics. *Ethnic groups* are culturally distinct. The two kinds of groups, of course, overlap. Among immigrants in Milwaukee, Wisconsin, ethnic categories (i.e., German, Italian, Irish, and Polish) defined by surname and by origin of grandparents showed differences in frequencies of certain genes (Stevenson et al., 1983).

The United Nations has recommended use of "ethnic group" as a comprehensive term, and "race" is no longer recommended, as in the UNESCO Statements on Race (see Montagu, 1960). The concept of biological race, however, may have some *limited* usefulness in physical anthropology (Baker, 1967; Howells, 1971) as well as in clinical medicine, epidemiology, and public health (Watts, 1981). The concept of race, although imprecise, has utility in descriptive epidemiological studies that may yield etiologic hypotheses to be explored by more detailed studies. Many health surveys, including the U.S. National Health Interview Survey, include questions on self-assessed race and ethnic identification (see Chapter 4).

From the viewpoint of the biological anthropologist, the adjective "racial" may be convenient because some biological traits predominate in some groups and help to distinguish geographic groups (Lasker and Tyzzer, 1982). The concept of *clines*, however, may prove even more meaningful in physical anthropology and epidemiology. Clines are geographic gradients in traits such as skin color and HLA (human leukocyte or major histocompatibility complex) phenotypes or other genetic polymorphisms. Continued discovery of such geographic gradients in key characteristics, such as genetic traits related to adaptations to malaria, indicate that the need to rely on "racial" groups will diminish as the methods of population genetics define the features of human biological adaptation. Population genetics, for example, has clarified the origin and molecular nature of sickling mutations in world populations, indicating that these mutations arose separately in populations in West Africa versus other parts of Africa and Asia

(Kan and Dozy, 1980), presumably in response to the same selective force (i.e., malaria). It is worth noting that many scientists including health workers mistakenly believe that sickling disorders are restricted to "Africans" or "blacks" (see Chapter 5.)

Thus, the use of racial groups may be an interim solution to the problem of describing human variability, with reference to disease patterns. This point will be discussed later with regard to other reasons for retaining the use of racial and ethnic categories in epidemiologic studies.

The major races of man (i.e., Caucasoid, Negroid, and Mongoloid) differ slightly in the frequency of known genes, such as those determining blood groups and certain proteins (see Chapter 3). These broad racial labels indicate little of the variety of adaptations of each major race in any large geographic region such as a continent or subcontinent with many ecosystems (Lasker and Tyzzer, 1982). The African continent provides a good example of such diversity, one basic division being between north and south of the Sahara. Other divisions include Khoisan language groups (now mainly in South Africa), Bantu expansionists, various East and West African populations, pygmies and pygmoids, and Nilotes (Hiernaux, 1975; Franklin et al., 1981) (see Chapter 3). Racial classifications have attempted to address this intraracial diversity by the use of subcategories (Chapter 3).

Racial groups are "evolutionary episodes" (Hulse, 1962) that change continuously and over relatively short periods of time owing to migration and intermixture. Estimation of the amount of intermixture is the task of physical anthropologists. Over long periods of time (i.e., generations), these estimated levels of admixture are subject to change.

Analogous with the problem of discerning racial variation in the presence of clines or geographic gradients in frequency of traits is the difficulty in distinguishing racial or ethnic differences in disease from apparent differences related to geographic (latitude) variation. This geographic variation may reflect environmental factors or clines in traits or gene frequencies, usually of unknown nature. Examples are North–South gradients in multiple sclerosis and Hodgkin's disease, and gradients for various cancers in China. Geographic patterns in disease may transcend racial and ethnic boundaries, as in adaptations to diseases ubiquitous in large geographic areas. Thus, apparent racial/ethnic concentrations of disease must be distinguished from broader geographic patterns.

What constitutes an *ethnic group* is sometimes difficult to define, and definitions shade into more loosely aggregated populations characterized by similar cultural characteristics such as dietary habits. These culturally distinct groups are regarded as subgroups of racial categories. "Ethnic" groups, however, may also exhibit certain genetic differences (e.g., in frequencies of HLA types). There is confusion regarding the definition of certain groups such as "Hispanics," and there is a lack of consensus on the choice of an appropriate label (Yankauer, 1987; Trevino, 1987). "Hispanics" do not constitute a racial grouping but comprise heterogeneous subgroups differing in geographic origin and cultural factors. These subgroups may be both culturally and biologically distinct (see Chapter 3).

In the *Harvard Encyclopedia of American Ethnic Groups* (Thernstrom, 1980), the list of features characterizing ethnicity includes common geographical origin, language, religious faith, cultural ties (e.g., shared traditions, values, symbols, literature, music, and food preferences), and shared political interests regarding the homeland. Social anthropological compendia of world cultures include hundreds of groups, and Murdock (1981) has recorded sociocultural-political characteristics for 563 societies.

Religious groups may be culturally distinct with regard to age at marriage and personal habits such as diet and use of tobacco and alcohol. These groups may be both culturally and to some extent biologically distinct because of a tendency to marry within the group (as in Jewish groups; see Chapter 3). The 17th-century philosopher Spinoza noted the social function of religion (e.g., Judaism) which involves not only moral principles but rules for social organization, marriage, diet, and other practices such as circumcision (as in the Torah or Mosaic law) (Allison, 1987). Ethnicity among left-wing American Jews, based on origin and background, was cultivated by symbolic representations including stories, poems and songs, Yiddish humor, dances, and a sense of shared social concern or responsibility toward all people (Schwartz, 1984). In contrast, "ethnicity" is diminishing among American Catholics of European ancestry (Alba, 1981), and this group is no longer significantly different from others in contraceptive behavior.

Recent interest in epidemiologic studies of religious groups has increased because of their relevance to studies of social networks and social support (Idler, 1987; Jarvis and Northcott, 1987; Najman et al., 1988), as well as cultural practices, in relation to health. Such diverse groups as Parsis, Moslems, and Seventh-Day Adventists, have been included in epidemiologic studies, as discussed later.

In summary, the concept of "racial" or biologically distinct groups may be of some limited use in physical anthropology and epidemiology. "Ethnic group" is often used instead of "race" as well as in a more limited sense of a culturally distinct group. It is difficult to define some groups as either culturally or biologically distinct, while others are distinct both biologically and culturally. There is some agreement that major "races" or groups with limited biological distinctiveness exist, but others regard such groups as either artificial creations or components of broader (clinal) patterns. A classification of these major racial groups is provided in Chapter 3. In this book we will often use the comprehensive label "racial/ethnic" to reflect the different uses of these terms and the difficulties in delineating a specific group as culturally and/or biologically distinct.

USE OF RACIAL/ETHNIC GROUP CONCEPTS IN EPIDEMIOLOGY

Disease patterns vary geographically or across different countries, and some of these countries differ in racial/ethnic composition. Epidemiologic studies of disease rates across different countries, as well as within a country, may provide clues regarding causation of disease. These causes may be environmental factors involving personal habits that differ in frequency among racial/ethnic groups. The proliferation of atlases dealing with geographical patterns of disease, sometimes including consideration of racial/ethnic groups, indicates the growing interest in describing these patterns. The main impetus lies in broadly delineating the potential scope of environmental influences in disease causation—for example, with regard to cancers and cardiovascular diseases.

Racial and ethnic differences in disease may exist within the same small geographic area, leading to speculation regarding causal factors associated with these groups. Obviously, not all ethnic groups have been studied intensively with regard to disease patterns, but the value of such studies is abundantly clear. In Singapore, for example, age-standardized incidence rates for total cancers are much higher in Chinese than in Malays or Indians. Cancer of nasopharynx is high in Chinese while cancer of the mouth is high in Indians (Shanmugaratnam et al., 1983). Such environmental factors as smoking and chewing of tobacco (i.e., personal habits) may be involved in these differences, as discussed in this book. Microenvironments may differ by racial/ethnic group within the same macroenvironment, and these differences may help to explain differences in disease patterns.

A few other examples will suffice. Religious–ethnic groups in Bombay, India—including Moslems, Christians, and Parsis—differ in customs and habits, as reflected in differences in incidence rates for specific cancers (Jussawalla et al., 1985). Numerous studies have also been conducted on diverse groups in Jerusalem defined by ethnic group, country of origin, and religious practices. In Los Angeles, California, striking differences in mortality rates among racial–ethnic groups (e.g., blacks, Hispanics and Anglos) (Frerichs et al., 1984) provide impetus for studies of explanatory factors.

Racial and ethnic differences in certain diseases may be due largely or entirely to differences in socioeconomic status (SES) and environmental factors associated with SES. Other differences transcend SES and reflect not only cultural differences but social stresses, prejudices, and social inequalities. Thus, another reason for compiling statistics on disease by racial and ethnic group is to substantiate such socioeconomic inequalities and the effects of discrimination on health. The prime example is apartheid in South Africa, but racial discrimination in the United States may result in health inequalities that are greater than those predicted by SES alone. In large urban areas of the northeastern and north central United States, residential segregation of blacks from Anglos (i.e., non-Hispanic whites) has not decreased in recent decades even in middle-class areas (Massey and Denton, 1987). The U.S. black–white gap in urban underemployment has also increased among young adults in recent years (Lichter, 1988).

Data for adequate evaluation of racial inequalities in economic opportunities and health may not exist. As noted in the United Nations publication *Apartheid and Health* (WHO, 1983), data on health status and disease frequency by racial group in South Africa are inadequate. Sources of error in South African statistics on cancer include uncertain population sizes and large numbers of deaths among blacks certified as due to "ill-defined" causes (Wyndham, 1985). Reliable data on mortality among South African blacks are needed for public health planning, as noted by health researchers in South Africa (Botha and Bradshaw, 1985; Botha et al., 1988). In the United States data quality is much better than in South Africa, but there are still few studies that attempt to separate the effects of socioeconomic differences and other social inequalities on racial differences in the frequency and course of disease. Some examples of these analytic studies will be discussed in this book.

It is the author's view that the concept of biological race has some value despite its limitations and should be maintained as long as it is useful. Hopefully racial prejudices will be abolished through social progress. In U.S. surveys antiblack prejudice (defined by attitudes regarding segregation and intermarriage) has declined in recent decades, especially in the South, due to a birth-cohort effect (Firebaugh and Davis, 1988). Amalgamation will increase even further the genetic and biological overlap between "races." Black–white amalgamation in the United States may take a considerable amount of time (Heer, 1967), while in Brazil there is a strong trend toward black–white admixture (Azevedo et al., 1983).

As noted earlier, racial differences in disease may be explained by a wide variety of factors—socioeconomic, sociocultural, biological, and genetic. Whatever the explanations for racial differences, there is increasing recognition of the need for targeting education and prevention programs to certain racial/ethnic groups, such as U.S. blacks, with regard to cancer, coronary heart disease, hypertension, tuberculosis, and AIDS (acquired immune deficiency syndrome).

Epidemiologic studies of certain ethnic–religious groups that differ culturally may provide clues regarding disease causation. The need for more extensive data on ethnic differences in disease is becoming more widely recognized. Maps showing the geographic locations of 11 major ethnic groups in the United States (Morin et al., 1984), defined by county of origin, may be used in the planning of various types of epidemiologic studies. These 11 countries or groups of countries with "similar economic and social characteristics" include "British" (from England, Scotland, and Wales); "Irish" (Ireland and Northern Ireland); "Scandinavian" (Norway, Sweden, Denmark, Finland); "German" (West Germany, East Germany) "other Middle European" (Netherlands, Switzerland); "Polish" (Poland); "Czechoslovakian" (Czechoslovakia); "Russian" (Russia, Lithuania); "other East European" (Austria, Hungary, Yugoslavia, Romania); "South European" (Greece, Italy, Portugal); and "Latin America" (Mexico, Central and South America) (Morin et al., 1984). While one could argue with the definitions of these categories, from an anthropological perspective, their use provides a basis for more definitive epidemiologic studies that could benefit from the input of both cultural and physical anthropologists.

Morin et al. (1984) noted that the ethnic map for "Latin Americans" obscured high concentrations of Puerto Ricans in the large population of New York City and that recent influxes of such groups as Cubans, although settling in areas with already high concentrations of "Latins," presented problems in enumeration. The need for studies on the health of various U.S. "Latin American" or "Hispanic" groups has only recently been recognized. Mexican-Americans were earmarked as an understudied population from a public health perspective (Hazuda et al., 1983). Studies of cancers and other chronic diseases, such as gallbladder and cardiovascular diseases, or risk factors for these diseases in Mexican-

Americans and other Hispanic groups have appeared recently. The delineation of cultural factors independent of SES in diabetes and cardiovascular risk factors in Mexican-Americans is one example of the relevance of such studies (Stern et al., 1984). Sources of data on health and health-related factors in U.S. Hispanics have expanded greatly in recent years (see Chapter 4), and disease patterns will be discussed in this book.

Surnames as an indicator for Mexican-American and other Hispanic ethnicity have been used in health research, and the use of parental surnames also has been advocated (Hazuda and Stern, 1986). Surnames have wide utility in anthropological research, including the delineation of ethnic groups in large American cities (Stevenson et al., 1983) and Asian ethnic groups in England (Nicoll et al., 1986). The use of surnames in investigating affinities of groups has been summarized in a special issue of *Human Biology* (Gottlieb, 1983) and by Lasker (1985).

Racial and ethnic groups may differ in their cultural patterns of attitudes toward illness, as reflected in delay in seeking medical care and stage at diagnosis of disease. Again, these differences may simply reflect socioeconomic factors or may be independent of SES, and it is the task of epidemiologic studies to provide explanations (see Chapter 2). The status of ill (including "mentally ill") persons and the elderly may differ across ethnic groups, with effects on the outcome of disease. Differences in perception of illness and in interactions with practitioners in selected ethnic groups, including blacks in America, are of interest to medical anthropologists (Harwood, 1981). Medical anthropologists are also becoming increasingly interested in describing and explaining racial/ethnic differences in disease.

The interrelationships of the disciplines of biomedical anthropology, social anthropology, medical anthropology, and epidemiology (Fig. 1.1) will become evident in this book. Increased fruitful collaboration among epidemiologists, biomedical anthropologists, and medical anthropologists is to be expected. Fundamental to such collaboration is a shared foundation in epidemiological methods needed for delineating racial/ethnic differences in disease and in interpreting these differences. We now turn to brief consideration of these epidemiologic methods.

EPIDEMIOLOGIC STUDY DESIGNS

The first step in the epidemiologic method is the description of disease prevalence according to characteristics of person (or "host"), place, and time. This book is concerned with one broad characteristic of person—namely, racial or ethnic group. "Place" is also considered herein, because certain geographical boundaries may contain a predominant racial/ethnic group. Geographically related patterns must be distinguished from racial/ethnic patterns. As noted above, racial/ethnic differences in environmental/cultural factors and disease risks may exist within the same geographic area. Other apparent racial/ethnic differences in disease prevalence, however, may be part of a broader pattern—for example, genetic polymorphisms and genetic diseases related to adaptation to malaria (see Chapter 5). Time changes in disease rates in different countries and among racial/

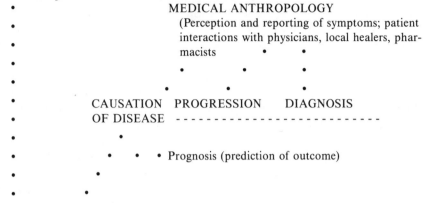

SOCIAL ANTHROPOLOGY
Cross- and within-culture studies of sexual habits; marriage and reproductive patterns; smoking, alcohol, and drug use patterns; dietary habits and food preferences; acculturation processes and sociocultural interactions)

                              MEDICAL ANTHROPOLOGY
                              (Perception and reporting of symptoms; patient interactions with physicians, local healers, pharmacists

                    CAUSATION   PROGRESSION   DIAGNOSIS
                    OF DISEASE -

                          • • • Prognosis (prediction of outcome)

EPIDEMIOLOGY • • • • • • • • BIOMEDICAL ANTHROPOLOGY
(Search for causes through descriptive   (Human biological variation in relation
and analytic studies; studies of disease   to disease: age, sex, race/ethnic group,
outcome and severity; factors contribut-   body build, genetic variation, biochemi-
ing to adverse outcomes and death)   cal and physiologic variation)

Figure 1.1   Interrelationships of epidemiology and anthropology.

ethnic groups also should be considered in evaluating the role of environmental factors in disease.

The results of *descriptive* studies of disease prevalence may lead to the formulation of hypotheses aimed at explaining racial/ethnic differences. Testing of these hypotheses involves *analytic* epidemiologic studies.

Descriptive Studies

Descriptive studies involve calculation of *rates* of disease that are specific to an ethnic or racial group. These rates, which will be used throughout this book, include *incidence* rates, the number of newly diagnosed cases of disease recognized during a specified time period (such as a year) divided by the population at risk during that time period; *prevalence* rates, the number of cases of a given disease on hand during a specified time period, regardless of whether they were first diagnosed during that time period; and *mortality rates*, the number of deaths occurring during a given time period (often 1 year) divided by the estimated population at risk (often at the midpoint of the time interval). *Proportional mortality and incidence ratios* are not rates, because the total population at risk is not involved in their calculation, but rather the proportion of deaths or incident cases attributed to a given disease. These proportional *ratios* are often used when the population at risk cannot be estimated—for example, in developing countries.

Populations defined on the basis of racial/ethnic group usually differ in their age and sex composition. Thus disease rates to be compared must be *specific* for age and sex, or they must be *adjusted* ("standardized") to provide an overall rate that takes into account the age and sex differences in the populations.

Age standardization involves either the "direct" or "indirect" method, described in basic texts such as Hill (1971) and Colton (1974). In the direct method, age-specific rates in the populations under study are applied to a standard population with a known age distribution. The standard population may be the entire U.S. population as determined by censuses (e.g., for 1980) or some other population more appropriate for worldwide comparisons; various standard world or European populations have been used. The proportions of persons in each age group in the standard population are simply multiplied by the age-specific disease rates for each racial/ethnic group and then summed to provide a summary estimate adjusted for age differences in the groups. Examples of these rates and their calculation will be provided later. It should be emphasized that age-standardized rates are summary statistics, and the age-specific rates themselves should be examined to assess consistency of patterns in differences (across age groups) between two or more groups.

Although Henry Clay remarked that "statistics are no substitute for judgment," statistical analyses are an essential element in the process of analysis and interpretation of epidemiological data. In epidemiologic studies, results are often incidence or prevalence rates, which are proportions. These rates can be expressed with confidence limits calculated either on the basis of the normal distribution or the Poisson distribution, the latter for small numbers as numerators. Handy reference tables are available for help in computing such confidence limits (e.g., Haenszel et al., 1962; Lilienfeld, 1967). The trend away from reporting results (e.g., differences between rates) simply as levels of "statistical significance" toward providing probability (p values) and confidence limits on rates or on the difference between two rates is commendable. Differences between two rates (proportions) can be analyzed statistically by methods, such as chi-square tests, familiar to social scientists (Snedecor and Cochran, 1967). In epidemiology, *ratios* of rates in two groups are often important.

"Ecologic" studies involve statistical *correlation* and *regression* methods. In regression the investigator is examining what happens to a dependent variable ("y," or a rate of disease) as one or more independent variables ("x") change. Independent variables include data on populations regarding such factors as composition of food or water. These population data are usually national or regional levels of consumption, available from other surveys, but new survey data may be included. Some examples, to be discussed later in this book, include salt intake with regard to hypertension, fat consumption in relation to breast cancer or other cancer sites as well as cardiovascular diseases, and fiber content of foods in relation to rates of cancers of the large bowel and cardiovascular diseases. In ecologic correlation studies, the proposed causal factors are examined at the group or population level as opposed to the individual level (see following section).

The main problem in interpreting ecologic studies is that many factors other than the one (or ones) being studied may differ among the populations with different disease rates. Thus, some ecologic studies have attempted to control for these other variables by various statistical methods. In *multiple linear regression* several or "n" variables ($x_2 \ldots x_n$) are involved including potential *confounders* that "confound" or complicate the attempt to evaluate the effect of one specific factor (independent variable x_1) on the rate of the disease under study. Confounders are variables associated with both the main independent variable of interest (x_1) and with the dependent variable (y) or disease rate.

As with all multivariate procedures, the results of multiple linear regression depend on the specific independent variables included and on the intercorrelations between these variables. Statistical methods to quantify the degree of confounding between variables in linear regression are important in the interpretation of ecologic studies. In a recent methodologic study, for example, the association between amount of protein consumed and the risk of coronary heart disease (CHD) may be attributed to the association between protein and fat intake (Hartz et al., 1988). The importance of type and amount of fat consumed in explaining population differences in CHD rates will be discussed in Chapter 7.

Multivariable methods are used to test for independent effects of variables and interactions between variables or risk factors in analyses of rates of disease. Similar methods are used by physical (or biomedical) anthropologists and by epidemiologists. Recent advances and applications of multivariate statistical methods in physical anthropology have been presented in Van Ark and Howells (1984). Multivariable statistical methods in epidemiology are mentioned in the next section, with reference to analytic studies.

Analytic Studies

The distinction between descriptive and analytic studies is not clear-cut. The ecologic studies described above resemble analytic studies, but the latter usually involve more intensive data collection including both disease rates and risk factors; also, risk factors are assessed at the individual level by direct measurement or interview. An extensive methodologic literature is developing with regard to the interpretation of ecologic versus analytic studies (e.g., Richardson et al., 1987).

Analytic studies may include racial/ethnic group as a variable along with various potential or known risk factors associated with the disease under study. *Cross-sectional* or prevalence studies involve the determination of disease prevalence and the measurement of risk factors in a defined population at a given point in time. Associations between risk factors and the disease can be assessed by comparing the prevalence of disease in subgroups defined by the presence or absence of risk factors (such as race/ethnic group or other qualitative factors) or by specific levels of quantitative risk factors. Stratified analyses, along with multivariate procedures, can be used to assess the independent effects of a given risk factor by controlling for the effects of other factors. Again, confounding must be assessed.

Stratification of data, by socioeconomic status (SES) or SES-related variables such as income or education, is a useful method in analyses of disease rates in racial/ethnic groups. *Interactions* may be detected between race/ethnic groups and SES in disease; that is, racial/ethnic differences may exist only within one SES stratum (e.g., the lowest). Evidence for such interactions provide valuable clues regarding disease causation. Examples of interaction will be discussed later in this book.

Cohort or incidence studies begin with the identification of a defined population or population sample free of the disease of interest at the start of the study. Data on various risk factors or other attributes are measured or determined in all members of the study cohort, who are then followed over a period of time in order to determine the incidence (i.e., number of new cases) of disease. The incidence rate (defined above) is compared in subgroups of the cohort defined by their attributes measured at the start of the study. Since all cohort members were free of the disease of interest at the start of the study, this longitudinal or prospective approach is relevant to the understanding of the development of the disease and the influence of antecedent factors.

In cohort studies the relative risk is equal to the incidence rate in the exposed group divided by the incidence rate in the nonexposed group. A classic paper on methods of analysis for follow-up studies by Harold F. Dorn, well known in epidemiology in connection with cohort studies of smoking and mortality among U.S. veterans (see Kahn, 1966), appeared in the journal *Human Biology* in 1950 (Dorn, 1950). Numerous examples of relative risks will be provided in this book.

Experimental studies resemble cohort studies in involving follow-up of individual persons to determine outcome, but an intervention or experimental procedure is involved in one group while another group serves as a control. Examples of interventions are diet and excerise programs, and the outcome may be a risk factor (e.g., serum cholesterol or cholesterol fractions) or disease. Such studies are often done in high-risk populations such as specific countries or targeted groups including racial or ethnic groups.

Case-control studies involve the identification of a group of persons with the disease under study, and a comparison or control group without the disease. Associations between the disease and the presence or absence of various factors, or levels of quantitative variables, can be evaluated statistically (see later). Risk factors compared in cases and controls usually involve recall of past events or habits. Careful attention must be given to the accuracy of such information, by using validation procedures based on independent records, and to recall bias or selective recall in diseased persons. Despite these considerations, case-control studies can be an efficient and cost-effective first approach for the study of certain potential risk factors in most diseases that are rare and would require large cohorts and long follow-up for investigation.

The test of association used in case control studies, the chi-square test, is well known. The measure of association is the *relative odds* or *odds ratio*. The usual fourfold table (Table 1.1) may also be used in stratified analyses, in which the table represents one stratum (e.g., age group) "*i*," where $i = 1, 2 \ldots I$ or the total number of strata. The relative odds or odds ratio is simply:

No. of cases with characteristic	divided by	No. controls with characteristic
No. of cases without characteristic		No. of controls without characteristic

or $(a_i/c_i)/(b_i/d_i)$, or $a_i d_i/b_i c_i$.

If the characteristic or exposure is smoking versus nonsmoking, the odds of smoking versus not smoking among cases is compared to the odds of smoking versus not smoking among controls, as if smoking were the number of "successes" in a statistical experiment involving probabilities. In reporting the results of case control studies, it is important to present confidence limits (say 95 percent limits) on the odds ratio that are based on the samples sizes; formulas to be used can be found in epidemiologic texts (e.g., Lilienfeld and Lilienfeld, 1980).

Under certain assumptions, relative odds in case-control studies can represent *estimates* of relative risk of disease in exposed versus unexposed persons. For example, the controls should represent an unbiased estimate of the characteristic under study among the entire nondiseased population from which they are drawn. *Relative risk*, or the ratio of actual rates of disease in two groups, can be calculated only in a prospective or cohort study, where rates of disease can be compared in groups of persons with and without the characteristic (or exposure) under study.

Extensions of simple chi-square tests are ubiquitous in the epidemiologic literature. Prominent among these tests is the Mantel–Haenszel chi-square test for summarizing associations across multiple strata (e.g., age strata). These tests involve the weighting of stratum-specific odds ratios (Table 1.1) using various formulas based on the sample sizes in the strata—the marginal totals ("n_{1i}," etc.) and the grand total ("n_i") (see Kleinbaum et al., 1982). If cases and controls in a case-control study were not matched on age, for example, a summary estimate of relative odds across all age strata would be needed. Applications of stratified analyses include adjusting for the effect of potential confounding variable (e.g., amount of alcohol vs. amount of smoking) on disease risk.

Stratified analyses become difficult when several risk factors or exposures are being examined across several strata such as age groups. As an alternative, multivariate methods have become widely used, especially *logistic regression*,

Table 1.1 Analysis of Results in a Single Stratum ("i") of a Case Control Study

Characteristic or exposure	Cases	Controls	
Present ("1")	a_i	b_i	$a_i + b_i + m_{1i}$
Absent ("0")	c_i	d_i	$c_i + d_i + m_{0i}$
	$a_i + c_i = n_{1i}$	$b_i + d_i = n_{0i}$	$n_i = $ total

A stratum may be defined on the basis of sex, age group, or level of any factor (see text).

which is similar to the linear discriminant function used for classifying an individual into one of two populations (see Kleinbaum et al., 1982; Lee, 1986). In logistic regression the independent variables may be categorical or continuous, the latter including actual individual measurements of physiologic or biochemical variables. Examples of the use of these methods will be given in discussing specific diseases.

STRATEGIES FOR COMPARING RESULTS OF DIFFERENT STUDIES

The ultimate goal of descriptive and analytic epidemiologic studies is the elucidation of disease causation. In experimental studies the goal is the reduction in disease risk through manipulation of the "web of causation," a term used by MacMahon and Pugh (1970). In this book many individual epidemiologic studies of diseases in specific countries or racial/ethnic groups will be compared and contrasted. For a specific disease such as coronary heart disease, the association of disease risk with specific risk factors can be considered in (1) a study within a single population or racial/ethnic group, to assess odds ratios or relative risks associated with these factors; (2) comparing two or more *separate* studies, in different populations or racial/ethnic groups, assessing a similar risk factor(s); and (3) a *single* study of multiple populations or racial/ethnic groups in a defined geographic area or (rarely) in several geographic areas.

A study of risk factors for a specific disease within a single population or racial/ethnic group, without reference to other studies, does not tell us about differences between populations in terms of rates of disease or possible explanations for differences. Such studies are of value, however, within the population in terms of planning programs to reduce the level of that disease in the population.

Comparison of the results of several independent studies, each within a defined population (i.e., country or racial/ethnic group), will indicate either consistency or apparent lack of consistency in associations. If the associations are consistent—for example, increased risk of coronary heart disease (CHD) associated with increasing levels of serum cholesterol—then differences in CHD risk between the populations may be due to differences in distribution of the risk factor (i.e., serum cholesterol). That is, one population may have a higher mean serum cholesterol level than the other population, possibly due to a more proximal cause such as composition of the diet.

The *range of variability* in the putative causal factor may be different in the populations compared, making it more difficult to show a consistent association. If the dose response relationship is not linear (i.e., does not follow a straight line), or risk increases greatly at a threshold level of the risk factor, differences in the range of variability in the risk factor may be especially important. That is, if there are few persons in one population having a level of the risk factor that is sufficiently high to be associated with increased risk of disease, then an association may not be detected.

Thus lack of significant associations between a specific risk factor and a given disease *within* a population does not preclude a role for that factor in explaining differences in disease rates *between* or across populations. Indeed this is the basis for expanding the already existing data base for worldwide variation in cardiovascular diseases and cancers. The assumption is that very low rates (risks) of specific diseases, such as cancer at a specific site, can be achieved through environmental modification—for example, reduction of intake of dietary components such as sodium, potassium, and certain fatty acids to ranges of levels seen in low-risk countries or in given racial/ethnic groups within countries. The expanding data base on cancer rates worldwide, including racial/ethnic groups within countries (Chapters 4 and 8), and the increasing number of descriptive and analytic epidemiologic studies indicate interest in reduction of cancer rates in high-risk areas through environmental manipulation. Another underlying assumption in this effort is the genetic similarity of human populations— the small amount of genetic heterogeneity across populations versus within populations (see Chapter 3).

Studies across populations, as in ecologic correlation studies, take advantage of the often wide variation in such factors as dietary constituents. These different populations are sometimes regions of the same country, or (more often) different countries comprised of different major racial/ethnic groups. In analytic studies within a country, where cases and controls in a case-control study are derived from the entire country, regional variation in diet or other characteristics is often involved. If racial or ethnic group is included as a separate variable in analysis, then an association with ethnicity independent of dietary factors suggests that risk factors other than diet may be involved.

Apparent lack of consistency in associations between specific risk factors and a specific disease in studies in two or more different populations may be due to several factors. Some are statistical in nature, while others involve the nature of the causal relationship (i.e., the dose response relationship) and the behavioral and/or biological variability in the populations. Statistical reasons relate to the sample sizes involved in the studies, and the study design (e.g., case-control vs. cohort); the calculation of statistical power involves a different formula for each study design (Schlesselman, 1982). Two studies of the same design (e.g., case-control) but differing in sample size will have different power to detect an association of the same strength (i.e., at the same odds ratio).

Large-scale analytic studies of a specific disease involving more than one racial/ethnic group and including a wide range of potential risk factors are rather rare. These studies allow comparisons of the groups in terms of consistency of associations with risk factors (i.e., risk factor "profiles") or in the *strength* of the association (i.e., relative risk or odds ratio). Also, the independent effect (if any) of ethnicity can be tested when all *known* risk factors are controlled in the analysis. Some examples of these large-scale studies, in cardiovascular diseases, will be discussed later. Migrant studies are especially interesting because of genetic similarities, established by anthropological studies, between migrants and *sedentes* (i.e., groups remaining in the homeland), and lack of sufficient time for large genetic changes in the migrants. Comparisons of disease rates by generation (e.g., foreign born vs. U.S. born) can be especially rewarding, with regard to delineation of environmental factors.

Differences in associations between specific risk factors and a specific disease across different populations may argue for *causal heterogeneity* of the disease.

Considerable work has been done in genetic epidemiology suggesting *genetic heterogeneity* in specific diseases, such as "adult-onset" (i.e., non-insulin-dependent) diabetes mellitus and certain cancers. That is, different genetic associations are found in different populations or racial/ethnic groups. Differences in the strength of associations between a specific risk factor and a specific disease, if real and not due to chance, also suggest differences in causal mechanisms that may operate through physiological or biochemical pathways. One must be cautious in examining evidence for heterogeneity because of the statistical considerations mentioned above. "Lack of evidence" for an association between a specific risk factor and a disease may be related to small samples sizes and low statistical power to detect a real association if it in fact exists.

CONCLUSIONS

Using the epidemiologic methods and statistical analyses described above, numerous studies have considered racial/ethnic groups either as a variable of primary interest or as a potential "confounder" in studies of other factors. Confounding variables are associated both with the main exposure variable of interest and with the disease under study. Thus, racial/ethnic groups are often considered in analyses of epidemiologic studies, because these groups are associated with socioeconomic status, and it is important to determine if risk of a disease is related solely to socieconomic status or to independent sociocultural factors.

Racial/ethnic groups are broad characteristics of person or host, and their utility in epidemiologic studies has been demonstrated. Their inclusion in epidemiologic studies of disease may provide clues to more definitive factors that may explain apparent differences in disease rates or manifestations of disease. Often, however, countries comprised of either one or a few racial groups, or regions within a country including many racial/ethnic groups are compared without regard to heterogeneity in racial/ethnic groups. More rarely, although increasingly, studies involve disease rates and risk factor prevalence in multiracial/multiethnic settings, including both descriptive and epidemiologic designs. Use of migrant groups (see Chapter 2) has a long history in epidemiology and anthropology, and comparisons of migrants with populations in the "homeland" as well as in each generation within the migrants provide important clues to disease causation.

Although an individual's racial and ethnic identification is itself not usually modified (except for religion), associations, between disease and racial/ethnic group can provide clues to associations with other factors that explain the associations and can be modified to prevent the disease. Categories of explanations for associations between racial/ethnic group and disease are described in the next chapter and are discussed throughout this book.

2

Interpretation of Racial/Ethnic Differences in Disease

It is much easier to describe racial/ethnic differences in disease than to definitively explain these differences. Attempts at explanations must be made, however, if such associations are to lead eventually to development of hypotheses concerning disease causation.

MacMahon and Pugh (1970) have provided a checklist of possible explanations to be considered in interpreting results of epidemiologic studies including those dealing with racial/ethnic groups. A modification of this checklist is shown in Table 2.1. Consideration of these explanations is useful in interpreting the results of descriptive epidemiologic studies and in formulating hypotheses to be tested by analytic studies. Also, in the analysis of analytic studies these explanations may be kept in mind in suggesting specific variables to be analyzed and in suggesting even more specific hypotheses to be tested by future studies. These categories will now be described briefly, and a few examples provided. In subsequent chapters dealing with specific diseases, these explanations will be discussed in more detail.

ERRORS OF MEASUREMENT

The first category of explanations relates to inaccuracies in epidemiologic data on morbidity and mortality. The extent of these inaccuracies may vary by racial/ethnic group in the same area or different areas. The first issue is the completeness of reporting of disease, regardless of the quality of the data reported. Worldwide, *completeness* of morbidity data is best for cancers, including data from cancer registries that cover entire populations, and certain infectious diseases. Even data on these diseases are not uniformly available for all countries and racial/ethnic groups within countries (see Chapter 4). In most of Africa, for example, conclusions about the incidence and prevalence of chronic diseases must be tentative because they are based on hospital admissions rather than registries or community surveys.

Mortality data are more completely reported but in developing countries completeness is always open to question, and accuracy is a major issue. Mortality rates may be infrequently updated by developing countries. Availability and

Table 2.1   Categories of Explanations for Reported Differences in the Frequency of Disease Among Racial and Ethnic Groups

I. Errors of measurement

Inadequate data or insufficient information, based on "clinical impressions" or hospital admissions

Differential access to medical care and diagnostic facilities

Differential use of available facilities; differences in reporting due to cultural factors or to difference in the severity of disease

Differing fashions of diagnosis (e.g., in death certification)

Problems of diagnosis associated with racial or ethnic group

II. Differences between groups with respect to more directly associated demographic variables

Age differences in the groups compared

Differences in socioeconomic class and occupation, and secondary factors associated with these differences (see III)

III. Differences in environment

Climatic differences and their effects. Geographic variation in disease frequency (as in multiple sclerosis)

Nutrition or diet

Differences in personal customs or habits (e.g., reproductive and nursing habits; use of tobacco and alcohol; and differences in sexual practices)

Differences with respect to personality development, family dynamics, interpersonal relationships, and role behavior; differences in patterns of psychosocial "stress" or acculturation

IV. Differences in body constitution

Anatomical differences; differences related to rates of growth and development

Physiologic and biochemical differences. These may be influenced by environmental factors (e.g., diet, exercise) and genetic factors

V. Genetic differences (e.g., blood groups, HLA-types)

Genetic differences among races or ethnic group may be due to consanguinity, differences in mutation rate, natural selection (differing selection pressures), random genetic differences due to founder effect and isolation

This table is based in part on lists presented by MacMahon and Pugh (1970) and McKusick (1967).

accuracy of the *denominator* is one consideration. The lack of adequate periodic censuses in developing countries and problems in age estimation (see later) affect mortality rates. In morbidity studies of hospital admissions, the reference population "at risk," which is needed for calculation of rates of disease (Chapter 1), is usually unknown in terms of its age and sex distribution and/or is not representative of the entire population at risk.

Adequate mortality data by cause of death are not available for many developing countries, where death registration is incomplete. In developing countries, and to a lesser extent in rural areas of developed countries, a large proportion of deaths are attributed to unknown or ill-defined causes. In South Africa, for example, underregistration and misclassification of deaths among blacks are a major problem for epidemiologic studies. The South African mortality pattern, with *ill-defined conditions* as well as infectious diseases as major causes (Botha and Bradshaw, 1985; Susser et al., 1985; Wyndham, 1985), resembles that of developing nations. Official South African health statistics exclude the so-called "independent" bantustans, or national states, which are impoverished underdeveloped areas representing the legacy of apartheid. Limited data on these areas indicate that as many as 53 percent of all deaths in Africans are classified as "symptoms, signs, and ill-defined conditions" (Botha et al., 1988) in the *International Statistical Classification of Diseases, Injuries, and Causes of Death* (ICD).

The ICD is a manual periodically revised by the World Health Organization (e.g., WHO, 1977). Included in the ninth revision were 17 categories of diseases, conditions, or causes of death from category I for "infectious and parasitic diseases" to XVI for "symptoms, signs, and ill-defined conditions" and XVII for "injury and poisoning." Codes involve four digits, but the three-digit code usually indicates a specific disease and is the most meaningful for comparative purposes; the fourth digit may indicate a specific disease, a disease subtype (such as "acute" or "chronic"), or an anatomical location.

In comparing rates of disease across populations, accuracy in the numerator is a major concern. Mortality data are usually based on the assignment of a single "underlying" cause of death as reported on the death certificate, while other diseases or "contributory" causes of death on the certificate are less frequently coded. The history of procedures involved in the assignment and coding of the underlying cause of death in the ICD coding system makes fascinating reading (WHO, 1977).

Comparisons of mortality rates by specific categories of cause of death are influenced both by the quality of diagnoses recorded by physicians on the death certificate and by the consistency in application of coding rules in assigning the underlying cause of death. Even for developed countries, inaccuracies in certification are important in comparing regional death rates. Studies of the *reliability* of death certificate diagnoses and underlying cause of death have been conducted within countries and across countries. "Reliability" refers to the agreement between the death certificate and hospital records. Validity refers to the agreement between these records and autopsy findings, which provide the most definitive diagnoses of diseases present at death and causing or contributing to death.

In a comparison of death and hospital records within a developed country (i.e., Vermont in the U.S.), 72 percent of all records agreed at the level of the three-digit code in the ICD; degree of agreement declined with age and varied significantly by cause of death (i.e., by three-digit code) and hospital of death. While agreement for "stroke" was high, there were considerable discrepancies by subcategory or cerebrovascular diseases (see Chapter 7). In developed countries inaccuracies in cardiovascular diseases, especially ischemic (coronary) heart disease and type of cerebrovascular disease, as cause of death make comparisons across geographic areas or populations difficult (Dobson et al., 1983). In the United States, death certificates may be especially inaccurate for certain racial/ethnic groups. One example is cardiovascular disease in U.S. blacks, where hypertensive disease may be misclassified as coronary heart disease (see Chapter 7).

Morbidity data are subject to similar but greater inaccuracies regarding completeness and accuracy. *Reporting* of existing disease may differ by racial/ethnic group, reflecting socioeconomic and sociocultural differences. Tolerance of the mentally ill may vary by racial and ethnic groups; in some tribal societies, tolerance is reportedly higher. Hospitalization rates for mental disorders may thus also vary (see Chapter 9).

Reporting of symptoms is subject to a complex interaction among such variables as pain perception, sociocultural attitudes about illness, and physician–patient interactions. These variables are of interest to medical sociologists and medical anthropologists (Harwood, 1981), as noted in Chapter 1. The reporting of health-related behaviors, such as visits to physicians or personal health practices, is also influenced by sociocultural factors. Data from national health surveys in the United States (see Chapter 4), for example, suggest that certain "Hispanic" groups may have a tendency to self-report positive health behaviors or "yea-say" on questionnaires (Aday et al., 1980; Richardson et al., 1987).

Access to medical care and hence the probability of diagnosis of existing disease also differ by racial/ethnic group. The true prevalence of disease will be distorted by such inequalities in access. In South Africa, for example, the vast majority of the black population has no (or very poor) access to medical care (Moosa, 1984; Susser, 1983). The United States is the only developed country other than South Africa that does not provide uniform, guaranteed access to medical care (see later). Such disparities may contribute to apparently higher *morbidity* in the privileged groups but may also increase *mortality* through lack of proper diagnosis and treatment in the underprivileged (Himmelstein and Woolhandler, 1984). Differences in access to medical care are largely due to socioeconomic differences among groups (as discussed later).

An estimated 37 million Americans have neither private health insurance nor access to state health benefits (Hiatt, 1987), and, not surprisingly, minorities (including blacks) and other lower-income groups frequently lack such coverage (Ries, 1987a). On April 12, 1988, the Massachusetts State Legislature passed landmark legislation mandating health insurance for an entire state population. An estimated 10% of the Massachusetts population, or 600,000 persons, without previous coverage will receive health insurance through their employees or pay for insurance on a sliding scale based on personal income. Such legislation may have long-term implications for improving health among minorities and other lower-income groups. Health insurance coverage in Hawaii is also nearly complete.

Black–white disparities in average number of annual *physician office visits* have disappeared in recent U.S. surveys of adults (i.e., the National Health Surveys), and attention has turned to *quality* versus quantity of care. Data on routine health *screening examinations* from the U.S. National Health Interview Surveys (NHIS) of 1973 and 1982 (see Chapter 4) indicate that whites were more likely than blacks to have even had eye exams and glaucoma tests, while black–white differences in certain other tests (e.g., breast exam, Pap smear, and routine physical) were small (Dawson et al., 1987). Data are also available on frequency or recency of tests (Bloom, 1986), which show recent improvements in frequency of regular examinations such as blood pressure and cervical cancer screening among blacks. Results of the 1987 cancer control survey of the NHIS show less knowledge and use of all cancer screening tests (except Pap smears) in blacks versus whites (Anon., 1988d), but analyses by socioeconomic level have not yet been presented.

The NHIS also showed that non-Hispanics were more likely than Hispanics to have ever had all of the screening procedures studied (including breast exams), and Mexican Americans had lowest frequencies of glaucoma tests and electrocardiographs (Dawson et al., 1987). Lower socioeconomic status among Hispanics is undoubtedly involved (see Chapter 4).

Adequate access to health care, such as medical insurance and residence near health-care facilities, may reduce or eliminate apparent racial/ethnic differences in frequency of various health-related practices or examinations. In a group of Hispanic women in Los Angeles having adequate access to health care, for example, use of breast cancer screening services was similar to that reported for Anglo women (Richardson et al., 1987) (see Chapter 8).

Utilization of available facilities may differ by racial/ethnic group. Use tends to be lower in some black populations and higher among certain Jewish groups, but differential access and utilization are often difficult to separate. Diarrheal disease due to *Campylobacter jejuni* (see Chapter 6), for example, may appear more frequent in Jews than in non-Jews, because the former may tend to consult a physician more often when mild or moderate illness occurs (Rishpon et al., 1984). Another example is the infrequent use by U.S. blacks of available community mental health centers in predominantly white areas. Lower rates of physician *contacts* (including telephone) in black versus whites in the U.S. National Health Survey, which held at all levels of family income except the highest (Ries, 1987b), require further examination in terms of sociocultural factors. Greater use of emergency rooms rather than private physicians among blacks and Mexican-Americans than among Anglos in a West Dallas community (Gurnack, 1985) has implications for quality of diagnosis and medical care, but underlying socioeconomic differences may be involved.

In the United States, the effects of race and lack of insurance coverage on medical care (Hayward et al., 1988) and *hospital utilization* are evident in hospitalization rates for specific chronic conditions such as hypertension and diabetes mellitus (Yelin et al., 1983). Differential hospital utilization may involve socioeconomic and/or sociocultural factors, as discussed later in this book.

In a 1982 U.S. national survey, Hispanics resembled blacks in having higher levels of *dissatisfaction* than whites with their most recent medical visit (Andersen et al., 1986). Satisfaction with previous health-system encounters may influence receptivity to preventive health practices.

AGE AND SOCIOECONOMIC STATUS

Age

Age-specific or age-standardized rates are needed in comparing populations that differ in age structure, as noted in Chapter 1. As an extreme example, the apparent rarity of certain cancers in African populations in the early literature was related to the small proportion of older persons, who are at higher risk for most cancers. In the United States, the age distributions of the black and white populations differ, and age-standardized or age-specific rates are needed (see Chapter 1); an example of the calculation of age-standardized rates (i.e., death rates) is given in Chapter 4.

The need for age-standardized rates is now widely recognized, as evidenced in comparisons of cancer incidence in which rates are standardized to various estimated "world populations" (e.g., Waterhouse et al., 1982; Parkin, 1986; WHO, 1987). Examples of such age-standardized rates are provided throughout this book. The age distribution of many populations is uncertain, however, especially at older ages—for example, blacks in South Africa (Wyndham, 1985), in other parts of Africa, and in the Caribbean (Mitacek et al., 1986). Even in the United States, census data used for denominators in rate calculations are subject to undercounting of blacks and Hispanics; young black male adults (35–54 years) are especially underrepresented (U.S. Vital Statistics, 1987).

Socioeconomic Status

Access to and utilization of medical services including hospitals and neighborhood health centers are often related to socioeconomic status (SES), as noted earlier. Even if access is comparable, comparability of mortality or health in racial/ethnic groups living in the same area is not assured. A prominent example concerns black–white disparities in childhood mortality in Boston (Wise et al., 1985), where access to medical care (including neighborhood health centers) is great. The underlying determinants involve socioeconomic and environmental factors that must be elucidated and addressed through preventive programs. The elucidation of such determinants, as noted in Chapter 1, is a major purpose of epidemiologic studies of racial/ethnic groups.

Ethnic groups in the same community may differ in SES. Comparisons between U.S. blacks and whites, for example, should consider SES when possible, but individual data on socioeconomic indicators are rarely available. Approximations are often based on group data, such as average incomes available for census tracts of residence in the U.S. census. Number of years of education is available on death certificates of individual decedents in the United States, and education of parents is recorded on birth certificates (see Chapter 4). Critical discussions of the use of variables to describe SES in specific studies will be provided later.

Interestingly, SES and health care disparities in U.S. blacks and whites affected health and mortality in the past. A study of a black cemetery in Arkansas, dating from around the turn of the century, disclosed skeletal evidence for malnutrition, chronic pulmonary disease, and osteoarthritis; the last may have been related to hard physical labor (Rose, 1985).

The importance of SES variables in explaining black–white difference in rates of many diseases has been demonstrated by numerous studies. In a classic study in the United States, Kitagawa and Hauser (1974) noted great differences in death rates for whites and "nonwhites" (especially blacks) and viewed these disparities as evidence of the underprivileged status of the latter. Studies in Alameda County, California, have been particularly informative. In a survey of residents in an economically depressed area in that county, health status was more strongly associated with income than with race (Satariano, 1986). In that same county more than one third of the total excess deaths among blacks could be attributed to "preventable deaths," and SES-related inequalities in access to and/or quality of health services may have been a major factor (Woolhandler et al., 1985).

Worldwide and especially in developing countries, SES may be difficult to assess and include in epidemiologic studies because of the lack of census and other data from population samples or uncertainty regarding the best indicator of social class in surveys. Using data from community health surveys in Jordan and Lebanon, Zurayk et al. (1987) have suggested that the average education score of the family may be a useful indicator of social class that predicts morbidity and accessibility to medical care in certain developing countries. Further testing of this approach is needed in other countries. In developed countries such as the United States both education and income should be considered in analytic studies (as discussed in subsequent chapters), since education may be associated more strongly with such health-related variables as obesity (Flegal et al., 1988).

Racial/ethnic differences in disease prevalence may be found *within* lower-SES groups. Such *interactions* between SES and race (i.e., U.S. blacks vs. whites) have been reported for various diseases. This research approach involving testing for interactions (Chapter 1) provides interesting leads for further investigation regarding explanations related to environmental factors. The effects of low SES, and especially poverty conditions, on total mortality may be profound and not totally explained by health-related behaviors (such as smoking) and access to medical care, suggesting a role for the social and physical environment in poverty areas (Haan et al., 1987).

DIFFERENCES IN ENVIRONMENT

The predominant role of socioeconomic status in explaining racial/ethnic differences in disease patterns actually operates through environmental influences associated with SES. These factors include crowding, poor nutrition and sanitation, and social stresses as well as inadequate medical care (discussed earlier). Differences in environment between ethnic and racial groups may also include personal customs and habits, other cultural factors related to social support and acculturation (especially in migrant populations), diet, and work environment. Indeed, these sociocultural differences between groups are the main reason for interest in racial/ethnic groups in epidemiologic studies. It is often not clear, however, whether sociocultural factors operate independently of SES in explaining racial/ethnic differences in disease.

In Los Angeles, SES levels are similar in the Hispanic and black populations, but mortality rates from certain chronic diseases are considerably lower among Hispanics (Frerichs et al., 1984). Racial/ethnic differences apparently not related to SES suggest that other factors, such as personal habits (e.g., smoking, diet, and reproductive patterns) or sociocultural patterns, are involved.

Personal Habits and Customs

Patterns of use of *tobacco* and *alcohol* vary among countries comprised of different racial/ethnic groups as well as among racial/ethnic groups within a country. Data on use of these drugs is often available from population surveys (see Chapter 4) or special studies, and these data are important in assessing racial/ethnic differences in a variety of diseases and causes of death or injury (as discussed later). In the United States for example, the proportion of current smokers is highest among young adult black males, while smoking in certain Hispanic groups, previously infrequent, has been increasing.

Of current interest in anthropology are differences in alcohol use across cultures and culture areas, and the uncertain role of genetic differences regarding racial differences in alcohol sensitivity (Heath, 1987) (see Chapter 9). According to the World Health Organization, for example, heavy consumption of alcoholic beverages, at >15 liters per adult per year, is characteristic of certain Western and Southern European countries, and other developed countries (including North America, the rest of Europe, New Zealand, and Australia) also have high levels (i.e., 10–15 liters per year). In contrast, with a few exceptions, annual consumption is lower in Central and South Americans and parts of the Caribbean, while adults in parts of Asia, Africa, and Oceania consume <5 liters per year. Differential use of various drugs other than tobacco and alcohol, including oral contraceptives and illicit drugs, is also relevant to interpretation of disease patterns among racial/ethnic groups. Sociocultural factors in drinking patterns in tribal and other societies are of particular interest to social anthropologists.

Other personal factors concern *sexual habits and reproductive patterns* in racial/ethnic groups. Age at first intercourse, number and type of sex partners, and reproductive patterns reflected in distribution of age at first marriage and pregnancy vary by religious and racial/ethnic group and are relevant to risks of various infectious and chronic diseases. Again, it is often difficult to distinguish apparent racial/ethnic or religious differences from socioeconomic differences, but sociocultural influences are involved in some cases.

The cross-cultural study of human sexuality is enjoying renewed vigor in anthropology, especially regarding extramarital sexual practices, homosexual behavior, and the social status of prostitution (Davis and Whitten, 1987). Such information is relevant to studies of disease patterns including viral diseases such as AIDS-related conditions, as discussed later. Regarding AIDS, the lack of cross-cultural data on homosexuality (Davis and Whitten, 1987) is noteworthy; even in the United States surveys of homosexual and bisexual behavior are few in number (Cameron, 1988). Quality of data in surveys on sexual behavior, including representativeness of samples and accuracy of responses, is of major concern, but the best available data are needed for interpretation of disease patterns and projections of disease occurrence.

Marriage patterns, family organization, and marital residence patterns have been documented for many ethnic groups (Murdock, 1981). Patterns of exogamy and endogamy, and resulting level of inbreeding in offspring, are relevant to studies of differences in diseases involving genetic factors. Examples of groups with relatively high rates of consanguineous marriages include the Old Order Amish, Japanese, "Dravidian" groups in southern India, Brazilian groups, and certain populations in the Middle East. Consanguineous marriages are still common in South India, especially among Hindus, with significant variations both within and between regions (Lukacs, 1984). In Moslems of Calcutta, some groups have a prevalence of first-cousin marriages as high as 29% (Basu, 1985). The extent of cousin marriages, especially of males with their father's brother's daughter, in the Middle East is the subject of debate. In general less than 10% of marriages may be consanguineous (Digard, 1986), but estimates are as high as 25% in some areas. In contrast with India, demographic surveys indicate that the proportion of consanguineous marriages is declining in younger married couples in Japan (Imaizumi, 1986) and in Beirut, Lebanon (Khlat, 1988).

Theoretical (i.e., predicted) effects of both inbreeding and the opposite tendency toward admixture or "hybridization" of groups vary according to the duration of the marriage patterns and assumptions used in genetic models. Some examples of research findings will be discussed later in this book.

Breast feeding and lactation patterns, which vary by culture, are relevant to various diseases and conditions in women and infants, as discussed later.

Sources of data on diet and exercise are discussed in Chapter 4. International correlations between age-adjusted rates of cancers and various dietary data were mentioned in Chapter 1. Some of the countries compared are composed of only a few predominant "racial" groups, but dietary patterns may vary within each country, reflecting socioeconomic, climatic, and soil conditions and sociocultural factors. Methodologically, the development and validation of food frequency questionnaires for dietary history data have facilitated analytic epidemiologic studies (Block, 1982). Examples include vitamins, fats, and cancer-related agents. A noteworthy specific example relevant to cancer studies is recent work on nitrosamine estimation from questionnaires on food and alcohol consumption (Howe et al., 1986), although nondietary sources of nitrosamines (e.g., from cigarette smoking) also must be considered (Preston-Martin et al., 1986). Nitrosamines may be involved in the causation of various cancers (see Chapter 8).

A potential area of increased collaboration between social anthropologists and epidemiologists (Fig. 1.1) concerns ethnic differences in food preferences and attitudes regarding the health effects of foods. In Oaxaca, Mexico, for example, preferences and attitudes regarding the sweetness level of beverages were compared within and between communities by using solutions of known sugar concentration (Messer, 1986).

The potential importance of traditional cultural attitudes regarding obesity are beginning to be recognized (Wright and Whitehead, 1987). Among small, non-European cultures limited anthropological data suggest that "plumpness or moderate fat" is the ideal female "body type" in the majority (Brown and Konner, 1987). In U.S. black females, studies are needed on cultural influences on concern about overweight (Kumanyika, 1987). Among U.S. gypsies, cultural attitudes apparently equate obesity with personal power (Thomas et al., 1987). Such attitudes may persist in the future, as in Aldous Huxley's vision (in *Brave New World*) where "Gammas Deltas and Epsilons had been conditioned to associate corporeal mass with social superiority" (Huxley, 1946, p. 43). Meanwhile further cross-cultural studies are needed on perceptions of and attitudes regarding overweight.

There is interest in developing simple methods for assessing levels of physical activity in epidemiologic studies, including questions on the number of "sweat episodes" per week (Washburn et al., 1987). The role of physical exercise and physical fitness in physical and mental health has become a major worldwide research issue. Differences in diet and exercise habits are relevant to overweight and obesity, discussed later, which in turn are risk factors for many diseases. Dietary and exercise habits are also discussed later with reference to studies of migrants.

Other Cultural Factors

Social support and *acculturation* mechanisms in racial/ethnic groups, within SES category, have been explored for such diseases as hypertension and depression. To cite one example, within-neighborhood ethnic differences in risk factors for cardiovascular disease and diabetes mellitus between Mexican-Americans and Anglos in San Antonio, Texas, could be due to cultural factors and degree of acculturation, which are under investigation (Stern et al., 1984).

Degree of acculturation is a variable, albeit difficult to define, that is being increasingly studied in relation to population differences in disease rates and risk factors for diseases. The concept of acculturation has a long history in anthropology (Beals, 1962), and the classic definition in the 1936 memorandum of Redfield et al. is often cited—that acculturation encompasses "those phenomena which result when groups of individuals having different cultures come into continuous first-hand contact with subsequent changes in the original culture patterns of either or both groups." The emphasis on process and the reciprocal or two-way nature of acculturation in early definitions is noteworthy, as is Beals' (1962) assessment of the need for quantification to objectively determine relative rates of acculturation.

In U.S. Hispanic groups, acculturation scales have been developed on the basis of language use, friendship patterns, and media sources as well as individual and parental birthplace. These scales have been used, for example, in the U.S. Hispanic Health and Nutritional Survey (or HHANES) (see Chapter 4) and in a study of knowledge and behavior related to cardiovascular diseases in San Diego, California (Vega et al., 1987). Results of the latter study suggest that immigrants should be targeted for education programs regarding exercise and diet.

The acculturation process involves a number of variables such as diet, exercise, and cultural and psychological aspects (see discussion of migrant studies, next section). Education and SES-related variables must be carefully controlled in studies of degree of acculturation as explanations for racial/ethnic differences in disease. In Los Angeles, for example, indices of cultural assimilation had little effect on preventive health behaviors (e.g., physical examinations, Pap smears, and screening for breast cancer) after age and education were controlled in multivariable analyses (Marks et al., 1987).

The effects of acculturation processes on disease patterns depend in part on the duration of contact, and studies of disease have included groups with relatively long contact (e.g., Maoris of New Zealand and Australian aborigines) as well as shorter contact (e.g., Melanesian groups, Micronesian migrants, and certain Hispanic groups in the U.S.). Examples of major multidisciplinary studies of acculturation that have assessed relationships with disease are the Solomon Islands Project of Harvard University (Friedlaender et al., 1987), the Samoans Project (Baker et al., 1986), and the Peru–Cangallo Project of Amerindian migrants from rural to urban areas of Peru (Richman et al., 1987). The Peru Project includes an acculturation scale with 21 items on language, customs (i.e., food, music, and clothes), ethnic identity, sociability, and perceived discrimination.

Migrant Studies

Consistently low or high disease rates in two racially similar groups living in different countries (and hence in different environments) may suggest that genetic factors are involved in their unusually low or high rates. Lack of such consistency may suggest the operation of environmental factors. Such comparisons are often difficult to interpret, however, because groups compared, such as American and "African" "blacks," actually differ slightly in genetic composition (see Chapter 3).

Migrant populations may resemble their parent populations in genetic makeup but are exposed to different environmental influences after their migration. These groups also may maintain, to some extent, certain habits and customs after migration. Studies of migrant groups are useful in attempting to distinguish host and environmental influences and in defining the operation of broad environmental factors. Results of migrant studies have reinforced our image of racial/ethnic groups as nonstatic in biological and cultural makeup. This plasticity is due to the processes as acculturation; intermarriage (with gene flow) also occurs among groups with acculturation. Human plasticity, shown long ago for body size and anthropometric characteristics, has also been demonstrated for disease risk. Examples of the use of migrant studies are discussed in this book with reference to specific disease categories, especially cancers and cardiovascular diseases.

Work Environment

Racial/ethnic differences in work environment may be involved in differences in disease risk. Such occupational differences may reflect more basic socioeconomic factors and discrimination. U.S. blacks, for example, may be exposed to hazardous working conditions more often than whites, but the pattern is complex and requires further study (Robinson, 1984). Specific work hazards more common in blacks may include exposure to high temperature, dusty conditions, noise, and infectious diseases. Overall, observed black–white differences in exposure to hazardous jobs do not appear to be explained completely by education and experience (Robinson, 1984). In occupational epidemiological studies, data are often not presented by racial/ethnic group, so that differences in mortality and morbidity cannot be evaluated. Some examples of international studies of the effects of work environment on specific diseases are discussed later (Chapter 8).

Other Environmental Differences

Other environmental influences may differ quantitatively across countries or geographical areas, and hence levels of exposure are associated with racial/ethnic groups. These environmental factors include altitude, temperature, latitude and longitude, hardness of drinking water, exposure to sunlight and background radiation (ionizing and nonionizing), and air and water pollution. On the other hand, cultural patterns may directly influence exposure. With regard to sunlight, for example, ethnic differences in behavior in work and leisure, including clothing worn, may affect susceptibility to various diseases such as skin cancer and vitamin D-related disorders (as discussed later).

Interest in such environmental influences in explaining disease patterns by person and place can be traced to Hippocrates, the father of epidemiology and medicine, as in his work, *Airs, Waters, Places.* Environmental influences such as climate affect microorganisms responsible for disease in man, but sociocultural factors are often important in transmission of these disease agents (as discussed in subsequent chapters).

DIFFERENCES IN BODY CONSTITUTION

The term "constitution" is used here in the sense of *phenotype*, not in the restricted sense of genetically determined features. Body constitution includes anatomic, biochemical, and physiologic characteristics that are determined in complex ways involving interactions between environmental and genetic factors.

Although body constitution is considered as a separate category among the explanations for racial/ethnic differences in disease risks, population differences in body constitution may be due to complex interactions between underlying environmental differences related to socioeconomic status (SES) and sociocultural influences (discussed earlier) as well as to genetic factors. Body size and rates of physical or somatic sexual maturation, for example, may be influenced by dietary factors early in life. Thus, racial/ethnic differences in these aspects of body constitution may be due to underlying differences in SES and culturally influenced eating behaviors. Associations between these constitutional factors and disease rates, in turn, may reflect underlying differences in SES and sociocultural factors.

Obesity and the *anatomical distribution of body fat* are involved, in part, in explaining racial/ethnic differences in risk of chronic diseases—for example, among U.S. blacks, whites (Anglos), and Hispanics. The tendency for U.S. black women to gain more weight with age than other groups, with resultant effects on blood pressure and cardiovascular disease risk factors, is now well documented (as discussed later). The underlying mechanisms, however, for such racial/ethnic differences are poorly understood (Kumanyika, 1987). Recent years have witnessed an increased interest among physical anthropologists in describing and explaining population differences in the amount and distribution of body fat, due in part to the growing evidence for relevance to disease (Bailey, 1986; Polednak, 1987c).

Associated with body weight and height in a complex manner, related to rates of physical maturation, is sexual maturation as reflected in *age at menarche*, or first menstruation. This biological characteristic has long been of interest to physical anthropologists, especially with regard to the explanations for long-term trends in age at menarche in different populations. The Northwest–Southwest (higher to lower) gradient or cline in average menarcheal age in Europe, for example, has not yet been explained by environmental factors known to be associated with this characteristic (Danker-Hopfe, 1986). In Great Britain average age at menarche is 13.3 years and is higher in northern England, Wales, and Scotland, even after controlling for social class differences (Mascie-Taylor and Boldsen, 1986). Some populations in circumpolar regions have late average age at menarche—for example, 13.8–14.3 years in some Alaskan Eskimo groups (Milan, 1980). This gradient could represent the influence of some other environmental factors, proximate in time, or a genetic factor representing the results of past adaptations or gene flow between populations. The epidemiologic association between earlier age at menarche and risk of female breast cancer, especially in premenopausal age groups, in various populations has led to increased interest among anthropologists in population differences in age at menarche.

Racial/ethnic differences in body constitution relevant to disease include *anthropometric* differences in body height and in proportions of limbs, reflecting growth patterns modulated by environmental and genetic influences. *Physiologic* and *biochemical* differences relevant to disease include such variables as blood levels of cholesterol (and its components), other blood parameters, and blood pressure, again reflecting complex interactions between environmental and genetic factors.

GENETIC DIFFERENCES

It is appropriate that genetic differences between racial/ethnic groups appear last in our list of explanations for differences in disease. As noted in the next chapter, the genetic overlap between racial groups is great. Approaches to the study of the role of genetic factors in explaining racial/ethnic differences in disease are summarized in Table 2.2. Genetic epidemiology is a relatively new subdiscipline, but the interface with physical anthropology (i.e., population genetics) is obvious—that is, in terms of methodologic approaches.

Table 2.2 Some Approaches to the Study of the Role of Genetic Factors in Explaining Racial/Ethnic Differences in Disease

1. Comparisons of the degree of familial aggregation in a specific disease across different racial/ethnic groups
2. Studies of genetic polymorphisms
   a. Descriptive studies or correlations of frequency data (e.g., blood groups, HLA types) with rates of disease
   b. Comparisons of associations with disease within specific racial/ethnic groups, independent of other known risk factors
   c. Examination of consistency of associations between specific traits (e.g., an HLA type) across racial/ethnic groups
3. Studies of degree of racial admixture as a risk factor for a specific disease, independent of other factors or interacting with other factors

Often the first step in genetic epidemiologic studies of disease involve data on family history of the disease under study. Positive family history for a specific disease usually reflects complex interactions between shared genes and shared environments. It is the task of genetic epidemiologic studies to delineate these factors and to evaluate the likelihood of specific genetic models or modes of inheritance. Comparisons of the degree of familial aggregation of specific diseases, especially cancers, in different racial/ethnic groups are being used to crudely assess differences in genetic susceptibility and/or differences in environmental exposures.

Descriptive and analytic epidemiologic studies can be used to address the role of differences in frequencies of genetic factors such as HLA (human leukocyte or histocompatibility antigens) in explaining racial/ethnic differences in disease. Studies of HLA antigen frequencies in various populations (see Chapter 3) in relation to variation in disease may suggest a role for genetic factors in etiology, to be explored by more detailed studies. HLA phenotypes or genotypes have been associated with an increasing number of diseases (Tiwari and Terasaki, 1985). Especially prominent in the list of HLA-associated diseases are those involving immune or autoimmune mechanisms as well as certain cancers involving infectious agents (and hence immune responses).

In most diseases studied, however, susceptibility is influenced by complex interactions between or among HLA or HLA-linked genes, other (non-HLA) loci, and environmental factors (e.g., infectious agents). Thus, racial/ethnic differences in diseases associated with HLA phenotypes may be difficult to explain by recourse to differences in HLA phenotype/genotype frequencies alone. Multivariate analyses of diseases in a multiracial/ethnic setting are needed to determine whether racial/ethnic differences in disease are related to differences in HLA factors or are independent of these factors.

Persistence of racial/ethnic differences in disease in groups with the same HLA phenotypes argues either for other genetic factors or for environmental influences. Consistency in associations between specific HLA types and a specific disease suggests genetic homogeneity in causation across populations. Inconsistency of HLA disease associations across racial/ethnic groups provides evidence for heterogeneity in causation of the disease (mentioned in Chapter 1) and the possible interaction with environmental factors (see also Thomson, 1983). The validity of this general approach has been confirmed by subsequent studies of HLA-associated diseases, as discussed later. The same approach of looking for consistency in associations between specific genetic markers and a specific disease can be expanded to other genetic polymorphisms (see Chapter 3). This comparative approach is analogous to that used in assessing the relative strength of family history as a predictor of a specific disease across racial/ethnic groups.

The estimation of degree of racial admixture in "hybrid" human populations has long been of interest to physical anthropologists, although methodologies have been developed by geneticists (e.g., Elston, 1971; Charkraborty, 1986). Recent research on degree of admixture and risk of disease has demonstrated the need for collaboration between human geneticists and epidemiologists. Such studies provide *general* clues to the role of genetic factors in disease, to be investigated by more detailed studies.

CONCLUSIONS

It should be obvious that the categories of explanations for racial/ethnic differences in disease discussed earlier are not mutually exclusive but provide a framework for interpreting results of epidemiologic studies.

The challenge to epidemiologists is to find why racial and ethnic differences in disease exist and to separate the overwhelming influences of underlying socioeconomic differences from "ethnic" (i.e., sociocultural) factors. Regarding sociocultural factors, there is a need for an expanded data base on cross-cultural differences in use of tobacco and alcohol (independent of or interacting with socioeconomic status), sexual habits, and attitudes toward overweight and "obesity" (as defined by various criteria). Epidemiologic studies may also disclose rarer occurrences where explanations for disease patterns involve biological or genetic differences. Biological explanations include physiological–biochemical and morphological differences among racial/ethnic groups. Body build or anthropometic differences among racial/ethnic groups, such as anatomical distribution of body fat and the strength of its association with disease risk across populations, have received renewed attention. These biological differences themselves represent complex interactions between environmental and genetic influences that are often poorly understood.

Genetic differences among racial and ethnic groups (see Chapter 3) are important in two respects. First, they must be taken into account as a potential confounding factor in examining associations between genetic factors and disease—for example, in studies of the association between human histocompatibility or HLA types and disease (Thomson, 1983; Tiwari and Terasaki, 1985). If cases and controls in a case-control study are not matched for ethnic group and differ in ethnic composition, spurious associations between disease and HLA types could result. Second, such associations between HLA types and a specific disease may not hold across all ethnic groups, and this may provide clues to heterogeneity of causation (as discussed later). In such comparisons across groups, statistical issues must be carefully addressed.

The major theme of this book concerns the interface between epidemiology and physical or biological (including biomedical) anthropology (Figure 1.1). The delineation and measurement of racial/ethnic differences in biological factors, including morphological, physiological, and biochemical characteristics, and genetic factors defined by population–genetic studies have been the task of physical anthropologists. Before turning to the description of racial/ethnic differences in disease occurrence and prognosis, some recent findings on the physical anthropology of selected groups are discussed in the next chapter.

3

Physical Anthropology
of Racial/Ethnic Groups

This review will highlight some recent findings from studies on the physical anthropology and population genetics of selected racial/ethnic groups. In our discussion of racial/ethnic differences in disease this background information should prove useful. A synopsis of methods for estimating degree of racial admixture is also included as a prelude to later discussions of admixture in relation to disease risk. Readers interested in the physical anthropology of racial/ethnic groups should consult standard physical anthropology texts (e.g., Lasker and Tyzzer, 1982) or works on human races (Garn, 1971; Osborne, 1971; Brues, 1977).

Most racial classifications, as noted above, recognize at least three major groups—white, black, and Mongoloid or Oriental (or Oriental/American Indian) (Brues, 1977). The number of additional groups recognized varies considerably. All classification schemes are arbitrary and temporary, as new genetic evidence becomes available and as the groups themselves change over generations. A modification of Garn's (1971) system is presented in Table 3.1, which is based on some of the evidence reviewed in this chapter. Many of these groups are discussed in this chapter, and the locations of some groups are shown in Figures 3.1 and 3.2.

A general conclusion that has emerged is that genetic variation per gene locus is smaller among the major races than among groups or persons within the same race (Nei and Roychoudhury, 1972, 1974, 1982; Chakraborty, 1984). Genetic distance measurements using Nei's technique are based on gene frequencies for blood group and serum protein loci that are "polymorphic"—that is, at least two alleles or alternate forms of a gene at a specific locus are present with a population frequency of >1 percent (Livingstone, 1980). Nei's method calculates a "mean standard genetic distance" based on the probability of different alleles existing over all loci examined in samples of persons from the two populations. The ratio of *interracial* (i.e., black–white) to *intraracial* codon differences, for example, was about 7–10 percent, but results varied with the specific loci compared (Table 3.2). Thus, the majority of genetic variation in the human species lies within races rather than between races, but the use of multiple genetic loci permits classification of individuals into major racial groups (Jorde, 1985).

A few examples of intraracial genetic heterogeneity will be cited. Within Mexican Indian tribes, gene diversity at 14 loci is about 95 percent versus only

Table 3.1 A Classification of Racial Groups

Geographical races	Local races	"Isolated" local races

Amerindian	North American
	Central American
	Caribbean (original inhabitants such as
	  Arawaks)
	South American
	Fuegian
		Eskimos and Aleuts;
		Reindeer Chuckchi and N.
		  Athapascan speakers;
		Algonkian speakers

Polynesian	Includes Maori of New Zealand	
Micronesian		
Melanesian–Papuan		Many locally differentiated groups
Australasian		Aborigines and Tasmanians
Asiatic	Turkic[a] Tibetan Northeast (Japan, Korea) Han Chinese Mongolians Zhuang in China Southern Chinese; Thailand, Vietnam, Philippines, Taiwan Extreme Mongoloid, Ainu Malay-Borneo cluster Pacific Negritos Semai Senoi of Malaysia	
Indian	"Hindu" (North) "Dravidian" (South)	A very large number of local races, "tribes," microraces
European	Northwest European Northeast European Alpine[a] Mediterranean[a] Iranian[a]	Lapps Icelanders
African	East African West Africans and Bantu-speaking groups San Khoi	Pygmy Zulu, Swazi, Venda, etc.

"Admixed" groups[b]	U.S. Hispanic populations including
	  Mexican-American (Amerindian–Cau-
	  casian)
	U.S. blacks
	Black Caribs
	Chileans
	Northern Brazilian groups (European–
	  Indian)
	Southern Brazilian groups (European–
	  African)
	South African "coloured"	

Modified and expanded from Garn (1971).

[a]Groups recognized by Garn but with (at present) little or no evidence for genetic separation (see text).

[b]This group has been expanded from Garn's list. The designation "admixed" is, of course, rather arbitrary, because all "races" are admixed (see text). However, the groups in this category have *major* contributions of genetic material from two or more other "racial" groups.

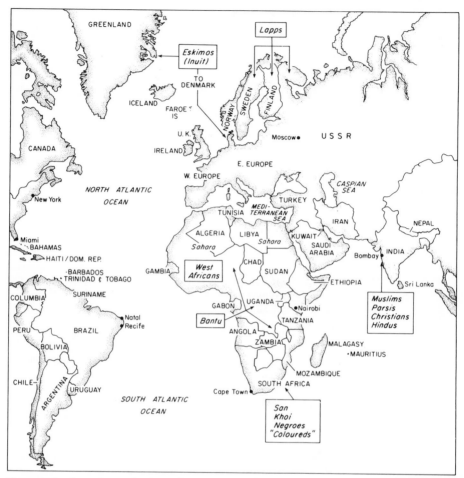

Figure 3.1. Locations of selected countries and racial/ethnic groups discussed in the text: The Caribbean, South America, Europe, Africa, the Middle East, and India.

about 5 percent intertribe (Roychoudhury, 1975). while intertribal variation in gene frequencies associated with the ABO blood group system in India is only 1.6 percent (Rajanikumari and Sizkumari, 1987), it is higher for other genetic polymorphisms demonstrated by modern techniques (see later). A large number of genetic studies in various populations demonstrate genetic heterogeneity in gene frequencies within populations. Obviously, genetic diversity within major racial groupings varies with region. This variation may be due to such factors as the size of the founder populations, which determines the probability for "founder effect" or chance peculiarities in gene frequencies. Other factors include adaptation via natural selection, and historical migration patterns with resulting gene flow (i.e., exogamy, or extragroup marriage vs. endogamy, or intragroup marriage, see below).

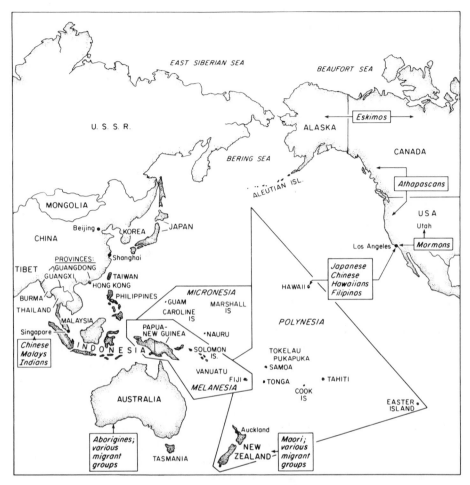

Figure 3.2. Locations of selected countries, regions (i.e., Polynesia, Melanesia and Micronesia), and racial/ethnic groups discussed in the text: the United States, the Pacific, and the Far East.

Before discussing some specific racial/ethnic groups, the genetic markers used in studies of population affinities will be reviewed briefly. Studies of genetic markers involve both the products of genes as expressed in phenotypes such as blood groups and, more recently, the genetic material (i.e., DNA) itself.

BLOOD GROUPS, SERUM PROTEINS, AND HISTOCOMPATIBILITY ANTIGEN TYPES

Anthropological genetic studies over recent decades have produced a vast amount of data on gene allelic frequencies for many populations, especially for *blood*

Table 3.2 Distances Between Races and Heterozygosity Based on Blood, Blood Groups, and Protein Enzymes

	Racial comparison		
Genetic criteria	Caucasoid vs. Mongoloid	Mongoloid vs. negroid	Negroid vs. caucasoid
Blood group loci			
No. of loci	18	17	17
Average heterozygosity	0.303	0.283	0.317
Average genetic distance between races	0.064	0.194	0.056
Protein enzyme loci			
No. of loci	38	40	41
Average heterozygosity	0.210	0.202	0.217
Average genetic distance between races	0.025	0.065	0.067

groups, red cell enzymes, and certain *serum proteins*—as compiled by Mourant et al. (1976), Tills et al. (1983a), and Roberts and De Stefano (1986).

Blood Groups

Some selected data on blood group frequencies in major racial groups are shown in Table 3.3. *ABO* and *Rh* blood group typing should be familiar to all readers because of their use in testing compatibility for blood transfusions. Fisher's explanation (in 1943) of the genetics of the Rh system involved three closely linked gene loci each occupied by a pair of alleles; each gene produces its own antigen. Rh typing involves testing for antigens by using five antisera (i.e., antibodies) designated at C, D, E, c, and e; "anti-d" is not known to exist. Genetically, each person inherits a gene complex of *haplotype* (e.g., cDE) from each parent. Both the Fisher-Race notation (using the three gene loci) and the Wiener notation (e.g., R° for cDe, and r for cde) are used for the haplotypes.

In blood group typing, blood samples are obtained and red cells are extracted by centrifuge for introduction into tubes containing antisera (i.e., antibodies) to the antigens being tested. Agglutination (clumping) of red cells containing specific antigens is then examined visually. Recent developments, however, have simplified procedures for ABO and Rh testing through the use of dispsticks (or immunobinding assays) which can be used with one drop of blood obtained from a finger prick sample (Plapp et al., 1986).

One must distinguish between frequencies of individual *genes* (or *alleles* at a given locus) and *genotype* frequencies, which determine the blood group substances on red cells—for example, genotypes OO (manifested as blood group O), AO, and AA (group A), BO and BB (group B), and AB (group AB). Noteworthy is the high frequency of the O *allele* of the ABO system in Amerindian groups (Table 2.2), especially some South American Indians (i.e., 100 percent), as discussed later with reference to maternal–fetal blood group incompatibilities (Chapter 9). The O allele is also frequent in Iceland (i.e., about 75 percent vs. about 62.5 percent for the world). Because of the high frequency of O, A is rare or

Table 3.3 Populations with High Gene Frequencies for Certain Selected Blood Group Alleles

A	B	O
Europe (Scandinavia)	Central Asia	South and Central America
Asia Minor	North India	North American Indian
American Indian (Western North America)	West Africa	Northwest Europe
Lapps (A2)	Hottentots	Southwest Africa
Eskimos	(Khoi)	Australia
		Arabia
		Basques

Rh (Selected variants only)

cDe (R⁰)	cde (r)	CDe (R¹)	Diego	Duffy (a–,b–)
Africa	Basques	Southern Europe	Mongoloid	African, U.S. blacks
Melanesia	Arabs	Mediterranean	Amerindians	
Central Asia		East Asia, Pacific	(not Eskimos)	
		Pakistanis	South Amerindians	

Duffy (Fyᵃ)	Kell
Europeans	Arabia
Indian	
Amerindian, Eskimo	
Australian aborigines	
Lapps	

Abstracted from data in Mourant et al. (1976), Tills et al. (1983), and other sources. For the Rh system, both notation systems (i.e., Fisher-Race and Wiener) are shown.

absent in Central and South America but more frequent in North American Indians (reaching 25 percent in the Blackfoot) and in Eskimos of Alaska and Greenland. The A gene is actually two major types in Europeans (i.e., A_1 and A_2), and additional subtypes exist in other populations. The A_2 gene is especially frequent among the Lapps of northern Scandinavia, a group discussed later.

Secretion of blood group antigens A and B in water-soluble form is controlled by a separate dominant gene (Se) which has been localized in the human gene map. Group O sectors secrete another antigen (H) which is controlled by a gene inherited independently from the ABO locus.

"African" markers include the cDe or R⁰ variant of the Rh blood group system and a variant of the e antigen called eˢ of VS (Sistonen et al., 1987a). Although two systems of nomenclature exist for the Rh system, the Fisher or three-allele notation system is most commonly used. The cDe complex, more properly called Dce in order of the discovery of these antigens, is uniformly preponderant in Africa south of the Sahara Desert. While the cde complex or r (with Rh-negative phenotype, because of the absence of the strongest or D antigen) is very low in the Japanese and Ainu (see below), it has a frequency of about 20 percent in southern Africa, reaches 40 percent in most Caucasians (e.g., British), and is most common among the Basques of the Pyrenean area of Europe and the Bedouin of the Sinai Peninsula.

Another important African marker is the Fy a–, b– phenotype or the absence of alleles Fy a and b of the *Duffy* system, first described in a man named Duffy. The *Diego* blood group is a marker of Mongoloid affiliation and is common among Amerindian groups. The presence of the Diego (Di^a) allele in certain Black Carib groups in the New World (see below) reflects an Amerindian contribution.

Some blood group types are nearly "universal" such as the Co^a of the *Colton* system, where 96 to 99 percent of various white groups are a-positive and in one study none of 1,706 U.S. blacks were a-negative; among whites about 7.4 percent are Co^b-positive (Mourant et al., 1976). Some additional comments on blood group frequencies are made later in this chapter, with reference to specific racial/ethnic groups.

Serum Proteins

Serum proteins include haptoglobins, transferrins, and gamma globulins, but only the latter will be emphasized in this text, because frequencies of some types have been associated with certain diseases. Since this is not a work on population genetics or physical anthropology of racial groups, it is not feasible to summarize much of the recent work on genetic markers; the reader is referred to the compendia cited above and some specific examples of racial groups discussed below.

Briefly, we note that conventional electrophoretic methods for differentiating serum proteins and red cell enzymes have been augmented by isoelectric focusing techniques which increase discrimination of protein variants. Electrophoresis made possible the study of genetic heterogeneity of specific proteins or their genetically determined varieties known as isoenzymes, as first demonstrated for abnormal hemoglobins. Amino acid substitutions in enzyme systems could be demonstrated by their differences in migration rate when exposed to an electric current in a suitable supporting medium (such as starch or cellulose acetate). In isoelectric focusing, use of a pH gradient allows greater differentiation of proteins (Papiha, 1986).

Examples of isoenzyme systems extensively studied electrophoretically in various populations are the serum protein *Gc* (or group-specific component) phenotypic subtypes and the red cell enzyme *PGM* (phosphoglucomutase) variants (Dykes et al., 1983), which have been useful in revealing apparent clusters of population groupings. The genes controlling production of various Gc and PGM types have been mapped in the human genome (McKusick, 1987–88). Gc is a serum protein (specifically, an alpha-2 globulin) synthesized in the liver and involved in the transport of vitamin D and its derivatives. Also synthesized in the liver are the "iron-binding" proteins called *transferrins*, and isoelectric focusing has also demonstrated numerous polymorphisms (Kamboh and Ferrell, 1987). More work is needed on the significance of these genetic variations in terms of disease and natural selection. Gc polymorphisms have been used in studies of population affinities and in some associations with specific diseases (as discussed later). Transferrins (TF) appear to play a role in immune regulation, and there is increased interest is associations between TF subtypes and various diseases.

Epidemiologically another noteworthy protein, with polymorphisms demonstrated by isoelectric focusing, is *alpha-1 antitrypsin*, or protease inhibitor (Pi). Population differences in frequencies of several alleles at this locus have been described. Several "rare" genes (e.g., Pi^Z) have been associated with Pi deficiency and with chronic lung and other diseases (as discussed later).

Genetic markers in human *immunoglobulins* have been studied in diverse populations. Human immunoglobulins (Ig) are composed of heavy and light chains and include various classes (IgG, IgM, etc.). The IgG heavy chain (or *Gm*) and light chain (or *Km*) immunoglobulin markers have been most extensively studied (see Steinberg and Cook, 1981; Tills et al., 1983a). Examples of recent studies include those in Chinese populations (Matsumoto et al., 1986), Jewish groups (Stevenson et al., 1985), and groups in West Bengal, India (Chakraborty et al., 1986). Some of these data are mentioned below in descriptions of specific racial/ethnic groups.

HLA Types

Excluded from the compilations cited above were *HLA* (*leukocyte or histocompatibility*) *antigens*. The human HLA system corresponds to the major histocompatibility complex (MHC) of other animals. Human HLA antigens, originally discovered on leukocytes, are coded by closely linked loci (on chromosome 6) called A, B, and C (collectively, called class I) and Class II or D and its subdivisions DR, DP, DQ, and DZ. These loci are highly polymorphic or variable in human populations, with a growing number of antigens identified (i.e., more than 100 as of this writing). The alleles are designated by numbers and/or letters at each locus—HLA-A1, A2, Aw24, etc. (see Table 3.4 for examples). The phenotypes or antigens expressed in an individual depend on the "haplotypes" or blocks of alleles inherited from each parent; hence each person has two alleles at each locus, which may or may not be different.

Genes for *complement components* (e.g., C4 and C2) are closely linked to the HLA complex on the same chromosome (i.e., number 6). These class III region molecules or serum proteins of the MHC are also involved in immune responses, and extensive human polymorphism has been shown for the C4 alleles. As with other polymorphisms, their value lies both in population genetics and in studies of disease associations (as discussed later).

International workshops on HLA have reported data on frequencies of specific HLA types (i.e., both phenotype and allele frequencies) in the major races and in certain geographic areas, although data are often based on small sample sizes (Terasaki, 1980; Tiwari and Terasaki, 1985). Separate reports of studies on HLA type frequencies in various human populations have recently begun to appear in the literature—for example, in Beijing, China (Yiping and Changxing, 1985), other groups in China (T. D. Lee et al., 1988) and among Nigerians residing in London (Okoye et al., 1985).

Some results of studies on HLA phenotype frequencies are summarized in Table 3.4 for selected HLA loci that have shown racial differences in frequencies of phenotypes. Some interesting differences in HLA phenotype frequencies are

Table 3.4 Some HLA Antigens That Show Differences in Frequency of Phenotypes Among the Major Races or Racial/Ethnic Subgroups

Antigen	African black	American Black	Nigerian[a]	European Caucasian	N.A. Caucasian	Jews (Ashk.)[b]	Mexican-American	Amerindian	Japanese	Chinese[c]	Chinese[d]
A1	4.9	6.5	4.4	27.5	25.7	20.9	18.8	2.9	1.0	6.5	6.8
A2	20.3	27.3	27.2	45.3	46.6	40.3	44.3	60.3	43.2	60.8	50.1
A3	11.9	14.2	18.4	21.9	26.0	16.3	5.9	2.9	1.1	11.2	6.4
Aw24	17.5	5.7	—	18.2	12.8	19.4	25.9	41.9	58.5	32.7	—
B7	21.7	17.0	14.0	16.8	18.7	7.8	6.0	1.5	11.4	6.5	5.1
B8	8.4	5.8	0.0	15.7	17.1	8.5	6.8	2.9	0.2	2.8	1.9
Bw51	1.4	2.7	—	13.9	9.3	6.2	13.1	43.5	15.9	—	—
Bw58	30.1	20.3	15.8	2.2	2.2	6.2	2.4	0.0	1.7	—	—
Cw1	1.4	0.1	0.0	8.1	6.0	7.0	1.2	20.3	32.1	11.2	27.5[e]
Cw3	16.1	17.5	15.8	19.1	22.6	7.8	19.1	62.3	46.5	68.2	59.8
DR2	20.3	28.5	38.8	25.1	25.3	17.3	14.8	46.3	36.0	—	25.8
DR3	37.0	31.6	12.6	20.4	22.2	13.5	16.0	6.0	3.2	—	24.4
DR4	12.3	9.6	0.9	18.3	27.3	24.1	28.4	47.8	41.4	—	25.1
DR5	18.1	24.8	32.0	19.5	19.4	39.0	27.3	3.0	4.3	—	17.3
No. in sample (approx.)		138	323	103	2499	1,013	127	84	67	884	2,441

Other Sources: Terasaki, 1980; Tiwari and Terasaki, 1985.

[a]From a study of a group of Nigerians living in London Okoye et al., 1985. Data on Nigerians in southwest Nigeria were similar (N = 12): 38% DR2, 23% DR3, and 0% DR4 (Macdonald et al., 1986).

[b]Ashk.: Ashkenazic or European Jews (see text).

[c]Chinese in Beijing, China (Yiping and Changxing, 1985).

[d]Randomly selected Chinese from 9 ethnic groups in 14 locations, including Beijing (T. D. Lee et al., 1988).

[e]For the Beijing subgroup, the frequency was 11.2%, or identical to that reported by Yiping and Changxing (1985).

evident across the major racial groups. In general there are some similarities between American blacks and certain African populations studied and among "Oriental" groups (i.e., Chinese in Beijing and Japanese groups) (Table 3.4). An "Oriental" marker, frequent in Amerindians and Oriental groups, is BW54. B27 (not shown) is common in Amerindians but not in Chinese.

Among 100 southern Chinese in Hong Kong (Hawkins et al., 1987), however, DR5 antigen frequency was 33 percent (or lower than in Japanese), DR4 was 26 percent (lower than in Japanese), and DR2 was 38% (similar to Japanese). The statistical reliability of these percentage estimates is dependent on the sample sizes (see Chapter 1). Larger samples studied throughout China show some variability in DR antigen frequencies among the ethnic groups; in Beijing DR2 (at 37.4%) is similar to Hong Kong and to Japan, while DR3 and DR5 are more frequent.

Our discussion has been limited to single HLA antigen phenotypes. Populations frequencies of certain HLA haplotypes, or sets of alleles as inherited in a block from each parent, have been compared for HLA A, B, and DR loci (Bodmer et al., 1987). Very few haplotypes were limited to a single population among 13 European groups and several other racial/ethnic groups compared. The A1, B8, DR3 haplotypes was the most frequent in 10 of the 13 European populations studied but was also present (at >1 percent) in all other population samples except the Japanese. The reader should be cautioned regarding sample sizes, however, which were only 27–35 in some groups and largest for Japanese (i.e., 536). Six haplotypes for these three loci were found only in Caucasoid versus Mongoloid or black populations. In China A1-B8 is uncommon, while Bw46-Cw1 is characteristic of all ethnic groups (T. D. Lee et al., 1988). Some of these haplotypes have been associated with certain diseases, and their use in epidemiologic studies is expanding.

HLA-DR phenotype differences are of particular interest because of associations between these phenotypes and various diseases related to immune or auto-immune responses. The HLA-DR4 phenotype, for example, is associated with rheumatoid arthritis in some populations, and its frequency is low in some black populations. The HLA-DR5 phenotype, associated with certain AIDS-related cancers, is slightly higher in some black groups (Table 3.4). These HLA associations with disease are discussed in subsequent chapters.

HLA antigens are important for tissue typing in organ transplantations, in studies of disease causation, and as one polymorphic system useful in assessing affinities of populations. Regarding population affinity studies, the recent use of DNA probes or restriction fragment polymorphisms (see below) has shown even greater population differences within the HLA genes.

Restriction Fragment Length Polymorphisms

Recent advances in the application of recombinant DNA technology include the use of *restriction fragment length polymorphisms* (RFLPs). These techniques allow comparison of the genetic material itself (i.e., DNA), rather than gene products such as blood groups, proteins, and HLA antigens, and the inferred genotypes (described above). RFLPs represent sites dispersed throughout the human genome, identified by bacterially produced enzymes that attack these specific ("restriction") points, and their presence or absence is inherited in a simple Mendelian manner. Work on DNA polymorphisms in humans began with the beta-globin gene cluster (on chromosome 11), involved in the synthesis of the beta chain of hemoglobin, and has expanded to other loci, including the alpha-globin gene cluster on chromosome 16, and more recently to mitochondrial DNA (as well as nuclear DNA). Recent surveys in China have shown differences in the frequencies of DNA polymorphic (i.e., variable) sites in the beta-globin gene cluster (Zeng and Huang, 1987), and other population differences based on small samples have been reviewed by Summers (1987).

RFLPs have been studied in several racial groups—especially Western Europeans and American blacks, and Chinese—but the enormous variability in the presence or absence of particular restriction sites is already apparent (Cooper and Schmidtke, 1986; Zeng and Huang, 1987). These RFLPs may themselves often represent regions of the DNA that do not code for proteins, but they may be tightly linked to another gene that is involved in a specific disease. A flowering of studies on the applications of RFLPs is expected, regarding population affinities, associations with diseases (and hence the role of natural selection in maintaining some of these polymorphisms), disease causation (via other genes closely linked to RFLPs), and prevention of genetic diseases through improved identification of carrier parents (see Chapter 5).

Conclusions

In summary, all of this genetic information is useful in characterizing human populations and in studying the effects of gene flow (migration) and genetic drift, as well as natural selection. The importance of natural selection, or differential mortality and differential fertility, in explaining population differences in frequencies of many of these markers is poorly understood. Associations between various diseases and blood groups and serum proteins have been reported, and some examples are discussed later. In explaining variation among populations in HLA types, population migration is believed to be more important than natural selection, but many associations between HLA and diseases have been reported (Tiwari and Terasaki, 1985), as discussed later. It seems probable that variation in HLA frequencies across populations represents in part the balance between selection involving various infectious and weaker selection involving autoimmune-related disorders and cancers.

On the basis of nonrandom distributions of Gm allotypes, there is indirect evidence for natural selection (Propert and Balkan, 1986). Interactions between HLA antigens and Gm immunoglobulin types may be involved in susceptibility to certain diseases, such as insulin-dependent diabetes mellitus (Tait et al., 1986). There is also increasing interest in population variations in polymorphisms of vitamin D-binding protein factor Gc, or group-specific component (Constans et al., 1985), and in associations between these proteins and diseases, such as diabetes mellitus in Polynesians (see Chapter 9). Thus, population differences in frequencies of alleles at these loci must eventually be considered in interpretation of differences in disease frequency (as discussed later).

ESTIMATION OF DEGREE OF RACIAL ADMIXTURE

The degree of racial admixture is a variable used in epidemiologic studies of disease (Chapter 2, Table 2.2). Racial variability in gene frequencies for certain blood groups and serum proteins, outlined above, has been used for estimation of degree of racial admixture in specific "hybrid" populations (as listed in Table 3.1). In general, there is a high degree of concordance between admixture estimates based upon serologic data versus those using skin color. Other characteristics used for admixture estimation include dental characteristics (i.e., odontometrics and odontological traits) and dermatoglyphics (i.e., finger and palm print patterns). Some specific examples of the use of these methods will be discussed.

A high degree of concordance between admixture estimates based on skin color variation as measured by reflectometry, or the amount of light reflected by the skin after exposure to a controlled light source, and serologic data has been shown for black Carib and Creole groups in Belize, Central America (reviewed by Crawford, 1983). Although the mechanism of skin color inheritance in man is not understood, evidence suggests that the skin colorimetric data yield consistent admixture estimates (Korey, 1980). Skin color has also been used in studies of admixture in Mexican-Americans, as noted below.

The state of the art of admixture estimation, excluding anthropometric/morphologic data, has been reviewed by Chakraborty (1986), who emphasized the need for data on ancestral populations. This same need is evident in studies of migrant populations, whether from an anthropological or an epidemiologic perspective (as discussed later). Chakraborty also discussed reasons for discrepancies in estimates of admixture in certain groups and cautioned that use of morphological traits may be misleading because of the uncertain genetic basis of these traits. The most extensive, albeit inconsistent, data on admixture are for U.S. blacks, Icelandic and Jewish populations, and some Hispanic and South American Indian populations.

Estimates of the amount of admixture of various American black populations, however, have varied considerably (see below). Uncertainties in estimation of degree of racial admixture are due to changes in estimates of the original African ancestral gene frequencies, variations in gene frequencies throughout U.S. black populations, and the influence of natural selection on gene frequencies. Even the Duffy blood group system, which has been assumed to provide the best estimates (Reed, 1969), may be subject to selection due to malaria present in Charleston, South Carolina, blacks (Livingstone, 1980). Chakraborty (1986) has reviewed these data, which show white admixture as low as 4 to 8 percent and as high as 40 percent, depending on the gene loci used; however, southern blacks consistently show lower admixture estimates than nonsouthern blacks.

In a preliminary survey of a population with an unknown extent of admixture between two or more ancestral groups, certain genetic markers known to differ greatly in frequency between or among these groups may be useful. Table 3.5 shows an example of the level of precision in estimation of phenotypic

Table 3.5 Theoretical Example of Error in Estimation of Blood Group or Serum Protein Frequencies in a Sample of 300 Blacks, Relevant to Admixture Estimation

Characteristic	Estimated frequency	Error in estimate $(+/-)$[a]
Blood group O	65–75% (West Africa)	~5.5%
Blood group R^o (cDe)	60–70% (West Africa)	~6%
Duffy, negative	90% (West Africa)	~3.5%
Serum protein $Gm^{z,a;b}$	54% (U.S. blacks)	~5.8%

[a]With 95% conficence.

A simple random sample of a given population is assumed.

frequencies of certain genetic markers that might be obtained in a preliminary survey of a population with uncertain degrees of black–white admixture in a U.S. black group. The a priori estimates are based largely on West African data, or the estimated "homeland" population for U.S. blacks. As the quantity of information on frequencies of genetic markers increases, previously accepted rules are modified. Thus, the $Gm^{z,a;b}$ immunoglobulin marker was believed to be "African," but foci in Melanesia and Central Asia have been reported (Szathmary, 1981).

The distinction between degree of admixture and overall genetic resemblance between groups should be emphasized. Percentage of "admixture" does not indicate genetic overlap, because as we have noted, the average genetic distance between the major races is quite small (Table 3.2).

Later in this book some examples will be given of studies of specific diseases in which the use of degree of racial admixture has helped to elucidate the possible role of genetic factors in these diseases and to propose explanations for racial differences or changes in racial differences over time (due to increasing admixture).

SOME RACIAL/ETHNIC GROUPS

Various "Black" Populations

Studies on degree of white admixture in U.S. black populations were mentioned above (see Chakraborty, 1986), and it was noted that southern blacks show lower amounts of admixture than northern blacks. In fact, earlier estimates by Pollitzer (1958) showing less than 10% admixture in blacks in the rural South (Charleston, South Carolina) have been corroborated in an isolated black population of McNary, Arizona, derived from backwoods lumbering towns of the South (Wienker, 1987). The latter endogamous population, on the basis of skin color and serological data, has less than 5% European ancestry, due to social and historical factors.

Recent physical anthropological studies have focused on the black Caribs of Central America and the Caribbean and on various groups of South African blacks. These data are of special interest, because studies of various diseases have also been carried out in these populations, and examination of disease risk in relation to degree of racial admixture or genetic differentiation among these populations should provide clues to disease causation.

The *black Caribs* of the West Indies, on St. Vincent Island, are an amalgam between West Africans and the original Amerindian groups (see later); the Amerindian component includes both Awarak and Island Carib Indians. Analyses of frequencies of various blood groups and serum proteins show about 50% Amerindian genes in Island Caribs (in the Caribbean), while black Caribs in coastal communities of Central America have up to 80% African ancestry (Crawford, 1983). Studies of degree of admixture and risk of hypertension in these populations will be discussed later (Chapter 7).

Population genetic studies of other groups in the West Indies have been limited. In *Haiti*, the genetic contribution from African genes is strong (i.e., an estimated 80 percent), with some French and Amerindian contribution, on the basis of blood group gene frequencies—58 percent for R^o and only 2.3 percent Fy^a (Basu et al., 1976). Some epidemiologic data on cancers and other diseases among Haitians are mentioned later. In *Trinidad* surveys, the average Caucasian admixture estimate involving several loci, including certain Gc and TF subtypes (mentioned above), was 25 percent (Saha and Samuel, 1987). This is comparable to the average estimate for certain U.S. black populations, as discussed earlier.

In *South America*, the degree of contribution of African, along with Caucasian and Amerindian, genes varies considerably by region (see later under "South America"). For example, northeastern Brazilian localities could be classified as predominantly black, mixed, Indian, or white on the basis of phenotypic data and family names (Azevedo et al., 1982).

South Africa includes blacks or Bantus (a group originating from other parts of Africa), who comprised about 68% of the population in 1980, Cape "coloured" (an admixed group), whites (about 18%), Asians, and other groups. Studies of *South African black* or Bantu groups, using 24 genetic loci, show distinct subclusters such as the Zulu and Swazi versus the Venda and Sanagana-Tsonga (Hitzeroth, 1986). The *Khoi* (formerly "Hottentots") and *San* (formerly "Bushmen") groups, as well as the "hybrid" or "*Cape coloured*" groups are also somewhat distinct (see Nurse et al., 1985). The Khoi and San are related and share a common but remote ancestry with the Negroes; the cDe gene, for example, is common in both Khoi and San. Also, the Khoi are difficult to separate from "coloureds" except by genealogies. The San, including the !Kung, are the best known and largest group of hunter–gatherers remaining in Africa. The Khoi are known for their lighter skin color and tendency for fat deposition on the buttocks and thighs. Details on genetic markers in the Khoi and San may be found in Nurse et al. (1985), who were unable to find published data on the prevalence of diseases in these groups, and in Excoffier et al. (1987). We have noted the paucity of vital statistics data from South Africa.

Genetic distance, and genetic heterozygosity in relation to endogamy or marriage within the group, among South African populations have also been studied by Harpending and Jenkins (1973) and Harpending and Chasko (1976). Further studies are needed to delineate the roles of specific factors—such as migration, hybridization, natural selection, mating patterns, and genetic drift—in explaining these population–genetic patterns. In any event, the demonstration of genetic variability within the South African blacks will be important in the eventual understanding of disease patterns; that is, South African blacks cannot be regarded as uniform genetically. This recognition may prove relevant to the interpretation of data on disease frequency—for example, rheumatoid arthritis and its association with HLA types (see Chapter 9).

The Khoisan language family extends to Khoisanoid remnants in Kenya and Tanzania, while the *Bantu* family of languages is related to West Sudanic in the larger group of "Niger–Congo" languages. The Bantu-speaking populations are related to *West Africans* genetically as well as linguistically (Excoffier et al., 1987). Among West Africans the Senegalese are noteworthy in showing similar frequencies with Bantus in RFLPs of mitochondrial DNA (Scozzari et al., 1988) and for their inclusion in worldwide cancer incidence comparisons (Chapters 4 and 8). In reviewing linguistic and genetic evidence, Excoffier et al. (1987) recognized a clear distinction between the Bantu speakers and the *East African* groups, which include the Cushites and Ethiosemites—long recognized as showing certain Caucasoid as well as African characteristics. Studies of 46 blood group antigens in an East African Somali population, however, suggested only minor Caucasian admixture (Sistonen et al., 1987b). Historical factors, including migrations, along with founder effects and marriage patterns have contributed to the complexity of interrelationships among Sub-Saharan African populations. The cultural and sexual habits of these populations have recently been of special interest with regard to viral diseases (see Chapter 6).

Studies of RFLPs in regions of the beta-globin gene cluster suggest similarities between Bantu-speaking groups and in southern Africa and *Central Africa* (Ramsay and Jenkins, 1987). Although this evidence supports the genetic cohesiveness of Bantu-speaking groups, caution is needed in interpreting results based on only one or a few markers.

Within Central Africa, genetic variation among groups is considerable for the Fy^a allele, as in the rest of sub-Saharan Africa, while the R^o (cDe) allele frequency is surprisingly variable. Intragroup genetic heterogeneity, apparently greater than for negroid groups reported by Nei and Roychoudhury, may have resulted from exogamy practices by certain tribes (Spedini et al., 1983). Certain rather distinctive polymorphisms of antitrypsin and Gc systems have been described in the Congo populations of central western Africa (Pascali et al., 1986), including a high frequency of the Gc-1F variant and an apparently new Pi-S allele. Central Africa has been of major interest lately with regard to origin of the human immune deficiency virus (HIV) and related viruses (Chapter 6). *Pygmies* of the Central African Republic have also been studied extensively, including anthropological, physiological, and medical–nutritional characteristics; these groups are closer to each other, genetically, than to other African groups (Cavalli-Sforza, 1986). Thus, their long-recognized separation in many racial classifications (Table 3.1) is supported.

The island of *Mauritius* near Madagascar represented one of the few areas of Africa for which there are data on mortality including cardiovascular diseases (as discussed later). Owing to historical factors including importation of slaves by the French from Madgascar and the introduction of workers from southern India and China, Mauritius includes a variety of racial/ethnic and religious groups.

American Indians, Mexican-Americans, and "Hispanics"

Studies using gene frequencies at six loci in 23 populations have separated *aboriginal North American groups* from *Asiatic populations* (discussed later). More extensive studies using 42 genes at 14 loci—including ABO, Rh, MNS, P, Kell, Duffy, Diego, and Kidd blood groups—suggest two basic divisions in northern North American populations (Szathmary, 1981): (1) Bering Sea, including Reindeer Chukchi, all Eskimos, and (northern) Athapascan speakers; and (2) Algonkian speakers. The first group is genetically related to the Asiatics (discussed later), because of gene flow between two related populations or because of a common origin from Beringia, the land bridge to Asia that existed prior to the most recent rise of the Bering Sea. The Algonkian speakers are genetically more removed, possibly because of an earlier entry into North America (Szathmary, 1981).

Using linguistic and dental traits, as well as genetic data, Greenberg et al. (1986) recognized three indigenous New World groups—Amerind, Na-Dene (i.e., Athapascan-speaking groups including the Haida and Tlingit), and Aleut-Eskimo. The influence of European admixture, using gene frequency maps for seven loci, has been investigated in large numbers of North American Indian populations (Suarez et al., 1985a). The Eskimo/non-Eskimo dichotomy (Table 3.1) is preserved even when highly admixed populations are deleted from analyses. This finding is of interest in interpreting differences in disease frequency in these groups along with data on important environmental factors such as diet. In our discussion of differences in prevalence of diseases, such as cancer, data are available separately for some of these major groups (e.g., Eskimos and North American Indians).

Within *North American Amerinds*, genetic variation, reflected in blood group frequencies, among 74 Indian populations has been reviewed (O'Rourke et al., 1985), suggesting an association between polymorphism at these loci and climatic variation. The Diego (Di^a) antigen, as noted earlier (Table 3.3), is found almost exclusively in the "Mongoloid race" or the Asiatic and Amerindian races of most classifications. This antigen, for example, was present in all four groups of Indians from Oklahoma, although less frequent in Cherokees than in other groups (Kasprin et al., 1987). There is considerable variation in frequency of Di$^{(a+)}$, however, within the North, Central, and South American regions, and it is absent in Alaska and western Canada. These data have been used in various theories regarding the origin of Amerindians, which need not concern us here.

The Arawaks (or Tainos), mentioned earlier in connection with admixture with black Caribs, were the people first encountered by Columbus and had by then established an extensive trade network in the Caribbean area.

South American populations, as noted with reference to black populations, comprise various mixtures of Caucasian, Amerindian, and black components. In Brazil, for example, admixture studies indicate that northern and northeastern groups have important Amerindian contributions, whereas southern populations are predominantly black–white dihybrid. Founder effects and marriage patterns may account for these regional differences (Franco et al., 1982). In Chile, Europeans and Chilean "aborigines" (i.e., Amerindians) are the major components of admixture (Valenzuela, 1983); some cancers (e.g., gallbladder) common in Chile may be related to the Amerindian genetic component (see Chapter 8). *Central America* was the major route for the colonization of South America, and lower Central American and northern South American tribes are similar genetically (Barrantes et al., 1982).

Distributions of several genetic markers in *Amerindian Mexican* populations have been studied, but only recently have gene frequencies been reported for large urban *mestizo groups*. Using data on various blood groups and serum proteins on 510 students in Mexico City, Lisker et al.'s (1986) trihybrid model estimated the proportions of Indian, white, and black genes at about 56, 41, and 3 percent.

Mexican-Americans have been shown to represent a hybrid of native American and (more than 50 percent) Caucasian populations, on the basis of skin color data (Relethford et al., 1981; Gardner et al., 1984). These data have relevance to interpreting the accumulating evidence on differences in disease frequencies in Mexican-American groups versus other U.S. groups, and studies of degree of admixture in relation to disease among Mexican-Americans have also been informative (as discussed later).

The term "Hispanic" is used in this book, although there is no consensus on the proper terminology, such as "Latino" versus "Hispanic" (Yankauer, 1987). The major Hispanic populations include Mexican-Americans in the Southwest and California, Puerto Ricans and other Spanish-surnamed groups in New York City, and Cubans in Florida. There are few data on blood groups in Hispanics in Miami, but a study of 820 blood donors showed one $Di^{(a+)}$ and the frequency of Co^b (of the Colton system, mentioned earlier) was about half that in various "Anglo" groups (i.e., 4.6 percent vs. about 7.4 percent) (Issitt et al., 1987; Mourant et al., 1976). As with South American populations discussed earlier, Hispanic populations are diverse culturally as well as genetically, with contributions from European, African, and Amerindian sources.

Mongoloid (Oriental) Populations

Frequencies of genetic markers at 21 classical loci in a Taiwan aboriginal group have been compared with data from other Asian populations. Three major population clusters, with geographical proximity, have been suggested (K. H. Chen et al., 1985); northeast (Korea, Japan); southeast (south China, Thailand, Vietnam, Philippines, Taiwan); Malaya and Borneo; and Polynesians, Micronesians, and Melanesians. We shall discuss briefly some of these groupings, before turning to China—including its southern region, which is allied genetically with parts of southeast Asia.

Koreans and Japanese are of particular interest because of studies of diseases in migrants from Korea and Japan. Despite genetic similarities, interesting cultural differences exist, and migrant studies allow examination of both retention of habits and acculturation processes in Japanese and Koreans. Frequencies of HLA types among Japanese were discussed earlier.

An intriguing sideline in the history of physical anthropology concerns the *Ainu of Japan*, who were once regarded as "hairy" and "white" but have proved to be neither. The Ainu are regarded as either an indigenous group present before modern Japanese speakers arrived, or as sharing a common ancestry with other Japanese via the Neolithic Jomon Culture (see Kirk and Szathmary, 1985; Rouse, 1986). The Ainu of Hokkaido Island were included in the International Biological Program (IBP) studies of indigenous populations of the circumpolar region (Milan, 1980). The author is unaware of epidemiologic studies among the Ainu, although diabetes mellitus is said to be relatively infrequent (Milan, 1980).

The *Southeast Asiatic* cluster is of interest regarding both similarities and differences in disease patterns (e.g., for certain cancers such as liver and naso-pharynx), reflecting in part dietary factors. Epidemiologic studies of various diseases are most common in Taiwan, with some data also for Thailand, as discussed in subsequent chapters.

Malaysia includes West Malaysia (Malay Peninsula) and East Malaysia (Sarawak and Sabah in Borneo), with the capital being Kuala Lumpur in West Malaysia (not shown in Fig. 3.2). In West Malaysia the *Semai Senoi* of the central hills may represent the aboriginal inhabitants, but the history of this region is obscure. These putative aboriginals lack A_2 and cde (or r), unlike South Indians. They have a long history of interaction with Malays, and recurrent founder effects and migrations have apparently resulted in considerable genetic differentiation at the village level (Fix and Lie-Injo, 1975). Some studies of cancer (Chapter 8) have contrasted these various groups in Malaysia. The *Malay-Borneo* cluster includes groups in the Philippines, the Malay Peninsula and culturally related groups in *Indonesia*, whose language is derived from Malay. Indonesia also includes Chinese immigrants and various ethnic groups in Irian Jaya or West New Guinea (not shown in Fig. 3.2). The *Pacific Negritos*, found in a widespread area including West Malaysia, the Philippines and Andaman Islands, were recognized as an isolated "local race" by Garn (1971) and may represent a Proto-Malay population whose small body size represents an independent adaptation to rain forest with no genetic relationship to African populations (Coon, 1965; Kirk and Szathmary, 1985). Epidemiologic studies from Indonesia have been limited, but recent reports include blood pressure surveys (Chapter 7).

Singapore merits discussion because of the availability of epidemiologic data (especially on cancers) concerning its diverse racial/ethnic groups (Fig. 3.2). When "founded" in 1819, the island was uninhabited, but trade expansion led to immigration of Chinese (especially during 1925–29), who came to outnumber the predominant Malays of the region. Of Singapore's approximately 2.6 million inhabitants, about 76 percent are Chinese, 15 percent are Malays, 7 percent are Indians, and 2 percent are various other groups (see Huff, 1987, for a description of economic development). Extensive data on cancer incidence are available from Singapore (Chapter 8).

Polynesians, Micronesians, and Melanesians occupy peripheral positions both genetically and geographically in relation to modern Asian populations (Chen et al., 1985). The ultimate Asian ancestry of these Pacific populations is the subject of much speculation, as are the genetic relationships among Pacific groups.

Polynesians range in a triangle from New Zealand, which includes both the *Maori* and a small number of Polynesian Islanders, to Hawaii and Easter Island

(Fig. 3.2). New Zealand is of great interest because of the availability of data on disease rates in Maori and "non-Maori" (i.e., European and island Polynesian) populations; included are Mormon religious groups which are both Maori and non-Maori. Although a rather small number of genetic studies have been reported for the Maoris, significant differences in ABO (e.g., higher A), Rh (lower cde or r), and PGM polymorphisms have been reported relative to Europeans in New Zealand (Woodfield et al., 1987). Polynesians may have originated from a southern Mongoloid population but are now genetically distinct from Mongoloids and also from Australian aborigines and (to some extent) from Melanesians (see later). Other Polynesian groups of interest epidemiologically are native *Hawaiians*, *Samoans*, and *Tokelau Islanders*, including various migrant groups (as discussed later). Polynesians probably migrated from Asia (perhaps Southeast Asia) through Melanesia (i.e., Fiji) around 1000–2000 BC, settling in Tonga and Samoa and ultimately reaching as far as the Hawaiian Islands (north), Easter Island (east), and New Zealand (south).

Micronesians (Fig. 3.2) include the Chamorros of the Mariana Islands of Guam and Rota, who have been studied epidemiologically to a limited extent. Genetic affinities, including HLA types, have been shown between certain Micronesians and local groups of Japanese and Filipinos. Micronesians have been studied as a consequence of surveillance after accidental exposure to atomic fallout from bomb testing in the 1950s and as a result of an unusual occurrence of certain neurological diseases (as discussed later). *Nauruans* of Nauru Island (Fig. 3.2) have been studied extensively with regard to diabetes mellitus and other chronic diseases (Chapters 7 and 9).

Melanesians, including various *Papua New Guinea* groups (Fig. 3.2), are of interest because of widespread retention, until recently, of traditional tribal life styles and some distinctive health characteristics (Chapter 7). In general Melanesians are distinct genetically from Polynesians in blood groups and serum proteins (Blake et al., 1983) as well as HLA types (Kirk and Szathmary, 1985). The *Fiji Islands* of Melanesia, however, are of particular interest because of their strategic position with respect to Polynesian migrations, reflected in linguistic and genetic similarities between the Melanesians and Polynesians. Studies of globin gene markers (RFLPs; see earlier) suggest overlap between Melanesians of Papua New Guinea and Fiji, and Melanesians and Polynesians share some unique markers (Trent et al., 1988). In Papua New Guinea and the Solomon Islands, considerable genetic heterogeneity exists within small geographic areas, suggesting isolating conditions involving geographic barriers and mating patterns (see Friedlaender et al., 1987). Melanesian populations have long been of interest epidemiologically, with regard to changes in cardiovascular disease prevalence with acculturation (Chapter 7) and also concerning specific diseases such as genetic disorders in the *Vanuatu Islanders* (New Hebrides) (Chapter 5) and the virally induced neurological disease kuru in a specific tribe in the eastern highlands of New Guinea (Chapter 9).

A subject of long-standing debate has been the degree of genetic and biological separation between Austronesian (formerly called Malayo-Polynesian) language family, found from Sumatra and Taiwan through Indonesia and including an Oceanic branch, and the linguistically diverse Papuan group of most of New

Guinea and nearby islands (see W. W. Howells, in Friedlaender et al., 1987). The Austronesian groups may have originated from South China or Southeast Asia, perhaps some 7,000 years ago, and subsequently spread and differentiated genetically, as suggested by K. H. Chen et al. (1985) (see earlier). The degree of genetic and biological separation between Chen et al.'s "Southeast" Asiatic cluster (including South China), the "Malayo-Borneo" group, and other Pacific populations including Polynesians and Melanesians (mostly Papuan speakers) remains to be elucidated. Studies of DNA polymorphisms (RFLPs) in the Pacific are expanding and offer promise in helping to analyze the complex genetic interrelationships in the region. Some RFLPs in the HLA-DR found in Pacific islanders (i.e., Melanesians, Micronesians, and Polynesians) appear to be rare or absent in Caucasoids, while others are shared with Caucasoids (Kohonen-Corish and Serjeantson, 1986). These genetic data support previous observations on blood groups and serum proteins, showing only low levels of genetic admixture between Pacific populations (i.e., Melanesians and Polynesians) and Europeans (Blake et al., 1983). The influence of natural selection on genetic markers, via malaria in some areas of the Pacific (Chapter 5) and other diseases, complicates the interpretation of population affinities.

Brief mention will be made of the *Australian aboriginal* populations. Skeletal remains in Australia dating from about 25,000 BP are clearly *Homo sapiens* and share some features with Australian aboriginals (Day, 1986). The original inhabitants of Tasmania resembled the surviving Australian aborigines but were exterminated by Europeans in a 30-year period during the 19th century; the last "pure" Tasmanian aboriginal died in 1876 (Howells, 1977). The first systematic blood-group data collected on aborigines for 28 adjacent tribal isolates in Western Australia (Birdsell et al., 1979) showed considerable intergroup heterogeneity absence of A_2 but R^o as frequent (or more frequent) as in Eurasia; $Fy^{(a+)}$ reached a gene frequency of 96–100% (see also Table 3.3). On the basis of average population distances in five genetic systems (including ABO and Rh blood groups, Gm and HLA-A and -B), Australian aboriginals are a separate group that may have originated early (with Micronesians) (Excoffier et al., 1987) with whom they share a high frequency of Duffy[a] (Table 3.3). On the basis of small sample sizes, some differences in RFLP frequencies between aborigines and Europeans have been suggested (Summers, 1987). As with South African black populations, data on the health status of aborigines are rather limited (Thomson, 1984), although routine vital statistics may soon be available.

The South China area was mentioned earlier as part of a Southeast Asiatic cluster of genetically related populations. Modern mainland *China* comprises about 93% Han Chinese and more than 50 ethnic minorities, with different customs, dispersed over much of the Chinese territory. Hans originated in the area of the Yellow River but are now distributed all over China. Genetic heterogeneity has been shown for Mongolians from Inner Mongolia, Koreans from the Northeast, and Zhuang from Guangxi Province (in southern China) (Fig. 3.2), using genetic markers including PGM_1 (mentioned above) (Goede et al., 1984) and HLA types (T. D. Lee et al., 1988). Within these major clusters in China, more specific population groups have also been studied. In an analysis of serum samples from five populations in China, a south–north gradient or geocline was shown for Gm loci frequencies but not for Kml alleles (Matsumoto et al., 1986). Genetic heterogeneity in these and other loci (especially HLA) is relevant to the interpretation of cancer mortality and incidence data, although environmental and other ethnic-related factors are undoubtedly more important (as discussed later in this book). For example, an association between degree of urbanization and cancer risk has been reported (Haynes, 1986) with some north–south gradients in both (Chapter 8). Associations with HLA phenotype frequencies should also be explored in future studies.

The reader should recall a point made in Chapter 1 concerning the importance of clines or gradients in frequencies of traits or genes. Clines may be relevant to both physical anthropological studies in eventually supplanting "race" as a variable of interest (Lasker and Tyzzer, 1982) and in epidemiologic studies, or more importantly in the merging of the two disciplines to increase our understanding of disease causation. Additional data are needed on the physical anthropology and epidemiology of these various Mongoloid groups, especially smaller geographic subgroups within each population. Reports on HLA phenotype and gene frequencies in northern (Beijing) Chinese (Yiping and Changxing, 1985) and HLA antigen frequencies in normal controls in a study of insulin-dependent diabetes mellitus in southern Chinese in Hong Kong (Hawkins et al., 1987) need to be supplemented by additional studies. A major recent study included 2,441 "randomly selected" Chinese from nine ethnic groups in 14 locations, including Southern Han, Mongols, various southern minorities (including Zhuang) and Koreans; heterogeneity among these groups was found for the frequencies of many HLA antigens (T. D. Lee et al., 1988).

All of these genetic data are of special interest in view of the increasing number of epidemiologic studies on various diseases, including cancers, among these Mongoloid or Mongoloid-derived populations. Recently published atlases of cancer mortality in China are mentioned in the next Chapter and studies on various genetic and chronic diseases in different parts of China are reviewed later.

Indian Subcontinent and Sri Lanka

One major subdivision long recognized on the Indian subcontinent is the north versus south (or "Dravidian") separation (see Table 3.1). The complex, kaleidoscopic picture of historical invasions and migrations, and their effects on the gene pool, is evident here as in other areas such as South Africa. Studies in West Bengal using genetic variation in 12 systems has supported earlier anthropometric–somatoscopic evidence for the presence of Mongoloid, Caucasoid, and "proto-Australoid" racial elements (Chakraborty et al., 1986). Considerable genetic variation is evident among Indian groups, even within each region, as shown by studies of HLA types in a tribe in southern India (Papiha et al., 1983), degree of Gc heterozygosity within various tribes (Papiha et al., 1987), and variation in an enzyme polymorphism of human red cells (phosphoglucomutase-1) in Dravidian-speaking groups of South India (Reddy et al., 1986). The population of *Sri Lanka* is ethnically diverse including the Tamils with historical roots in southern India. Legendary linkages of the Sinhalese to East India have not been supported by genetic studies of 13 polymorphic loci which show no differences between the Tamils and Sinhalese (Saha, 1988).

The *Parsis* of Bombay were mentioned briefly in Chapter 1. This group originated from Persia (Iran) about 900–1,200 years ago and now show distinct patterns of marriage (i.e., endogamy) and reproduction. The colorful groups known as *gypsies* are mentioned here because they probably originated in northern India about 1,000 years ago and spread to Europe and the United States. Studies of blood groups and other genetic factors suggest an affinity between gypsies from northwestern India and those from Europe (Balgir, 1986). Genetic differentiation has occurred among gypsy groups owing to dispersal, inbreeding (within specific subgroups), and varying degrees of "hybridization" with local nongypsy groups. Nevertheless, these groups have attempted to organize internationally and to ensure their cultural identity (Liegeios, 1986). Gypsy groups in the United States are mentioned later, including some limited epidemiologic data on diseases.

Jewish Groups

Although populations sharing the Jewish religion do not constitute a major biological race, they are closer to one another than to their non-Jewish neighbors in various characteristics. Examples of such characteristics are the relatively high frequency of the "cDe" (or R^o) haplotype in the Rh blood group system versus other Europeans (although not as high as in Africa) and certain anthropometric characteristics with high heritability suggesting genetic control (Kobyliansky and Livshits, 1985; Sofaer et al., 1986). A study of immunoglobulin (Gm) types also indicates distinctive characteristics (Stevenson et al., 1985), suggesting that Jewish populations are derived from a common gene pool with minimal gene flow. The genetics of Jewish populations have been discussed in great detail by Mourant et al. (1978) and by Rothschild (1981).

Use of morphologic characteristics in admixture studies has been criticized by Chakraborty (1986), who also reviewed estimates of "gentile" admixture, which are inconsistent but generally quite high in various Jewish groups. Briefly, we note that European or Ashkenazic Jews tend to show higher rates of admixture than Oriental or African (Sephardic) Jews (Jorde, 1985). Further studies of Ashkenazim versus Sephardim groups would be interesting in view of differences in diseases between these major groups (discussed later).

Other Groups

Levels of genetic differentiation have been studied in various other ethnic groups. Briefly, all *European* populations appear to be closely related, probably reflecting high rates of migration and gene flow (Jorde, 1985).

An exception to the genetic homogeneity of Europeans is the divergent *Lapps*, an isolated local race (see Table 3.1, Fig. 3.1). The Lapps, who prefer to call themselves Samer and now inhabit the far north of Scandinavia and Kola Peninsula of the Soviet Union, may have originated from Russia. Aside from their high frequency of the A-2 allele of the ABO blood group (noted earlier), "pure" Lapp children attending "nomad schools" in Sweden had frequencies of Gc types (including a high frequency of the Gc-1F gene) significantly different from those of other Swedish groups and non-Lappish Finns (Beckman et al., 1988).

The *West Asian region* is essentially European-like biologically, with some African and Oriental admixtures, and includes several subgroups such as Arabia–Southern Afghanistan, Syria–Armenia–Central Afghanistan, and Iraq–Persian Gulf–Iran (Bowles, 1977). Although Garn (1971) recognized "Mediterranean," "Turkic," and "Iranian" local races, the degree of genetic differentiation among these groups is uncertain. In a study of 1,038 persons in Greek Macedonia using multiple blood group and serum protein markers, only small differences were observed from Turks, other Greeks, and Bulgarians, but the lack of genetic data on populations in the region was also noted (Tills et al., 1983b). The same RFLPs in X chromosome segments were found in both German and Turkish population samples, with no conclusive evidence of different allele frequencies (Schurmann et al., 1987).

The Maltese of the Island of Malta will be mentioned because of the availability of mortality data (Chapter 4). The earliest inhabitants of the Mediterranean island of Malta (south of Sicily) were Phoenicians, as reflected in the modern language and the name Malta (from Phoenician "Maleth"), but early European contact resulted in Europeanization of culture.

"Modest but definable" differentiation in blood polymorphisms (blood groups, red cell enzymes, and serum proteins) were reported in local groups within the relatively closed Iranian Christian groups, probably due to urbanization (in Tehran) and random factors (Akbari et al., 1986). The level of differentiation was similar to that found for interstate and intrastate subpopulations in India (Papiha et al., 1982) but less than that in the diverse populations of South Africa and South America. Some limited data on cancers in selected Iranian populations, especially those near the Caspian Sea, are discussed later (Chapter 8). However, extensive regional data on cancer and other diseases in these areas are not yet available (see Howe, 1986).

The degree of genetic differentiation is rather small among subpopulations of northwest *England*. In areas such as Great Britain, the extensively studied distribution of surnames shows that since the Middle Ages the population structure has been open, with "considerable opportunity for the exchange of genes among geographic areas" (Lasker, 1985). In another island population, *Iceland*, the unresolved controversies regarding the degree of "Nordic" admixture and the effects of possible heterogeneity of the early Nordic and Celtic settlers have been reviewed by Chakraborty (1986). Chakraborty also noted the probable effects of past epidemics, such as smallpox and plague, on frequencies of genes at heterogeneity and other loci. Some diseases more common in Iceland and the Scandinavian countries are mentioned later.

Several selected *U.S. ethnic groups* should be mentioned, in addition to Hispanics and U.S. blacks. Included are several religious/cultural or "ethnic" groups. The *Mormon* population of Utah increased rapidly after initial colonization in 1870 and is now genetically homogeneous, due to the large founding population and internal migration. Mormons resemble U.S. whites genetically but show some cultural differences including smoking habits, diet, and marriage patterns (Jorde, 1982; Jorde and Durbize, 1986). The *Hutterite Anabaptists*, in contrast, have only 15 surnames among geographic and endogamous subdivisions derived from Ukrainian immigrants. The Hutterites are an Anabaptist sect originating in the Moravian Alps (c. 16th century) who migrated to eastern and southern Europe and, in small numbers, to the United States and western Canada. Cancer patterns have been studied in the Mormons and Hutterites. *Seventh Day Adventists* are a religious group in the United States and Europe that is culturally distinct in terms of personal habits (e.g., diet and smoking), and thus the relative frequency of various chronic diseases in this group are of particular interest (as discussed later).

Other U.S. groups include more than 650,000 *Southeast Asian refugees* admitted since 1975, who show high frequencies of certain genetic conditions (Chapter 5) and infectious and parasitic diseases (see Chapter 6). Studies on reproductive outcomes and psychiatric epidemiologic studies also have been conducted (Chapter 9). *Haitian immigrants* have appeared over the past 25 years in several large cities and often maintain cultural traditions (Laguerre, 1981). These Haitian-Americans are of interest epidemiologically for several reasons, including the study of effects of previous environmental influences such as malnutrition in Haiti (the poorest Caribbean country), an apparent tendency to seek treatment at later stages of diseases (such as cancers), and in connection with the epidemic of AIDS-related diseases (as discussed later). *Gypsy* groups (see earlier) began to arrive in the United States about 100 years ago, and epidemiologic studies of families in Boston suggest high frequencies of certain chronic diseases (see later).

OTHER PHYSICAL ANTHROPOLOGICAL DATA

The above discussion has emphasized population genetics and has been limited to variation in frequencies of phenotypes related to genetic loci involved mainly in blood group, serum protein, immunoglobulin, and heterogeneity polymorphisms. Other research in physical anthropology concerns anthropometric and physiologic differences between populations. Brief mention has already been made of anthropometric and odontrometric characteristics in connection with estimation of racial admixture or population affinities.

Other anthropometric and physiologic characteristics that show differences among populations are related to disease susceptibility. Examples are level of obesity, anatomical distribution of body fat, density of bones, and various blood chemistry parameters. Table 3.6 shows some differences in selected characteristics found between certain "black" versus white populations, the two groups that have been studied most extensively.

Earlier surveys of noninstitutionalized children 6–11 and 12–17 years of age in the United States showed lower average skinfold measurements (an index of body fat) in blacks versus whites (Johnston et al., 1972, 1974). Recent interest has focused on differences in obesity among U.S. black and white children and adults, the adolescent development of abdominal fat (i.e., the male or "android" pattern)

Table 3.6 Some Selected Differences in Anthropometric, Physiologic, and Biochemical Characteristics in Black and White Populations

Higher in blacks	Lower in blacks
Density of bone	LDL cholesterol in blood[a]
HDL cholesterol in blood	Leukocyte count in blood
Fibrinolytic activity in blood	Hemoglobin concentration in blood
Testosterone in blood (males)	Lactase deficiency[b]
Red cell sodium concentration	Width of female pelvis
Blood pressure (U.S., parts of Africa)	Birth weight and gestation length
Intraocular pressure	
Body fat, adult females	
Lean body mass and density[c]	
Leg length	
Shoulder/hip breadth	

Modified and updated after Damon (1971, 1977).

[a]Low- and high-density lipoproteins are discussed throughout this book.

[b]Deficiency in the enzyme lactase is related to intolerance to lactose, also frequent in certain other groups (e.g., Japanese and Koreans) (Johnson et al., 1984). This condition is usually mild and is not discussed in this book.

[c]Due to denser and heavier skeletons (Schutte et al., 1984).

in U.S. blacks and whites (Baumgartner et al., 1986), and the possible role of adrenal androgens in explaining population differences in childhood growth (Zemel and Katz, 1986). Some of these racial differences in biological characteristics will be discussed later, with reference to interpretation of disease patterns.

The tendency for greater weight gain in U.S. black versus white adult females has been observed by several investigators (Khoury et al., 1983; Blair et al., 1986). According to the U.S. Health and Nutrition Examination Survey, the prevalence of "overweight," as defined by a weight/height index, reaches 60% among U.S. black women by age 45 years (see Chapter 4). Kumanyika (1987) has reviewed the literature on obesity in black women and noted the need for studies on cultural versus social class factors, including attitudes regarding obesity, as well as studies of diet during adolescence. There is evidence that the factors that contribute to the development of obesity in blacks (especially women) may differ from those involved in maintaining obesity once it is established. Data from the Bogalusa (Louisiana) Heart Study indicate that total fat and cholesterol intakes were greater in black than white children 6 months to 4 years of age, and this could influence eating behavior in later childhood and adolescence (Nicklas et al., 1987a).

Results of a study in a selected group of higher-SES women in Dallas suggest that black women have poorer cardiovascular fitness (on the basis of a treadmill test) than white or Mexican-American women, even after adjusting for greater body fat among blacks (Farrell et al., 1987). Thus intensive intervention programs may be needed for black women, aimed at improving fitness through exercise programs. Earlier Gartside et al. (1984) had concluded that weight reduction programs in obese black female *adults* should emphasize increased physical activity rather than reduced caloric intake, because of lack of black–white differences in caloric intake in adults. In summary, intervention programs should aim at reducing fat intake in black children in order to prevent the establishment of obesity in childhood or adolescence, while exercise programs may be more beneficial in reducing obesity once it is established in adult black women. This does not preclude studies on the role of exercise programs in children as an adjunct to dietary programs in obesity prevention.

Another group studied in recent years is the U.S. "Hispanic" population, comprised of several subgroups including Mexican-Americans in California and the Southwest and Puerto Ricans in the New York area. Earlier studies of Mexican-Americans were concerned with the effects of undernutrition on growth, while more recent studies have turned to overnutrition and excess fatness, along with shorter stature, in children (Malina et al., 1986). Recently available anthropometric data are from U.S. surveys, including the National Health and Nutrition Examination surveys (1971–73 and 1976–80) and the Hispanic Health and Nutrition Examination Survey (1982–84) (see Chapter 4). Special studies in select groups have confirmed the shorter stature of Mexican-Americans and also shown that the relatively longer lower extremities of blacks are not found in white or Mexican-American youths (Malina et al., 1987).

Extensive research has been carried out on body size, shape and composition among Japanese in Japan where changing habits of diet and exercise are influencing chronic disease rates—for example, for cardiovascular diseases and certain cancers. The secular or long-term trend for increasing stature, for example, may be ending (Kimura, 1984), while young adult women are becoming slimmer (Takahashi, 1986).

Comparative studies of height, weight, limb proportions, and amount and distribution of body fat in racial/ethnic groups are relevant to the interpretation of differences in the development of such diseases as hypertension, other cardiovascular disorders, and cancers. The relevance of these and other anthropometric and physiologic differences to racial/ethnic differences in disease will be discussed later.

Our discussion has turned from population genetic data obtained through special anthropological surveys to other aspects of physical anthropology that have been studied in large-scale health surveys in developed countries. Physical anthropological data obtained from health surveys, along with data on other risk factors in disease will be discussed in the next chapter.

CONCLUSIONS

The last decade has witnessed a major expansion of knowledge on the genetic differentiation of major racial groups and various selected populations. Some limited conclusions have been drawn regarding possible meaningful subdivisions of mankind and the extent of admixture in such areas as the Far East, India, the Caribbean, South Africa, and the United States. Methodologic difficulties and problems of interpretation of conflicting estimates of genetic differentiation and degree of admixture, however, are great.

The integration of all of these data on physical anthropology with descriptive and analytical epidemiologic studies on racial/ethnic differences in disease is obviously a major task, as yet barely begun. Some case control studies involving specific genetic characteristics, such as blood groups and HLA types, in different racial/ethnic groups will be discussed later. Attempts to consider the usefulness of genetic differentiation and especially degree of admixture in the interpretation of for racial/ethnic differences in disease will be discussed later in this book.

Now that we have considered some evidence from physical anthropology regarding genetic and other biological characteristics of racial/ethnic groups, we shall turn to sources of data on health and disease in these groups and comparisons of disease rates.

4

Some Sources of Data on Health and Disease

We have discussed the utility of racial/ethnic groups in epidemiology and described some anthropological characteristics of selected groups relevant to studies of disease. Some sources of information on morbidity and mortality in racial/ethnic groups will now be outlined. Also included are sources of data on nutrition and other risk factors for disease in the United States. These sources will be utilized later in discussions of specific diseases.

UNITED STATES

Mortality and Other Vital Statistics

In the United States, health statistics have traditionally been presented in routine statistical reports according to "white" and "nonwhite" groups. More recent reports, however, have included separate data (on numerators, if not rates) for various racial/ethnic categories, such as Japanese, Chinese, American Indian, blacks, and Anglo and Hispanic whites. There is also interest in diseases and other characteristics (e.g., birth weight) for subcategories within broad groupings, such as Indochinese refugees within the "Asian" group.

The annual *Vital Statistics of the United States*, Volume II (Mortality), Part A, includes *numbers* of deaths by sex for various groups defined by "race or national origin"—white, black, Indian, Chinese, Japanese, Filipino, other Asian or Pacific Islander, and "other." Death *rates* by age and sex, however, are presented only for whites and blacks. Starting with 1984, numbers of deaths from 72 selected causes were presented by Hispanic origin in 10-year age groups by sex for 15 reporting states (excluding New Mexico), for which data on Hispanics were judged to be at least 90% complete; these states account for only 45% of the total Hispanic population. Death rates for this subpopulation of Hispanics were not presented, and studies in specific states are discussed later. Obtaining national mortality data on the US. Hispanic population is a major priority, although regional data are also needed to explore regional differences within the broad "Hispanic" category.

There is concern regarding the quality of death certificate data on race and its comparability with census data. Reporting of black race on death certificates is accurate as shown for the United States and for New York State (Kitigawa and Hauser, 1973; Carucci, 1979). Denominators for death rates involve census data that have problems of undercounting of blacks, especially young adult black males. Spanish origin or "Hispanic" data on death certificates is generally less reliable. Country of origin (e.g., Puerto Rico, Mexico, and Cuba), however, has been used in mortality analyses for the entire United States (Rosenweig, 1987).

Age-specific mortality rates for U.S. blacks and whites can be compared from routinely published vital statistics data (Table 4.1). These published data involve use of codes for causes of death based on the latest revision of *International Classification of Diseases* of the World Health Organization (e.g., WHO, 1977). Some marked differences in mortality rates for specific diseases and age groups are evident, and these are discussed in more detail in subsequent chapters. Table 3.7 will be cited throughout the text; presently, it serves to indicate the type of mortality statistics available by age, sex, and race.

Table 4.2 shows an example of direct age standardization of death rates, for all causes, in U.S. blacks and whites for 1985. The total population of the United States, expressed as percentages by age group, is used as the standard population (see Chapter 1 for discussion of age-standardized rates). It is noteworthy that complete reliance on age-standardized rates, which is a summary measure, obscures the fact that the black/white ratio of death rates for all causes is highest in young adults (ages 25–54) and low at age 75 years and older (when death rates are highest). Also missed by age-standardized rates are variations in black–white differences in death rates by age group for certain specific causes, as discussed later.

Age-specific death rates are needed to evaluate the impact of mortality on life expectancy. Such concepts as "years of potential life lost" (YPLL) or "preventable mortality" are useful in demonstrating the impact of differential mortality by age and may be used for specific disease categories (Anon., 1986i). Obviously, important contributors to total YPLL and preventable mortality are deaths during the first year of life or infant mortality, which is also subdivided into neonatal and other categories (see Chapter 9). Infant mortality rates (per 100,000 live births) are presented in annual *Vital Statistics of the U.S.* reports for the racial groups listed above and also for 61 selected causes of death for white and black infants.

The National Cancer Institute has published atlases of mortality from cancers and other diseases for white and nonwhite populations in the United States, the most recent being that for whites (Pickle et al., 1987) (see Chapter 8). An updated version of an earlier atlas on cancer mortality in nonwhites (Mason et al., 1976) is due shortly.

Morbidity and Risk Factors

A major source of data on racial/ethnic-specific disease morbidity and risk factors for disease in the United States is the National Health Survey, established as a continuing program by congressional act in 1956, which includes the Na-

Table 4.1 Mortality Rates (per 100,000 population) from Selected Causes in U.S. Black and White Adults by Age Group (15 Years and Older) in 1985, Sexes Combined (Unless Otherwise Indicated)

Cause (ICD codes)	Age group (years)							
	15–24	25–34	35–44	45–54	55–64	65–74	75–84	85+
All causes								
White	92	108	181	472	1,219	2,772	6,407	15,757
Black	116	235	444	936	2,008	3,759	7,407	13,076
Tuberculosis (010–018)								
White	0.0	0.1	0.2	0.4	0.9	1.8	4.0	5.8
Black	0.2	1.0	2.3	3.9	5.2	7.0	12.4	22.5
Syphilis (090–097)								
White						0.1	0.2	0.4
Black				0.1	0.3	0.3	0.7	2.5
All cancers (140–308)								
White	5.5	12.8	43	161	438	829	1,272	1,595
Black	5.3	15.9	70	255	618	1,014	1,479	1,636
Breast cancer (174)								
White	0.1	2.8	17	47	84	110	140	179
Black	0.2	4.4	26	54	89	99	121	153
Oral cavity, pharynx cancer (140–149)								
White	0.0	0.2	0.6	3.4	9.4	15	17	21
Black	0.1	0.4	3.4	12	20	18	17	10
Digestive cancer (150–159)								
White	0.3	1.4	6.6	30	94	205	369	538
Black	0.7	2.8	13	61	160	282	450	555
Respiratory cancer (160–165)								
White	0.1	0.7	7.5	50	154	268	297	202
Black	0.2	1.4	15	82	217	295	288	201
Diabetes (250)								
White	0.2	1.2	3.3	7.1	22	54	120	211
Black	0.7	2.1	7.6	23	60	121	232	261
Hypertensive heart disease (402)								
White	0.0	0.2	0.8	3.5	10	24	60	157
Black	0.2	1.3	8.6	28	59	95	177	249
Ischemic heart disease (410–414)								
White	0.3	2.7	22	103	307	782	1,955	5,106
Black	0.7	5.6	37	137	371	792	1,685	3,238
Hypertension (401, 403)								
White	0.0	0.0	0.2	0.8	2.8	8.5	26	72
Black	0.1	0.5	2.5	7.4	16	31	65	119

Table 4.1 *(continued)*

Cause (ICD codes)	Age group (years)							
	15–24	25–34	35–44	45–54	55–64	65–74	75–84	85+
Cerebrovascular diseases (430–438)								
White	0.7	1.7	5.4	17	47	158	593	1,873
Black	1.4	5.7	22	59	130	315	791	1,514
Intracerebral hemorrhage (431–432)								
White	0.2	0.5	1.7	5.4	12	28	68	121
Black	0.6	2.3	11	24	33	44	83	109
Thrombosis (434.0–434.9)								
White	0.1	0.1	0.3	1.5	6.1	25	99	336
Black	0.1	0.3	1.4	4.9	18	45	120	241
Pneumonia (480–486)								
White	0.6	1.1	2.3	5.7	16	55	235	1,017
Black	0.9	4.3	11	19	37	78	240	615
COPD[a] (490–496)								
White	0.3	0.4	1.3	10	48	154	304	377
Black	1.4	1.7	4.0	15	46	99	171	175
Ulcer (531–533)								
White	0.0	0.1	0.3	1.3	3.3	8.9	25	65
Black	0.0	0.3	0.9	1.5	5.7	8.8	23	38
Chronic liver disease and cirrhosis (571)								
White	0.1	2.2	7.6	20	33	38	33	20
Black	0.3	8.1	28	41	46	37	25	13
Chronic glomerulonephritis (582–3, 587)								
White	0.0	0.1	0.1	0.2	0.6	1.9	5.0	14
Black	0.1	0.3	0.5	0.8	1.5	4.1	13	26
Renal failure (584–6, 588–9)								
White	0.1	0.3	0.8	2.0	6.9	22	66	189
Black	0.3	1.7	4.7	9.2	28	65	141	318
Motor vehicle accidents (E810–25)								
White	39	23	17	15	15	18	28	27
Black	20	22	21	18	21	18	25	18
Suicide (E950–9)								
White	14	16	16	17	18	20	26	20
Black	7.6	11	8.7	7.8	6.4	7.9	8.7	3.4
Homicide (E960–78)								
White	7.4	9.1	7.5	5.7	4.2	3.2	3.6	3.4
Black	40	55	43	28	21	16	13	13

Source: Vital Statistics of the United States 1985 (published 1988).

[a]Chronic obstructive pulmonary disease.

Where the rate is less than 10, it is shown to one decimal place.

Table 4.2 Calculation of Age-Standardized Rates for All Causes Combined in U.S. Blacks and Whites for 1980

| | Whites | | Blacks | | Standard population |
Age	Rate	Rate × SP	Rate	Rate × SP	in percent
15–24	92	22.3	116	28.1	0.242
25–34	108	22.9	235	49.8	0.212
35–44	181	26.4	444	64.8	0.146
45–54	472	61.4	936	121.7	0.130
55–64	1,219	151.2	2,008	249.0	0.124
65–74	2,773	246.8	3,759	334.6	0.089
75–84	6,407	281.9	7,407	325.9	0.044
85+	15,757	204.8	13,076	170.0	0.013
Total		1,017.7		1,343.9	

SP: Percent of standard population (total U.S. population) age 15 years and older.

tional Health Interview Survey (NHIS), the National Health Examination Survey (NHES, starting in 1959–62) and the National Health and Nutrition Examination Surveys (NHANES) Phases I (1971–74) and II (1976–80). The NHIS is a continuing annual nationwide survey by household interview of a probability sample of the civilian noninstitutionalized population; the sample in 1983 was approximately 41,000 houeholds with about 106,000 persons, and the response rate was high. NHANES is periodically updated, with resurveys scheduled for 1988–91 and 1992–94, and includes data on diet and serum and urine samples. Blacks and Hispanics were oversampled to provide more reliable data on these groups. The annual NHIS includes self-identification of race and Hispanic origin, so that results can be analyzed by race and ethnic group. The U.S. National Cancer Institute has conducted a special version of the NHIS that focuses on smoking and cancer prevention and on cancer control through screening for earlier detection of cancer (Anon., 1988d).

Special surveys include the Hispanic Health and Nutrition Examination Survey (HHANES), which focused on three subgroups of U.S. Hispanics— Mexican-Americans in the Southwest (mainly California and Texas); Cuban-Americans in Dade County, Florida; and Puerto Ricans in New York City. Data from HHANES have recently been released as "public use tapes" for researchers. These data include results of physicians' examinations as well as anthropometric and dietary survey results (see also Malina et al., 1986). National surveys of health and health practices of blacks and Hispanics include some special surveys of attitudes and practices regarding cancer and cancer screening, sponsored by the American Cancer Society.

In the United States a recent survey of adults conducted by the CDC found that black males 25–34 years of age had the highest smoking rate (45.9 percent) while younger black men had the lowest rate (14.3 percent). Overall, the smoking rate was slightly higher in black men (32.5 percent) than white men (29.3 percent) and among black versus white women (25.1 percent vs. 23.7 percent respectively) (Anon., 1987e). The average number of cigarettes smoked was lower in blacks, perhaps reflecting socioeconomic disparities. U.S. Hispanics once smoked less than Anglos or blacks, but this pattern has changed (Caetano, 1983; Marcus and Crane, 1985). Among schoolchildren in New Mexico, the prevalence of smoking was similar in Hispanic and non-Hispanic whites, and male Hispanics actually smoked more cigarettes per week (Greenberg et al., 1987). Thus, antismoking educational efforts are needed to help maintain the generally lower rates of certain cancers among these Hispanic groups (see Chapter 8). The same may be true for Amerindians.

As noted above, dietary surveys in NHANES includes data on intake of specific nutrients in blacks and whites, which are relevant to studies of racial differences in various chronic diseases including cancer. Detailed tables include data on mean and median intake of selected nutrients (e.g., total calories, protein, calcium, iron, and several specific vitamins) in blacks and whites by age, sex, and income (i.e., above vs. below the poverty level) (Abraham et al., 1977). The Pediatric Nutrition Surveillance System established by the Centers for Disease Control in 1974 and involving 33 states includes data on the prevalence of "short stature" and "overweight," based on national growth reference charts for children under 5 years old, in low-income families participating in various programs and clinics. Noteworthy were the high prevalence of overweight in Hispanic children after 11 months of age and the high prevalence of short stature among Pacific Islander children (Anon., 1987h).

Turning to morbidity data, the NHIS reports include current estimates of acute and chronic conditions and number and type of physician contacts by black–white race and (often) by income level within each race. Rates of limitation of activity due to chronic disease or impairment, defined as inability to carry out major activities of one's age group (e.g., school, housekeeping, or work) in blacks and whites decrease with increasing income level (Table 4.3). Black–white differences in limitation of activity are small within income level, but the racial difference in distribution of incomes leads to a slightly higher total rate in blacks (Anon., 1986j).

A comparison of average income levels of U.S. whites, blacks, and Hispanics from the 1980 census (Table 4.4) shows this disparity. Giachello et al. (1983) have discussed both the problems and opportunities involved in using 1980 census data for studies of health care needs of Hispanic populations, including the need for

Table 4.3 Data from the U.S. National Health Survey: Percentage of Population (All Ages) with Limitation of Activity Due to Chronic Conditions, by Race and Family Income

Race	All incomes	<5,000	Family income ($) 5,000– 9,999	10,000– 14,999	15,000– 24,999	25,000+	Ratio[a]
Total	12.7	26.6	20.6	12.9	8.4	6.0	4.4
White	14.5	30.9	23.7	14.6	10.2	9.0	3.4
Black	15.4	25.5	17.9	10.6	8.7	6.3	4.0
Other	9.1	23.1	14.1	8.3	5.7	4.3	5.4

Source: Anon. (1986j).
[a]Ratio of rate in lowest income to rate in highest income.

Table 4.4 Income and Poverty Characteristics by Racial/Ethnic Group in the United States, According to the 1980 Census

Family income ($)	White	Black	Spanish origin
Median	20,840	12,618	14,711
Mean	24,279	15,721	17,360
Persons below poverty level (%)	9.4	30.2	23.8
Total population	184,431,365	25,661,955	14,343,741

Hispanic identification items on birth and death certificates of all states. Native Americans (i.e., Amerindians and Alaskan Eskimos) are similar to blacks in income levels and percentage below the poverty level in the 1980 census.

NHANES included data on blood pressure and prevalence of hypertension (Drizd et al., 1986) and serum cholesterol in blacks and whites by age and sex, as discussed later. Also included were data on "overweight" and "obesity" using height, weight, weight/height ratio, and skinfold measurements for black and white adults by age and sex; poverty status is also considered in some analyses (Van Itallie, 1985). Most noteworthy was the high prevalence of overweight in black women (see Chapter 3 and later discussions of specific diseases), increasing from 30 percent at age 25–34 to 60 percent at age 45–54 years. Although poverty status is associated with overweight, the effect of race was independent of poverty status. Previously the NHES had involved noninstitutionalized children aged 6–11 and 12–17, and included skinfold (i.e., body fat assessment) data in blacks and whites (Johnston et al., 1972, 1974). Analyses of NHES and NHANES data covering 1960 to 1980 show that female black–white differences in body mass index (i.e., weight/height) at comparable educational and income levels have persisted over time (Flegal et al., 1988).

NHANES I included questions on sunlight exposure history and dermatologic examinations focused on the deleterious effects of sunlight exposure, showing a lower prevalence of skin damage in blacks versus whites (Engel et al., 1988).

Increasingly common are risk factor surveys in individual states in the United States. In Alabama, for example, telephone survey results largely paralleled U.S. trends in showing higher rates of hypertension, diabetes mellitus, obesity (especially in women), and smoking (men only), in blacks versus whites and little difference in alcohol consumption (Rabbani et al., 1987).

For *cancer incidence*, population-based registries in such multiethnic areas as New York State, Detroit, Illinois, California, and New Mexico continue to provide valuable data on incidence and mortality rates as well as on survival of cancer patients. Some of these registries are part of the U.S. National Cancer Institutes SEER (Surveillance, Epidemiology, and End Results) program, which includes about 13% of the population but is concentrated in areas with large minority populations, such as blacks (in Detroit and New Jersey), Hispanics in New Mexico and California, Amerindian groups, and Mormons (in Utah and California) and Puerto Rico and Hawaii. The National Cancer Institute also publishes data on cancer survival by racial and ethnic group, although not all ethnic groups are included (see Chapter 8).

The National Cancer Institute has published a useful summary on "Cancer Among Blacks and Other Minorities: Statistical Profiles" (Baquet et al., 1986) which includes comparisons of incidence, mortality, and survival rates by racial/ ethnic group. Cancers and other leading causes of death among minorities are discussed in a series of "Topics on Minority Health" published periodically in *Morbidity and Mortality Weekly Reports* by the Public Health Service, in response to a 1985 recommendation to the Secretary of Health and Human Services by a task force on black and minority health.

Important sources of data on black–white differences in chronic disease incidence and risk factors are special prospective community studies of cardiovascular disease. The Evans County (Georgia) study includes mainly rural, lower-SES blacks and whites while the Framingham (Massachusetts) study involves higher-SES whites and a small sample of blacks (in the Minority Study). The Bogalusa, Louisiana, Heart Study has focused on black–white differences in diet and cardiovascular disease risk factors in children. For other racial/ethnic groups the San Antonio Heart Study provides population-based data on risk factors for cardiovascular diseases and diabetes in Mexican-Americans and Anglos. Some results of these studies will be discussed later in this book.

INTERNATIONAL

Mortality

Mortality data are available for largely multiethnic and multiracial countries, and are periodically compiled in various sourcebooks (e.g., Alderson, 1981; Thom et al., 1985). Regional comparisons of total mortality rates and rates by major causes of death, however, are for large geographic areas such as Africa, Oceania, and East Asia. These areas are comprised of many racial/ethnic groups (Chapter 3). Total annual death rates, of course, are higher for Africa (i.e., 18.0 per 1,000) and the least developed countries (17.1 per 1,000) versus the world (11.3 per 1,000) (Hakulinen et al., 1986).

The World Health Organization's *World Health Statistics Annual* (WHO, 1987) includes mortality rates, age-standardized to an estimated "world population," for selected causes of death by sex for 52 countries. Table 4.5 shows rankings (calculated by the author) from lowest to highest for selected causes of death. The countries include a variety of racial/ethnic groups and may be classified in various ways. Table 4.5 has been organized in the following groups: Canada and the United States; the Caribbean; Central and South America; Britain; Ireland and Northern Ireland; Iceland; Scandinavia (Norway, Denmark, Sweden); Finland, France; Germany; other Middle European (Netherlands, Switzerland, Luxembourg); Poland; other Slavic (Czechoslovakia, Bulgaria, Yugoslavia); other Eastern European (Austria, Hungary, Romania); South European (Spain, Portugal, Italy, Greece); Malta; Mauritius (in Africa); Israel; Kuwait; Japan; Singapore; Sri Lanka; and Western Pacific (Australia and New Zealand). These groups may be compared with those for the United States, mentioned

Table 4.5 Selected Data on Annual Age-Standardized Mortality Rates (per 100,000) in 52 Countries, Compiled from Data in WHO (1987), and Ranked from Lowest to Highest Rates

Region/country	All causes Rate	All causes Rank	Infectious/ parasitic Rate	Infectious/ parasitic Rank	All cancers Rate	All cancers Rank
North America						
Canada	504.7	5	2.9	4	134.5	34
U.S.	563.7	15	7.2	28	132.2	31
Caribbean						
Bahamas	730.6	38	14.5	37	103.2	10
Barbados	596.2	22	15.8	38	111.1	18
Cuba	594.1	21	12.4	36	110.1	16
Dominica	807.4	45	30.5	48	157.7	49
Martinique	622.7	28	10.8	34	127.7	29
Puerto Rico	561.6	14	9.8	33	93.9	7
St. Vincent/Grenadines	889.1	49	22.0	44	111.3	19
Trinidad/Tobago	899.9	50	20.7	42	99.4	8
Central/South America						
Guatemala	1023.5	52	216.0	52	56.9	2
Argentina	683.5	35	22.9	45	118.5	24
Belize	707.2	37	55.9	50	58.6	3
Chile	739.8	39	26.3	47	122.9	27
Suriname	864.2	48	40.5	49	83.5	5
Uruquay	676.6	34	21.0	43	152.2	46
Britain						
England and Wales	586.9	19	3.2	7	150.0	45
Scotland	662.7	32	4.4	15.5	160.9	50
Ireland						
Northern Ireland	655.4	30	2.4	1	142.1	39
Ireland	664.5	33	4.7	18.3	146.1	43
Iceland	459.8	2	3.7	11	121.9	26
Scandinavia						
Denmark	585.2	18	3.5	9	155.6	48
Norway	522.6	8	4.7	18.3	121.6	25
Sweden	493.7	4	4.0	12.5	112.5	21
Finland	577.0	16	4.9	21	118.0	23
Northern Europe						
Belgium	600.3	23	4.6	17	153.0	47
Netherlands	507.2	6	2.8	2.5	145.8	42
Middle Europe						
Luxembourg	606.0	24	3.4	8	147.1	44
Switzerland	471.6	3	5.4	23	131.2	30
Poland	768.7	40	8.7	31	144.4	40
Eastern Europe						
Czechoslovakia	787.1	42	2.8	2.5	161.1	51
Bulgaria	784.3	41	6.5	26	107.1	13
Yugoslavia	801.4	43	17.5	39	112.3	20
Other Eastern European						
Austria	581.8	17	3.0	5	133.7	33
Hungary	855.9	47	6.4	24.5	172.8	52
Romania	829.6	46	9.2	32	101.6	9
France	519.4	7	6.8	27	138.5	36

Table 4.5 (continued)

Region/country	All causes		Infectious/ parasitic		All cancers	
	Rate	Rank	Rate	Rank	Rate	Rank
Germany, FRG	551.4	12	4.7	18.3	136.5	35
Germany, DDR	698.6	36	3.6	10	125.1	28
Southern Europe						
Portugal	616.5	26	7.9	29	106.3	12
Spain	531.4	10	8.5	30	110.7	17
Italy	591.6	20	4.0	12.5	141.9	38
Greece	525.2	9	4.4	15.5	109.5	15
Malta	611.8	25	4.2	14	115.8	22
Africa—Mauritius	913.4	51	23.4	46	71.4	4
Israel	557.9	13	11.6	35	105.4	11
Kuwait	662.6	31	18.6	40	89.8	6
Japan	418.1	1	6.4	24.5	108.4	4
Singapore	642.3	29	20.0	41	139.8	37
Sri Lanka	803.7	44	57.8	51	35.6	1
Australia	549.4	11	3.1	6	132.5	32
New Zealand	618.1	27	5.2	22	145.1	41

Region/country	All circulatory		IHD		Stroke	
	Rate	Rank	Rate	Rank	Rate	Rank
North America						
Canada	199.6	6	123.6	33	33.3	5
U.S.	240.3	24	134.6	36	35.6	6
Caribbean						
Bahamas	251.4	29.5	66.4	14	84.0	41
Barbados	249.1	28	50.3	10	83.3	40
Cuba	248.1	26	135.7	38	55.5	20
Dominica	327.7	41	34.5	5	73.3	34
Martinique	212.8	10	16.8	1	98.6	45
Puerto Rico	206.1	9	80.3	21	29.9	4
St. Vincent/Grenadines	336.4	42	40.8	6	67.6	29
Trinidad/Tobago	398.2	48	164.6	48	122.0	50
Central/South America						
Guatemala	119.4	1	30.4	4	27.0	2
Argentina	298.8	37	75.0	16	66.6	28
Belize	238.4	21	52.3	11	38.8	9
Chile	213.6	11	77.5	19	71.1	32
Suriname	251.4	29.5	90.6	24	65.8	26
Uruquay	239.6	23	82.3	22	76.8	37
Britain						
England and Wales	260.4	32	156.0	45	60.7	23
Scotland	302.8	38	184.2	51	75.5	35
Ireland						
Northern Ireland	309.9	39	190.2	52	69.2	30
Ireland	313.4	40	174.2	49	64.8	25
Iceland	201.8	7	135.4	37	38.6	8
Scandinavia						
Denmark	232.4	18	147.5	42	42.9	12
Norway	224.9	15	129.7	34	50.7	16
Sweden	235.4	20	146.8	41	42.0	11

Table 4.5 (*continued*)

Region/country	All circulatory		IHD		Stroke	
	Rate	Rank	Rate	Rank	Rate	Rank
Finland	280.6	36	163.1	47	62.5	24
Northern Europe						
Belgium	225.7	16	77.0	18	55.1	19
Netherlands	205.2	8	103.4	28	41.0	10
Middle Europe						
Luxembourg	258.9	31	86.6	23	90.4	44
Switzerland	181.7	5	68.7	15	36.9	7
Poland	364.3	44	75.6	17	47.7	14
Eastern Europe						
Czechoslovakia	394.6	47	179.2	50	115.1	49
Bulgaria	432.1	51	146.4	40	153.5	52
Yugoslavia	375.2	46	63.6	13	86.5	43
Other Eastern European						
Austria	264.2	34	95.7	26	75.5	36
Hungary	406.8	49	153.0	44	113.9	48
Romania	449.7	52	111.0	29	112.8	46
France	156.5	4	47.1	7	45.9	13
Germany, FRG	238.9	22	98.1	27	57.1	22
Germany, DDR	356.5	43	93.0	25	53.6	17
Southern Europe						
Portugal	232.6	19	48.5	8	125.5	51
Spain	220.9	12	49.7	9	77.5	39
Italy	248.8	27	78.7	20	70.5	31
Greece	223.0	13	57.3	12	85.9	42
Malta	370.7	45	149.5	43	77.1	38
Africa—Mauritius	424.3	50	131.4	35	113.0	47
Israel	224.1	14	114.9	30	48.5	15
Kuwait	276.6	35	120.2	32	27.9	3
Japan	150.3	3	24.9	3	66.1	27
Singapore	230.3	17	119.1	31	71.7	33
Sri Lanka	122.8	2	22.5	2	17.5	1
Australia	244.7	25	141.7	39	54.9	18
New Zealand	261.4	33	156.2	46	56.8	21

Region/country	Chronic liver		Injury		Motor vehicle		Suicide	
	Rate	Rank	Rate	Rank	Rate	Rank	Rate	Rank
North America								
Canada	7.3	20	45.9	21	14.9	33	11.3	30
U.S.	9.6	27	53.6	30	17.6	40.5	10.7	28.5
Caribbean								
Bahamas	16.3	39	65.8	46	11.2	23.5	0.7	3.5
Barbados	4.8	9	41.0	13	9.2	12.5	1.6	6
Cuba	6.4	16	67.7	47	—	—	—	—
Dominica	8.5	24	23.9	2	9.6	15	0.0	1
Martinique	12.6	32	53.8	31	15.6	35	4.1	12
Puerto Rico	24.7	48	53.3	28	15.8	36	10.0	26
St. Vincent/Grenadines	2.6	3	52.0	26	4.6	3	2.4	8.5
Trinidad/Tobago	13.5	34.5	62.6	40	17.3	39	8.6	22
Central/South America								
Guatemala	15.2	38	62.3	39	1.5	1	0.9	5

Table 4.5 (continued)

Region/country	Chronic liver		Injury		Motor vehicle		Suicide	
	Rate	Rank	Rate	Rank	Rate	Rank	Rate	Rank
Argentina	11.6	30.5	49.9	25	11.2	23.5	6.2	15
Belize	13.5	34.5	43.8	18	9.0	10	1.9	7
Chile	44.8	51	83.1	48	7.7	5	6.3	16
Suriname	20.1	44	101.0	51	27.4	48	29.1	47
Uruquay	6.4	16	44.9	19	7.8	6	8.1	21
Britain								
England and Wales	3.5	5	28.9	3	8.6	8	7.1	18
Scotland	5.4	12.5	42.2	16	10.8	20.5	9.3	24
Ireland								
Northern Ireland	3.6	5	41.2	14	12.0	25	7.2	19
Ireland	2.5	2	37.0	6	13.3	28	6.6	17
Iceland	1.2	1	38.4	8	10.0	19	12.3	33
Scandinavia								
Denmark	9.0	25.5	56.5	36	13.4	29	22.0	44
Norway	5.0	11	46.7	22	9.5	14	12.5	34.5
Sweden	4.7	8	42.1	15	8.8	9	14.5	38
Finland	6.5	18	65.1	45	10.8	20.5	22.6	46
Northern Europe								
Belgium	9.0	25.5	56.1	35	17.9	43	18.4	43
Netherlands	4.0	7	29.5	4	8.5	7	9.3	24
Middle Europe								
Luxembourg	13.4	33	54.0	32	20.6	45	10.7	28.5
Switzerland	7.6	21.5	54.4	34	14.2	32	18.1	42
Poland	8.4	23	63.0	43	12.7	27	11.8	31
Eastern Europe								
Czechoslovakia	14.2	37	63.0	41.5	9.6	16.5	15.7	39
Bulgaria	11.6	30.5	54.3	33	11.0	22	12.1	32
Yugoslavia	20.7	45	53.6	29	17.8	42	13.9	36
Other Eastern Europe								
Austria	19.3	43	61.3	38	16.3	37	22.3	45
Hungary	31.5	50	90.1	50	14.0	30	35.2	48
Romania	26.3	49	63.0	41.5	—	—	—	—
France	16.7	40.5	63.2	44	16.5	38	17.5	41
Germany, FRG	14.0	36	40.5	12	12.2	26	14.0	37
Germany, DDR	10.8	29	—	—	9.6	16.5	—	—
Southern Europe								
Portugal	22.0	46	59.6	37	22.3	47	7.4	20
Spain	16.7	40.5	36.0	5	14.1	31	3.8	11
Italy	22.3	47	38.8	9	15.1	34	5.7	14
Greece	6.7	19	39.9	11	18.7	44	3.2	10
Malta	4.9	10	16.1	1	6.0	4	0.2	2
Africa—Mauritius	18.4	42	49.2	24	2.0	2	2.4	8.5
Israel	6.3	14	43.2	17	9.1	11	5.4	13
Kuwait	7.6	21.5	47.2	23	27.8	48	0.7	3.5
Japan	10.0	28	39.8	10	9.2	12.5	16.9	40
Singapore	5.4	12.5	38.0	7	9.7	18	12.5	34.5
Sri Lanka	—	—	84.8	49	—	—	—	—
Australia	6.4	16	45.0	20	17.6	40.5	10.4	27
New Zealand	3.6	5	52.4	27	21.1	46	9.3	24

Table 4.5 (*continued*)

Region/country	Breast cancer (female)		Lung cancer (male)		Lung cancer (female)		Stomach cancer	
	Rate	Rank	Rate	Rank	Rate	Rank	Rate	Rank
North America								
Canada	24.2	36	55.0	39	18.3	44	5.8	5
U.S.	22.5	32.5	56.9	41	20.4	49	3.9	1
Caribbean								
Bahamas	25.0	38.5	24.1	12	1.1	1	7.8	15.5
Barbados	22.5	32.5	16.6	7	1.6	2	8.5	19
Cuba	14.3	12	38.2	22.5	13.6	41	5.7	4
Dominica	39.1	51	34.9	19	11.2	38	24.1	50.5
Martinique	22.3	31	10.2	4	6.2	19	14.7	41
Puerto Rico	10.5	6	15.5	5	6.5	23	8.7	20
St. Vincent/Grenadines	28.8	47	8.2	3	5.0	10.5	8.0	17
Trindad/Tobago	16.6	18	15.6	6	3.0	4	12.7	35
Central/South America								
Guatemala	2.3	1	0.9	1	2.0	3	16.5	46
Argentina	19.4	25	38.0	21	5.3	12	9.5	23
Belize	2.5	2	20.4	9	5.0	10.5	7.4	12
Chile	12.4	7	21.2	11	5.8	15.5	24.1	50.5
Suriname	7.1	4	6.4	2	6.1	17	5.9	6
Uruguay	25.0	38.5	53.0	37	3.7	5	12.1	33
Britain								
England and Wales	29.3	49	64.9	44	19.3	46	9.7	25.5
Scotland	28.9	48	76.7	49	26.1	51	9.6	24
Ireland								
Northern Ireland	27.6	45.5	59.3	43	14.2	42	9.8	27
Ireland	25.7	41	51.9	36	18.8	45	10.5	29.5
Iceland	32.9	50	44.9	26	25.1	50	22.6	49
Scandinavia								
Denmark	27.6	45.5	55.8	40	19.8	48	6.9	9
Norway	18.2	22	29.5	17	8.5	37	9.2	21.5
Sweden	18.1	21	24.9	14	8.2	34.5	7.8	15.5
Finland	16.7	19	53.1	38	6.2	19	11.1	31
Northern Europe								
Belgium	25.8	42	79.5	51	6.4	21	9.2	21.5
Netherlands	26.5	43.5	76.8	50	8.2	34.5	9.9	28
Middle Europe								
Luxembourg	23.3	35	72.8	48	6.2	19	8.3	18
Switzerland	24.9	37	48.8	32	6.7	25	7.6	14
Poland	15.1	14	66.3	45	8.4	36	16.2	44.5
Eastern Europe								
Czechoslovakia	19.1	24	72.7	47	7.6	31	14.6	40
Bulgaria	15.6	16	38.2	22.5	6.8	26	16.2	44.5
Yugoslavia	13.2	9	42.3	24	6.5	23	13.5	38
Other Eastern European								
Austria	22.2	30	46.5	28	8.1	33	13.2	37
Hungary	21.9	29	72.5	46	12.3	40	16.9	47
Romania	13.1	8	34.1	18	5.8	15.5	13.7	39
France	19.0	23	44.6	25	4.3	9	6.8	8
Germany, FRG	22.9	34	48.6	31	7.2	28.5	11.6	32
Germany, DDR	16.8	20	51.0	35	5.7	14	12.6	34

Table 4.5 (continued)

Region/country	Breast cancer (female)		Lung cancer (male)		Lung cancer (female)		Stomach cancer	
	Rate	Rank	Rate	Rank	Rate	Rank	Rate	Rank
Southern Europe								
Portugal	16.2	17	24.3	13	4.1	8	17.6	48
Spain	13.7	10	35.6	20	3.8	6	12.8	36
Italy	20.3	26	57.4	42	6.5	23	15.4	42
Greece	15.2	15	49.1	33	7.1	27	7.2	10.5
Malta	25.2	40	48.0	29.5	5.4	13	9.7	25.5
Africa—Mauritius	8.2	5	17.8	8	4.0	7	10.5	29.5
Israel	21.7	28	25.1	15	7.5	30	7.5	13
Kuwait	14.6	13	20.6	10	7.2	28.5	5.2	3
Japan	6.0	3	27.6	16	7.7	32	27.0	52
Singapore	14.2	11	49.9	34	19.7	47	15.9	43
Sri Lanka	—	—	—	—	—	—	4.2	2
Australia	21.2	27	48.0	29.5	11.5	39	6.5	7
New Zealand	26.5	43.5	45.7	27	15.2	43	7.2	10.5

Note: For countries with identical rates, the average of the ranks has been assigned.

above (Morin et al., 1984). Physical anthropological data on some of these populations were discussed in Chapter 3.

Worldwide coverage of age-specific mortality data by country, and especially by racial/ethnic group, is obviously incomplete. For many developing countries, such as Bangladesh, Pakistan, and Haiti, official mortality statistics are unavailable and/or unreliable owing in part to the large numbers of unrecorded deaths occurring in remote areas. In the WHO (1987) statistical report, data on Africans were limited to the ethnically diverse population of the island of Mauritius (see Chapter 3), U.S. racial/ethnic groups were not separated, and China was absent. European "local races" (rather uniform genetically) are overrepresented, along with a variety of Caribbean countries comprised of predominantly black populations or considerable mixtures of Europeans and blacks. The category Central and South America includes Belize (which includes black Caribs and Creoles) and Chile (with its Chilean local race). Japan includes one predominant racial group, but also Koreans (in the Northeast Asiatic local race; Table 3.1), while Singapore includes several racial/ethnic groups and Israel includes several country-of-origin groups.

Comments on the mortality data in Table 4.5 will be provided in subsequent chapters dealing with specific diseases. Noteworthy major patterns include high rates for infectious diseases and stomach cancer, but not other cancers, in Central and South America. Infectious disease rates are also high in the Caribbean, and high stroke rates in Trinidad are noteworthy. (The poorest Caribbean country, Haiti, is missing, but infectious diseases such as tuberculosis are known to be major causes of death.)

Low total age-standardized death rates (from all causes) but high rates for ischemic heart disease (IHD) and (ostensibly) higher suicide rates occur in Scandinavia (Table 4.5). The highest IHD rates, high lung and breast cancer, and low chronic liver disease rates are found in Britain, Northern Ireland, and Scotland. High male lung cancer rates prevail in Belgium and the Netherlands, and there are high rates for strokes, chronic liver disease, and stomach cancer in Portugal. Africa is represented only by the island of Maritius (off Madagascar), which has high rates for infectious diseases and cardiovascular diseases (specifically, strokes) but low cancer rates. France, Spain, and Italy are noteworthy for high rates for chronic liver diseases. Eastern European countries tend to have very similar total death rates and higher rates for stomach cancer, male lung cancer, and cardiovascular diseases; in fact stroke rates in Romania and Bulgaria are the highest of all countries.

Greece has higher death rates for stroke but lower rates for IHD, while Malta has higher IHD rates. Kuwait has low rates for all cancers, stomach cancer, stroke, and suicide, while Israel has lower rates for chronic liver diseases, accidents, and total cancers (including stomach). Japan has the lowest total age-standardized death rate, lower rates for cardiovascular diseases and IHD (but not stroke), and low rates for breast (but not stomach) cancer. In contrast, Sri Lanka shows low rates for stomach cancer and stroke. Singapore, with its diverse racial/ethnic groups, shows high death rates for female lung cancer. New Zealand, including European and Polynesian populations, has high rates for IHD, breast cancer, female lung cancer, and motor vehicle accidents; Australia also has higher accident rates.

Some of these same countries are also included in the MONICA (for "MONItoring of trends and determinants in CArdiovascular disease") Project of the World Health Organization (Tuomilheto et al., 1987; Tunstall-Pedoe, 1988). Interestingly the Far East is represented not by Japan but by Beijing, China. MONICA includes 117 "reporting units" in 40 centers in 26 countries, which report for a period of 10 years (starting in 1984) on population surveys and official statistics regarding trends in mortality and morbidity from IHD and cerebrovascular disease in defined communities. The extent to which trends are related to changes in known cardiovascular risk factors also will be evaluated. Age-standardized mortality rates, using a world population as a standard, for cardiovascular diseases in MONICA areas will be discussed in Chapter 7.

Atlases of cancer mortality have also been published for such areas as China (China Map Press, 1981; Li, 1980, 1982), West Germany (Becker et al., 1984), and Finland (Pukkala et al., 1987), among others.

Morbidity

Extensive health surveys are limited to developed countries. Data from the U.S. HANES surveys (mentioned above), for example, have been compared with surveys in Britain and Canada, in showing that the prevalence of overweight and obesity (defined by weight/height index) was highest in U.S. men and women (especially in women aged 45 to 54 years) and lowest in the British (Millar and Stephens, 1987). Differences in SES may underlie these differences in obesity, although the appropriate analyses have not been conducted.

International morbidity data by geographic area and ethnic group are most extensive for cancers and infectious diseases. For cancers, *Cancer Incidence in*

Five Continents is periodically updated; Volume IV (Waterhouse et al., 1982) contains data for 1973–78. Segi (1977) and his colleagues (Kurihara et al., 1984) and others have compiled data from *Cancer Incidence in Five Continents* (Volume IV) including rankings of cancer incidence rates by site and sex for each country and ethnic group within certain countries or cities. The regions covered by this compendium include those of multiracial/ethnic composition (such as Bombay, India) as well as specific groups in certain countries or regions of countries. The latest volume (Muir et al., 1987) includes 105 registries covering 187 populations or groups in 36 countries. Some populations with cancer registries included in Volume IV are rather uniform ethnically, such as Shanghai, China, and Dakar, Senegal. Most informative are separate data on racial/ethnic groups in the same geographic area—for example, Maoris, other Polynesian Islanders, and non-Maoris in New Zealand; blacks, Chinese, Hispanics, and Anglo whites in California; and Israeli groups of different geographic origin (see Chapter 8).

Cancers have become recognized as a major problem in developing countries as well as in developed, industrialized nations. Parkin et al. (1984) have provided estimates of worldwide frequencies by 24 geographic areas for 12 major cancer sites, using data from Waterhouse et al. (1982) and other sources on mortality rates and relative frequencies of cancer types. Each area, such as East Africa and the Caribbean, includes numerous ethnic groups, although data are also presented for areas comprised of fewer major racial or ethnic groups such as Japan, China, and Melanesia. Again using data from Waterhouse et al. (1982), as well as hospital-based tumor registries and mortality data, Howe (1986) has edited a monograph on geographic variation in cancer throughout the world (excluding mainland China), and Aoki et al. (1982) and Parkin (1986) have edited volumes on cancer in developing countries.

Multinational analytic studies of various cancers are being conducted, including case control studies of lung cancer in women (see Chapter 8). Future analyses may allow examination of consistency of risk factors such as passive smoking across racial/ethnic groups.

For infectious diseases, frequencies of diseases subject to international health regulations and other diseases under surveillance by the World Health Organization are reported periodically. Relevant periodicals include *WHO Weekly Epidemiological Record*, *World Health Statistics Quarterly*, *Pan American Health Organization Bulletin*, and *Bulletin of the WHO*. Such information, however, is often incomplete, and reporting is delayed. Diseases reported include plague, cholera, yellow fever, smallpox, influenza, malaria, poliomyelitis, and other infectious diseases (Anon., 1985a) (see Chapter 6).

For chronic diseases other than cancer, international and ethnic data are much less complete, being based on special surveys or ad hoc studies. A major longitudinal (cohort) study of coronary heart disease is the *Seven Countries Study* (Keys et al., 1980) (see Chapter 7). The same cohorts from seven countries have been used to examine cancer mortality (Keys et al., 1985). International studies on cholesterol levels and lipid fractions, or low- and high-density lipoprotein concentrations, in relation to diet have also been published (Lewis et al., 1986). Other examples of international, multiethnic studies are the WHO Myocardial Infarction Community Register Study and the WHO International Pilot Study of Schizophrenia (WHO, 1973). In China, along with cancer data (mentioned earlier), results of large surveys have begun to be reported for various chronic diseases such as "stroke" (see Chapter 7), and smaller-scale studies of mental disorders have emerged (see Chapter 9). A recent survey of hemoglobin disorders in China involved 900,000 persons in 28 provinces (Zeng and Huang, 1987; see Chapter 5), and other large-scale surveys have examined genetic eye diseases (Hu, 1987).

The World Health Organization publishes quarterly and annual statistical reports that include international comparisons of cardiovascular diseases (WHO, 1985) and surveys of various other diseases. The WHO has considerable interest in worldwide and regional disease patterns (Hakulinen et al., 1986) in view of its worldwide health goals for the year 2000.

OTHER SOURCES

Although the sources of data on morbidity and mortality mentioned above are used extensively in *descriptive* epidemiologic studies, in-depth *analytic* epidemiologic studies provide the most useful information on racial/ethnic differences in specific diseases and their possible explanations. These studies are often case-control in design (see Chapter 1), using the population-based cancer registries cited above for ascertainment of cases. Interesting examples include studies of various cancers in Shanghai (with its cancer registry) and other parts of China. Other case-control studies, too numerous to mention, involve hospital-based registries of disease, or often hospital series of cases that cannot be referred to a population. The consistency of associations between risk factors and disease in various countries, comprised of different racial/ethnic groups, can be compared in these case-control studies. Such comparisons must be made with caution, however, because of methodological and statistical issues.

Finally, inexpensive cross-sectional surveys in *developing countries* should be mentioned. One example involved postal questionnaires for follow-up of patients with chronic diseases seen at a hospital in northeastern Thailand. Trained local interviewers traveled to obtain information on nonrespondents and to check the consistency of mail responses (Sitthi-Amorn et al., 1986). Among the Parsis of Bombay, India, a questionnaire was developed for administration by trained lay health workers to rapidly screen for neurologic disorders (including stroke). Information provided in this inexpensive manner was followed up by analytic (e.g., case-control) studies, which identified hypertension as an important risk factor (Bharucha et al., 1987). Neurologic surveys in developing countries are increasing, as witnessed by reports in the journal *Neuroepidemiology*.

Citing some classical historical precedents including the work of Denis Burkitt in identifying a new ("African") disease now known as Burkitt's lymphoma (see Chapter 8), Fox (1984) has noted the value of conducting low-cost epidemiologic research in developing countries. Variation in estimated disease prevalence by altitude, climate, and local customs and habits can be noted by district health officers with the help of local social workers, nutritionists, and family planning workers. This work can be done despite the lack of information based on "high technology." Fox (1984) also hopes that every hospital in developing countries will develop a cancer registry. Despite the limitations of such data, often without adequate denominator (i.e., population) estimates, steps can be taken on the road to the eventual filling in of the blank spaces on the current worldwide cancer map.

CONCLUSIONS

Sources of data on mortality and morbidity in specific racial/ethnic groups include descriptive statistics provided either for the purpose of studying racial/ethnic differences or for comparisons of disease by "place" (i.e., country or other political/geographic unit). Comparisons of mortality data worldwide are subject to numerous pitfalls related to inaccuracies in numerator and denominator data, as well as differences in classifying and coding disease and causes of death (Chapter 2). Aside from infectious diseases and cancers, morbidity data are largely limited to developed countries and are most extensive for the United States, where surveys of systematic samples of the national population are conducted periodically.

Analytical epidemiologic studies are often designed in countries where descriptive statistics are available through cancer registries or ongoing special community projects. Case control versus cohort studies are often conducted because of cost considerations. Other studies, fewer in number, are prospective or cohort, such as the U.S. studies in Framingham (Massachusetts) and Evans County (Georgia) and the international Seven Countries Study of coronary heart disease rates and risk factors in various populations. In some of these studies, racial/ethnic group is included in multivariate analyses with risk factors for the disease under study. Thus, the independent contribution of racial/ethnic group, if any, can be estimated, and interactions between racial/ethnic group and other risk factors can also be analyzed. Examples of such analyses will be provided later.

Although analytic epidemiologic studies, especially of the case-control type, are being conducted and reported increasingly in developing countries and in such areas as China, many developing countries must rely on inexpensive cross-sectional surveys. Utilizing local personnel, such surveys can (inexpensively) provide information that may lead to selected analytical epidemiologic studies, mainly of the case-control type.

5

Single-Gene Disorders

Although "single-gene" or "simply inherited" disorders comprise only a small part of the burden of disease worldwide, our discussion of specific disease categories begins with this group. In anthropological history such genetic diseases, especially those related to abnormal hemoglobins (e.g., hemoglobin S and sickle cell anemia), achieved great prominence. Also many genetic diseases represent the outcome of adaptations of populations to infectious diseases (especially malaria), which are still the major causes of death in man (see Chapter 6).

A unique, large-scale follow-up study of about 1.2 million births (1952–83) in British Columbia has provided the best available data on the frequencies of a variety of "genetic disorders" including single-gene disorders in a Western population (Baird et al., 1988). Before the age of 25 years, single-gene disorders occurred in about 3.6 per 1,000 live-born persons, including 1.4 per 1,000 for disorders due autosomal-dominant genes, 1.7 per 1,000 for autosomal-recessive genes, and 0.5 per 1,000 for X-linked disorders. Multifactorial disorders, caused by interactions between multiple genes and environmental factors, were much more common (i.e., 46.4 per 1,000); included were various birth defects, diabetes mellitus, and mental disorders (see Chapter 9).

Although many of these genetic disorders are rare, the genes involved may be common—especially in the heterozygous state for recessive and codominant genes. Also the frequencies of many single-gene disorders reported for British Columbia do not apply for other populations comprised of different racial/ethnic groups. Worldwide the burden of single-gene disorders is considerable, especially for abnormal hemoglobins and thalassemias.

This topic departs from the organization of most of the remainder of this book, which is based largely on the World Health Organization's continuously revised *International Statistical Classification of Diseases, Injuries, and Causes of Death*—the "ICD" (WHO, 1977). The ICD system largely involves grouping by organ systems, but other groups are based on pathology (e.g., "neoplasms"), etiology or causation (e.g., "infectious and parasitic diseases"), and time or age of occurrence (e.g., "conditions originating in the perinatal period"; "congenital anomalies"; and "complications of pregnancy, childbirth, and the puerperium").

Table 5.1 presents a sampling of single-gene disorders more common in selected ethnic groups. Not all of these disorders are discussed here, but the worldwide variations are made apparent, reflecting local adaptations or historical factors related to marriage patterns in certain ethnic groups.

Table 5.1 Racial/Ethnic Differences in Single-Gene Disorders

Group	Relatively high frequency	Relatively low frequency
Ashkenazic Jews	Abetalipoproteinemia	Phenylketonuria
	Bloom's disease	
	Dystonia musculorum deformans	
	Factor XI (PTA) deficiency	
	Gaucher's disease	
	Niemann-Pick disease	
	Pentosuria	
	Tay-Sachs disease	
Mediterranean peoples	Familial Mediterranean fever[a]	Cystic fibrosis (CF)
(Greeks, Italians,	G6PD deficiency, Mediterranean type	
Sephardic Jews)	Combined factor V and VIII deficiency	
	(bleeding disorders)	
	Thalassemia (mainly beta)	
	HbS (HbAS, HbSS)	
Africans	G6PD deficiency, African type	CF
	Hemoglobinopathies (HbS, HbC)	Hemophilia
	Alpha and beta thalassemias, persistent	Phenylketonuria
	HbF	Wilson's disease
Melanesians	Alpha thalassemia	
Japanese, Koreans	Acatalasia	Alpha thalassemia
	Dyschromatosis universalis hereditaria	Phenylketonuria
	Oguchi's disease	
	G6PD deficiency	
Chinese	Alpha thalassemia	
	G6PD deficiency, Chinese type	HbE[b]
	Beta thalassemia (South China)	
(Thais)	HbE	
	Alpha and beta thalassemias	
	Combined HbE-thalassemia syndromes	
	G6PD deficiency	
Armenians	Familial Mediterranean fever	
Finns	Aspartylglucosaminuria	Phenylketonuria
	Von Willebrand disease (factor VIII	Cystic fibrosis
	deficiency)	

References: Expanded and updated mainly from McKusick (1967), Norio (1981), Rothschild (1981) and other sources.

[a]Also known as familial paroxysmal polyserositis.

[b]Low in China, except in Yunnan province (Zeng and Huang, 1987).

SOME RECESSIVELY INHERITED DISEASES

Cystic Fibrosis

Cystic fibrosis (CF) is the most common recessive-gene disorder. In the British Columbia study (Baird et al., 1988), CF was by far the most commonly occurring autosomal-recessive disease before age 25 years (i.e., 232.5 per million, or 0.23 per 1,000 births). The gene has been localized to the long arm of chromosome 7, and probes for several RFLP markers closely linked to the abnormal gene have been identified (e.g., various *met* loci, pJ3.11, and D7S8). The disease, classified among "other and unspecified disorders of metabolism" (WHO, 1977), involves mucus-secreting and sweat glands throughout the body.

CF is rare in Oriental groups (including those in Hawaii) and black populations (Table 5.1) but is relatively common in Caucasian groups, reaching an estimated incidence of at least 1 in 2,000–2,500 live births or higher in some populations (Meindl, 1987) and about 0.5 per 2,000 in the British Columbia study. In Israel CF appears to be about as frequent as in other Caucasian populations, especially among Ashkenazi families.

The heterozygous condition for the recessive CF gene is common (i.e., about 1 in 22 persons among Caucasians). The common occurrence of both CF and tuberculosis in Europeans and certain physiologic characteristics of the heterozygote carriers (who are clinically normal) have led to the hypothesis that the CF gene has been maintained by natural selection or selective advantage of carriers as an adaptation to tuberculosis (Meindl, 1987).

With regard to prevention of CF disease (in homozygotes), the use of probes for DNA polymorphisms (RFLPs; see Chapter 3) as markers or probes to identify parents who are asymptomatic carriers of the CF gene has improved prospects for prevention of CF disease. Extensive work is being done to identify a marker (or RFLP) that is very closely linked to the CF gene on chromosome 7. Reduction in the frequency of CF disease is worthwhile because of the seriousness of the condition, which involves chronic obstructive pulmonary disease and pancreatic insufficiency, although improved medical therapy has increased the proportion of patients surviving to adulthood.

A major research issue concerns the possibility of *genetic heterogeneity* of CF. This question has practical implications for genetic counseling in specific countries or racial/ethnic groups. In Italy all 12 CF families studied using the *met* locus suggested lack of genetic heterogeneity (Vitale et al., 1986). Genetic analyses of 47 Canadian and 13 Danish CF families confirmed previous observations that both *met* and D7S8 were closely linked to CF, and hence the same CF locus was involved. Subdivision of families by geographic region and ethnic background reportedly did not reveal any differences in linkage to these markers (Tsui et al., 1986). In the inbred Hutterite families, studies using DNA probes linked to the CF gene (including *met*H) suggested that the CF locus was the same as that involved in outbred populations (Ober et al., 1987). Studies in 19 Israeli families using three probes (including two *met* loci) close to the CF gene, however, reportedly disclosed one haplotype more frequent among Ashkenazi than among Sephardic families (Voss et al., 1987). This suggests a genetic difference in CF among Ashkenazi versus Sephardic families that could have implications in genetic counseling.

The ideal RFLP would be a unique identifier of the molecular difference that determines the abnormal gene. The basic gene defect in CF remains unknown. As an alternative method, a closely linked RFLP marker can be diagnostic of the presence of the (unknown) gene defect in many families. The occurrence of recombination between the abnormal gene and the linked RFLPs, or absence of segregation at linked markers in families, complicates genetic counseling. Recombination, which depends on the physical proximity of gene loci, also complicates studies of associations between RFLPs and disease susceptibility in populations.

Multiple marker methods are useful when no single, tightly linked marker is known (Clark, 1987). In Britain, 30 of 37 CF families were sufficiently informative, using multiple (i.e., four) probes, to permit prenatal diagnosis of CF (Harris et al., 1988). Meanwhile, the search for genetic heterogeneity in CF continues.

Phenylketonuria (PKU)

PKU, described in 1934, is due to an abnormality in a gene (on chromosome 12) controlling synthesis of the liver enzyme phenylalanine hydroxylase (PAH), which is involved in metabolism of the amino acid phenylalanine. PKU is the most common "inborn error" of *amino acid* metabolism, occurring in from 1 in 38,000 to 1 in 4,500 births in Caucasian groups. In British Columbia the risk (by age 25 years) as 64.1 per million births (or 0.64 per 10,000), which is lower than that for CF (described earlier), but the carrier of heterozygote frequency in Japanese, American blacks, and Ashkenazi Jews (Table 5.1) than in non-Jewish Caucasians. In Israel most Jewish PKU families are of either North African or Yemenite origin.

Population data on the frequency and combinations of different RFLPs in the PAH gene region are rather limited. In five apparently unrelated Yemenite Jewish families, however, use of nine RFLPs showed homozygosity for the same mutation (i.e., a deletion of one region of the PAH gene) (Avigad et al., 1987). The occurrence of this mutation in non-Ashkenazi (vs. Ashkenazi) Jews could reflect the geographical and genetic separation of these groups. In U.S. blacks, a low-risk group, use of eight RFLPs and PAH probes (i.e., cDNA, or complementary DNA) suggested the possibility of a different PKU allele in comparison with published data on other groups (i.e., Danes) (Hofman et al., 1987). In higher-risk groups, previous studies in the Danish population had disclosed that a mutation in the PAH gene was closely linked with RFLPs that could be used as markers for PAH alleles. DNA haplotypes within the PAH gene in 44 German families showed differences from those observed in the Danish population, suggesting genetic heterogeneity (Aulehla-Scholz et al., 1988).

Thus, at present there is more evidence for genetic heterogeneity in PKU than in CF, but more work is needed in both disorders. The limited data in Germany suggested that 70% of individuals at risk in that population might be suitable for prenatal diagnosis and carrier testing with available markers.

PKU is a paradigm for the importance of environmental (i.e., dietary) influences on gene action and its consequences. Mental retardation can be avoided in PKU individuals by restricting dietary intake of phenylalanine. Another issue in PKU research concerns the health risks to *non-PKU* offspring of mothers with PKU. High maternal levels of phenylalanine during pregnancy are associated with birth defects among non-PKU offspring. In the United States and Canada, a collaborative 7-year *prospective* study is in progress to evaluate the efficacy of maternal dietary control (i.e., a phenylalanine-restricted diet). In these higher-risk populations some 2,800 women have been estimated to be at risk for maternal PKU; to date, 1,285 women have been identified and 62 pregnancies followed, with rather high compliance with dietary restrictions (Friedman et al., 1987).

Rare Recessive Gene Disorders

Noteworthy in Table 5.1 is the high frequency of certain Mendelian or single-gene-related disorders among Jewish groups. The genetic diseases more common (or less common, as in the case of PKU) among Ashkenazic Jews are almost all recessively inherited, suggesting the role of endogamy and consanguineous mating. That is, expression of recessive traits in offspring requires the presence of the gene in both (heterozygous or carrier) parents. Endogamy is the tendency to marry within the group, resulting in limitation to that group of genetic material which originated by new mutations or was introduced by immigrants to the group. These recessive diseases more common in Jewish populations have been described in great detail elsewhere (Mourant et al., 1978; Goodman, 1979; Goodman and Motulsky, 1979; Rothschild, 1981; McKusick, 1983) and only a few are discussed here.

Tay-Sachs disease (TSD), due to a gene on chromosome 15, is about 10 times more common in Ashkenazi Jews than in other populations. The disease involves a partial or complete deficiency of one of several types of cellular (i.e., lysosomal) enzymes called hexosaminadases, which leads to accumulation of a substrate (i.e., gangliosides) in the brain. Hence TSD is classified with "cerebral degenerations" in the grouping of diseases of the nervous system and sense organs of the ICD (WHO, 1977). Interestingly, a disease clinically identical to TSD occurs in non-Jewish French Canadians in Quebec, but the specific genetic lesion involved appears to differ from that found in Jewish populations. Thus, a hypothesis of transfer of a gene by intermarriage may not be needed to account for the occurrence of TSD in the non-Jewish population (Myerowitz and Hogikan, 1986). This example of apparent independent origin of single genes with similar, but not necessarily identical, expression in terms of clinical disease is not unique. Other examples are discussed below.

Gaucher's disease, another recessively inherited metabolic disorder, is characterized by a deficiency of the enzyme glucocerebrosidase, which leads to accumulation of glucocerebroside in the reticuloendothelial system and sometimes in the nerve cells of the brain. The classic, or type 1, form does not involve the brain and is found primarily in Ashkenazic Jews. A subtype involving neurologic symptoms has been traced to a single base change in the DNA of the recessive gene (Tsuji et al., 1987). In *Niemann-Pick's disease* a recessive gene determines an enzyme deficiency that leads to accumulation of lipid, mainly sphingomyelin, in reticuloendothelial cells and in ganglion cells of the central nervous system; enlargement of the liver and spleen and mental and neurologic disturbances are involved. About 40% of cases are Jewish (McKusick, 1983).

Several hereditary bleeding disorders related to anbormalities in clotting factors are listed in Table 5.1. Classified under "coagulation defects" in the larger category of "diseases of blood and blood-forming organs" of the ICD (see Chapter 9), the relevant genes have been localized to specific chromosomes in recent years. Deficiency of one component of Factor VIII leads to Von Willebrand's disease, involving a gene on chromosome 12. Factor XI deficiency occurs mainly in Ashkenazic Jews, while factor VII deficiency occurs mainly in Iranian, Moroccan, and Iraqi Jews.

Although most of these hereditary clotting disorders involve only one clotting factor, combined factor V and factor VIII deficiency occurs, probably as an autosomal-recessive trait, in about 1 per 100,000 Oriental or Sephardic (i.e., non-Ashkenazic) Jews but not in Ashkenazic (i.e., European) Jews (Seligsohn et al., 1982).

Familial Mediterranean fever (FMF) is at least in some cases a genetic disorder, apparently involving a recessive gene. FMF occurs primarily in Sephardic (i.e., non-European) Jews, Armenians, "Arabs," and Turks (Table 5.1). Although more cases have been reported among Sephardic Jews, FMF also occurs in Ashkenazi Jews in Israel and the United States (McKusick, 1983). The metabolic disease tends to appear in the first 10 years of life, with fever, muscle pain, and bone and joint involvement. FMF often involves attacks of fever and the development of amyloidosis or increased serum levels of a specific protein (i.e., amyloid A protein). Hence the disease is classified as an "amyloidosis" in the grouping of "endocrine, nutritional, metabolic diseases and immunity disorders" of the ICD. Fever may be the only symptom of this enigmatic disease, also called "familial paroxysmal polyserositis," with amyloidosis as a complication (Armenian and Sha'ar, 1986). "Polyserositis" refers to the occurrence of inflammation of serious tissues including the pleura of the lung, the peritoneum, and joint articular surfaces. Although FMF has been included under recessively inherited conditions, its etiology remains uncertain.

FMF may also involve nephropathy (i.e., severe renal disorders), which varies in frequency by ethnic group. Among Sephardic Jews of North African origin living in Israel, drug treatment with colchicine (an alkaloid) leads to improvement in most cases of FMF nephropathy except those with advanced disease (Zemer et al., 1986). Thus, early recognition and treatment are necessary, involving awareness of the ethnic distribution of FMF.

It is possible that natural selection maintains the putative FMF gene through an adaptive advantage of the heterozygote in the Mediterranean area.

In general the *mechanisms* underlying racial/ethnic differences in genetic diseases include inbreeding and genetic drift (including founder effect) as well as natural selection (Chapter 2 and Table 2.1). We have already discussed the importance of endogamy or tendency to marry within the group. The level of consanguinity of parents, and the resulting "inbreeding" of offspring, depend on marriage patterns—that is, the proximity of the genetic relationship between marriage partners. The long-debated issue of the consequences of high levels of inbreeding on "deleterious genes" (i.e., diseases or conditions associated with single genes) involves opposite theoretical conclusions. While inbreeding in the short term would tend to increase the frequency of conditions caused by rare recessive genes, the long-term consequences might be a reduction in "deleterious genes" in the population. In South India, where consanguineous marriages have long been favored in traditional rural communities, however, surveys suggest that the frequency of various genetic diseases may not be low (Devi et al., 1987). Other studies on level of inbreeding, in relation to reproductive outcomes and birth weight, are discussed in Chapter 9.

Founder effect, rather than inbreeding or heterozygote advantage, may explain the high frequency of *severe combined immune deficiency disease* in a subgroup of Athapascan Indians (see Chapter 3) in Arizona and New Mexico (Murphy et al., 1980). Founder effect, the genetic consequence of one of a few founders or a very small founding population, may be especially relevant to Amerindians. Analyses of DNA (specifically, mitochondrial DNA) in southwestern Amerindian tribes suggests that these tribes were founded by small numbers of female lineages and the new mutations became fixed after their separation from Asia (see also Chapter 3). Founder effect has been suggested as an explanation for the relatively high prevalence of certain genetic diseases in isolated areas such as Finland (Table 5.1 and Norio, 1981), but a high prevalence in the original (not necessarily small) population may also be involved (O'Brien et al., 1988). Studies using RFLPs linked to disease offer promise.

The possible role of natural selection, through heterozygote advantage, was mentioned above. More conclusive evidence involves other disorders, to which we now turn.

G6PD DEFICIENCY, THALASSEMIAS, AND HEMOGLOBINOPATHIES

Many racial/ethnic differences in genetic disorders can be explained by the mechanism of natural selection via adaptation to malaria in Africans, Mediterraneans, Asiatics, and other populations. Included are the red cell disorders: *G6PD (glucose-6-phosphate dehydrogenase) deficiency* (abbreviated as G6PD⁻ or G6PDD); various *hemoglobinopathies* associated with abnormal hemoglobin (Hb) types (e.g, HbS, HbC, HbE, HbF, etc.); and the *thalassemias* (*alpha* and *beta*) or deficiencies in the alpha or beta chains of normal adult hemoglobin (HbA). These disorders, involving hemolytic anemias, are classified as "hereditary hemolytic anemias" in the broader grouping of "diseases of blood and blood-forming organs" of the ICD (WHO, 1977).

Homozygotes for some but not all of these alleles develop very serious diseases, such as sickle cell anemia and thalassemia major. While heterozygotes may be at an advantage in malarial environments, other genetic factors may modify these adaptations—for example, possibly HLA-related factors in malaria (Bayoumi et al., 1986).

The worldwide distribution of abnormal hemoglobins, thalassemias, and G6PD deficiency has been reviewed extensively in monographs by Tills et al. (1983a), Livingstone (1985), and Winter (1986). Our discussion will highlight the results of some recent research on the distribution and public health implications of these disorders.

G6PD Deficiency

G6PD deficiency (G6PDD), an X-chromosome-linked trait (see McKusick, 1983), is included under the category "hereditary hemolytic anemias" in the broader grouping of diseases of blood and blood-forming organs of the ICD. Because of its X-chromosome-linked basis, G6PDD is mainly of interest in human males, who are "hemizygous" (i.e., have the XY chromosome constitution) and hence have no normal allele to influence the expression of the gene on the X chromosome.

G6PDD is a disorder of the metabolism of glutathione, which protects red cells against injury by inactivating oxidants. G6PDD "affects" millions worldwide. It is the basis for sensitivity to certain oxidant drugs (e.g., the antimalarial drug primaquine) and is manifested clinically by hemolytic anemia. The Mediterranean variety of G6PDD involves chronic hemolysis of red cells even in the absence of the provocative exposure to certain drugs and foods (i.e., the fava bean).

Other higher-risk populations include various Asiatic groups (Table 5.1). A very large number of G6PDD variants have been described that vary in degree of enzyme deficiency, as tabulated by McKusick (1983). Variants with severe enzyme deficiency associated with hemolytic anemia have been reported in widely diverse populations.

Both the *Mediterranean* (*G6PDB⁻*) and *African* (*G6PDA⁻*) variants of G6PD deficiency have been shown to have increased frequency in the same geographic areas as the sickle cell (HbS) gene in Central and North Africa and in India and Turkey (Akoglu et al., 1986). Presumably, this co-occurrence represents a common genetic adaptation to malaria in these areas. Resistance to malaria among persons with G6PDD, however, may not be entirely at the red cell (erythrocyte) level; removal of sickled erythrocytes or G6PD⁻ erythrocytes damaged by parasites could enhance immune responses (Bayoumi et al., 1986).

It is believed but not demonstrated that *G6PD⁺* red blood cells provide a barrier to malaria parasites (*Plasmodia*), while *G6PD⁻* red cells containing parasites at certain stages of development may be removed from the circulation. G6PDD and malaria are associated geographically. In central Sudan, adults claiming resistance to malaria more often had G6PDD than malaria patients (Bayoumi et al., 1986), in agreement with the results of other case-control studies.

There is increasing interest in mass screening of newborns in populations at high risk or G6PDD, using a simplified method involving a fluorescent test on a spot of dried blood on filter paper (Solem et al., 1985). The high prevalance of G6PDD among Southeast Asian immigrants in the United States (Monzon et al., 1986) adds impetus to this interest. An estimated 10% of the more than 600,000 Southeast Asian refugees in the United States carry the G6PDD gene. Newborn screening programs for other conditions, such as beta thalassemias and sickle-cell disease, are discussed below.

Thalassemias

The word "thalassemia" is derived from the Greek for "sea," referring to the predilection of Mediterranean populations. Thalassemias are included under recessive phenotypes in McKusick's (1983) catalog of Mendelian traits and have been discussed in great detail in a separate monograph by Weatherall and Clegg (1981) that includes data on racial/ethnic differences in distribution and clinical expression. At the molecular level, thalassemias are caused by substitutions or point mutations involving single bases of DNA as well as by gene deletions (discussed later) or rearrangements. Descriptions of the chromosome (i.e., autosomal) locations of the genes involved in synthesis of the various chains of human hemoglobin can be found in various compendia on the human gene map (e.g., McKusick, 1983, 1986–87). The molecular basis of thalassemias has been described in a monograph edited by Stamatoyannopoulos et al. (1987).

Alpha Thalassemias

Alpha thalassemias are often due to the absence of normal gene(s) controlling synthesis of the alpha chains of normal adult hemoglobin. The alpha globin gene cluster on chromosome 16 contains three functional genes; one is embryonic, and two (alpha 1 and 2) are adult.

The alpha thalassemias are actually an extremely heterogeneous group of disorders. In the deletion forms clinical severity depends on the number of abnormal genes at the four loci involved (i.e., two from each parent). A minus sign is used to indicate the deleted gene(s); for nomenclature, see Weatherall and Clegg (1981) and Lehmann and Carrell (1984). Two major divisions are alpha^0 and alpha$^+$, characterized by the total or partial absence of synthesis of the alpha chain of normal adult hemoglobin. The gene haplotype, or genotype derived from one parent, for alpha^0 thalassemia is designated as "$--/$"; thus, the homozygote is "$--/--$" and the heterozygote "$--/$aa." The alpha^0 homozygote has hydrops fetalis, a fatal neonatal syndrome due to large amounts of abnormal (i.e., alpha chain-deficient) hemoglobin. The genotype "$--/-$a" is associated with a chronic hemolytic anemia (Hemoglobin H disease), while thalassemia "trait" involves the genotypes "$--/$aa" and "$-$a/$-$a" and is sometimes associated with mild anemia. The carrier, or genotype "$-$a/aa," is clinically normal.

For alpha thalassemias a genetic adaptation to malaria is suggested by the negative association between altitude and alpha thalassemia in New Guinea (Oppenheimer et al., 1984), where malaria is endemic. Direct evidence for red cell resistance to malaria, however, is lacking or conflicting; the same holds for beta thalassemias (discussed later). Alpha thalassemia, including hydrops fetalis, is common in the Guangxi Zhuang region of Southern China, bordering on Vietnam, and the possibility of some advantage (i.e., via natural selection) for the *heterozygote* and carrier states has been suggested (Zeng and Huang, 1987). It has been postulated that the "alpha$^+$" or "$-$alpha/$-$alpha" heterozygote with two affected genes, may be the oldest malaria protective trait. This genotype may have become common in the progenitors of all the Bantu-speaking peoples (see Chapter 3) before they left their area of origin in central Africa and migrated southward (Ramsay and Jenkins, 1984).

The specific DNA deletions involved in some types of alpha thalassemia have recently been characterized in terms of the length of the missing DNA segment as measured in kilobase pairs (1 kb = 1,000 bases in the DNA). The most common type of "alpha-2" (i.e., genotype aa/a$-$) deletion of 3.7 kb ($-$a$^{3.7}$) is caused by a crossover between the normal a1 and a2 genes, but several subtypes have been described depending on the location of the crossover. Some Melanesians and Polynesians with the $-$a$^{3.7}$ deletion have a predominance of one subtype ("type III") that is less common in other populations.

Clinical applications of this information should also be noted. Recognition of the fact that reduced hemoglobin levels in Polynesian neonates in New Zealand may indicate alpha thalassemia rather than iron deficiency anema may avoid unnecessary hematologic investigations and therapy by iron supplementation (Mickelson et al., 1985). Homozygotes for "alpha-thal. 2" with genotype $-a/-a$ (alpha$^+$) have reduced blood cell indices and anemia, but of course this anemia is not due to iron deficiency. In the Southwest Pacific (Melanesian) islands of Vanuatu (Fig. 3.2), high frequencies of such gene deletions which cause mild hemoglobinopathy may explain hypochromic anemias that do not respond to iron supplementation (Bowden et al., 1985).

The occurrence of "$--/aa$," formerly called "alpha-thalassemia 1," is high among Southeast Asian refugees in the United States (Monzon et al., 1986). In 52 members of 17 Laotian families screened for hereditary anemias, after ruling out iron deficiency, the "Southeast Asian" alpha-1 thalassemia or 20-kb double deletion ($--^{SEA}$) was found in 6, and the single "$-a^{3.7}$" deletion in 26; half of the latter heterozygotes had normal red cell indices (Titus et al., 1987).

Nondeletion forms of the alpha thalassemias also occur, alone or in combination with the deletion forms. Hemoglobin H, produced when α chain synthesis is greatly reduced, can be found in all of these various genotypes. Presence of a nondeletion gene defect alone involves reduced alpha-chain synthesis which can be associated with clinically severe hemoglobin H disease (Kattamis et al., 1988). Triplicated or additional alpha globin genes have also been found in various populations.

RFLPs described for the alpha gene cluster have been used in attempts to study population affinities and associations with selection due to malaria. Melanesians of Vanuatu appear to have the $-a^{3.7}$ type III form common in Fijians and Polynesians but not in other Melanesians (Trent et al., 1988). Malaria is endemic in Papua New Guinea but not in Fiji and Polynesia. An $-a^{4.2}$ deletion variety also occurs in Melanesia.

Although blacks have a high incidence of alpha thalassemia trait, the clinically severe forms of the disease are rare; the hydrops fetalis syndrome does not occur. This has been shown to be due to the nature of the gene deletion(s) among blacks, (Dozy et al., 1979) in that usually only one of the alpha-chain-controlling genes is deleted (i.e., $-a/aa$) or, more rarely, two genes (i.e., $-a/-a$ or $aa/--$). In other populations at risk for alpha thalassemia, the more severe forms of the disease are associated with deletions of additional genes (i.e., $--/-a$ or $--/--$) (Higgs et al., 1979; Weatherall and Clegg, 1981; Anon., 1982). The specific deletion in U.S. blacks involves the $-a^{3.7}$ defect type I, but RFLP studies suggest that some black families living in Georgia have an unusual "hybrid" alpha 2 gene probably originating as a double crossover with the alpha 1 gene (Gu et al., 1988). The complexities of the genetics of these conditions are beyond the scope of this book.

Beta Thalassemias

The beta globin gene cluster on chromosome 11 includes two genes functional in adults, one being the beta gene. Beta thalassemias, involving abnormal or deficient synthesis of the beta chains of normal adult hemoglobin, are common in the Mediterranean, Africa, the Middle East, and parts of the Far East—that is, in China and in Southeast Asia including Thailand (Table 5.1) but not in Japan. Of course these thalassemias also occur in members of ethnic groups derived from these areas who have migrated to other countries. Heterogeneity in terms of severity of deficiency of hemoglobin chains, as with alpha thalassemias, has been described (McKusick, 1983).

The two main categories are called beta$^+$ and beta^0 and usually involve partial or complete absence of beta chain production, respectively. The clinically important forms formerly called "beta thalassemia major" usually involve *homozygosity* for either the beta$^+$ or beta^0 gene; others are *compound heterozygotes* for both genes. The carrier states for either one of these genes are called heterozygous beta$^+$ and heterozygous beta^0 thalassemia. Older (clinical) terms like "thalassemia minor" or "minima" should be abandoned (Weatherall and Clegg, 1981).

Clinical findings in homozygous beta thalassemia are severe and usually manifested in the first months of life; even treatment with repeated blood transfusions has untoward effects including a severe transfusion-related hemolytic (or red blood cell destroying) anemia called Cooley's anemia. Thus prevention of the homozygous condition is an important medical goal, involving genetic counseling. Beta^0 thalassemia is rare in African blacks (Table 5.1) but not in nonblack groups in North Africa (especially Algeria). The beta$^+$ thalassemias include a "severe Mediterranean type" and a "mild Negro type."

The true heterozygous carrier for *only* beta$^+$ *or* beta^0, not in compound state in the same person, is probably clinically normal except for mild anemia in nonblacks (Weatherall and Clegg, 1981). A follow-up study of beta thalassemia heterozygotes in Italy could find no effect on survival or fertility among presumed heterozygotes (Canella et al., 1987).

The southwest Pacific archipelago of Vanuatu was mentioned earlier with regard to alpha thalassemias misdiagnosed as iron deficiency. More important clinically is the high frequency of homozygous beta thalassemia, a major cause of infant mortality in some islands of Vanuatu. The high heterozygote carrier rate of 20% may reflect both malarial selection and genetic drift in small, isolated island populations (Bowden et al., 1987), but this has not been established. Again, natural selection and genetic drift (or founder effect) are potential explanations for differences in disease rates among populations that may correspond to racial categories (Table 2.1).

Asymptomatic beta thalassemia heterozygotes or carriers can be detected by simple blood tests. Thus programs of public education of specific ethnic groups, population screening, genetic counseling, and prenatal diagnosis (and abortion) of homozygous affected fetuses can have a significant impact on the frequency of homozygotes in the population. In Cyprus these measures have led to an apparent decrease in homozygotes among births (Angastiniotis and Hadjiminas, 1981). In Britain, a similar program has also led to reduction in thalassemia major births in most at-risk groups (i.e., Cypriots, East Africans, Asians) except Pakistanis (Modell et al., 1984). The application of DNA polymorphisms has improved prenatal diagnosis of beta thalassemias, as shown in Asian Indians, Chinese, and various Mediterranean populations including Italians (see Carestia et al., 1987; Chan et al., 1987).

When mutations cannot be detected directly by restriction enzymes, a genetic probe may be used that is complementary to the normal or mutated gene. This probe is a short piece of synthetic DNA called an "oligonucleotide" because it includes a small number of nucleotides. It has become increasingly evident that prenatal diagnosis of some single-gene disorders requires determination of the type of molecular lesion causing the disease in a specific geographical area or even within special racial/ethnic or country-of-origin groups in the same area (McKusick, 1988; Saiki et al., 1988). Use of such probes, of course, requires knowledge of the exact nature of the gene defect responsible for the disease.

A large and growing number (more than 47 to date) of different mutations in and around the beta gene can cause beta thalassemia, and racial/ethnic groups vary in the types of mutants that predominate. Four specific mutations of the beta-globin gene, for example, account for about 80–95 percent of cases in Mediterranean–Sicilian populations. Beta thalassemia is common in southern China, especially in the Guangdong and Guangxi provinces. Most studies of Chinese beta thalassemia mutations have involved migrants to Hong Kong and other areas. The heterozygote frequency in Hong Kong may reach 6 percent. In 48 Hong Kong patients with homozygous beta thalassemia, probes for known mutation sites in the beta gene revealed that four specific mutations accounted for 87 percent of the beta thalassemia genes, mostly in the codon 41/42 region of the gene. The finding of the latter mutation in Taiwan and Thailand was also noted, the probable explanation being the similar genetic origin of these populations (Chan et al., 1987b) (as discussed in Chapter 3).

RFLPs were also characterized in Hong Kong, in order to develop a thalassemia control program including prenatal diagnosis (Chan et al., 1987). The same objective was shared by a group working in Guangdong province of South China. Zhang et al. (1988) found six different mutations in four different haplotypes among 40 patients with homozygous beta thalassemia; again, a deletions at the 41/42 codon was the most common mutation. Analysis of two or three RFLP sites was sufficient to identify the four haplotypes on which the mutations reside and allow the choice of probes for detecting the mutations (Zhang et al., 1988).

Other populations are now under study. Among 131 *mestizo* patients with homolytic anemia in northwestern Mexico, 28 hemoglobin abnormalities including 16 "thalassemias" were found (Ibarra et al., 1988). Included were six $beta^0$/beta, two $beta^+$/$beta^+$, as well as two $beta^0$/$beta^S$ (see below).

Noteworthy is the occurrence of beta thalassemias in other (non-high-risk) ethnic groups as a result of spontaneous mutation. This may reflect mutational "hot spots" in the beta globin genes (Chehab et al., 1986). Indeed, abnormal hemoglobins are well suited for analyses of mutation rates in human populations, but dominantly inherited hemoglobinopathies are most useful (Nute and Stamatoyannopoulos, 1984). More variants of human hemoglobin have been discovered for beta than for alpha chains. As originally suggested by Ingram (1963), who also identified (in 1959) the abnormality in the beta chains of hemoglobin S, mutations affecting alpha chains of hemoglobin are more likely to impair fetal survival, because these chains are produced at higher levels than beta chains during fetal development. Thus, alpha chain *diseases* arising by new mutations may be difficult to detect, because few fetuses survive with such defects (see Nute and Stamatoyannopoulos, 1984). The alpha-globin gene loci, however, are highly polymorphic, as shown by DNA polymorphism studies.

Abnormal Hemoglobins

Abnormal hemoglobins are extremely heterogeneous. The beta globin gene exhibits extensive polymorphism when digested with restriction endonucleases such as Hpa-1, which results in a fragment containing the beta globin gene. Both the beta A and beta S genes may be associated with Hpa fragments of different lengths (in kb) at varying frequencies in different populations. On the basis of these studies *mutations responsible for abnormal hemoglobin S*, involving single amino acid substitutions in the beta chain of adult hemoglobin, have arisen several times independently in human populations in central and western Africa and in Asia (Kan and Dozy, 1980; Roberts and De Stefano, 1986). African and Greek populations show the same 13 kb Hpa-1 fragment, but the ultimate origin of the HbS gene in these groups is unclear. The association of beta S with a 5.6-kb fragment after digestion with Hpa-1 in Saudi Arabia suggests either an independent origin or introduction by migrants from others parts of the world (El-Hazmi and Warsy, 1987). Other abnormal hemoglobins (discussed below) also have arisen independently through different genetic mutations in different populations. HbAS is of interest mainly with regard to genetic adaptation to malaria, and more practically in connection with screening of prospective parents.

The distribution of HbS worldwide, and within continents such as Africa, closely corresponds to the distribution of malaria—that is, equatorial Africa, the Mediterranean, parts of the Middle East, India, and Southeast Asia. The maximum frequency of HbS in Africa is around the equator, with moderate frequencies from Senegal to Kenya, while HbC (involving the same sixth amino acid position at one end of the beta chain) is limited to northwestern Africa. Other genetic adaptations to malaria have occurred in these areas, as discussed earlier. Both beta thalassemia (described earlier) and the HbS allele are common in the same areas (e.g., Sicily), and adaptation to malaria is believed to be the explanation. The uniform frequency of beta thalassemia in Sicily, but a South-North cline in Hbs frequency, has suggested that hypothesis that the former is more ancient than the latter (or G6PDD) (Barrai et al., 1987).

Direct evidence, as opposed to indirect evidence by geographic association, for malarial resistance is best for HbS, as noted earlier. There is evidence that either red blood cells carrying HbS are less viable for malaria parasites or the sickle-shaped red cells infected with parasites are preferentially removed from the circulation (Roth et al. 1978; Friedman and Trager, 1981). Although the HbS gene is common in parts of Africa, its low frequency in southern Africa may reflect the migration of populations prior to the establishment of malaria in Africa. As noted in Chapter 3, blacks or Bantus in South Africa migrated from other parts of the continent.

Screening programs for abnormal hemoglobins have been conducted in various parts of the United States, including New York State, where a special population screening program was conducted in 1972–74 (Janerich et al., 1973; Polednak and Janerich, 1975) and where testing of newborns for hemoglobinopathies has been mandatory since 1975 (Porter, 1979). In New York City, testing of parents of newborns with *sickle cell trait* (*HbAS*) has been shown to be useful in counseling the family and has led to the fetal diagnosis of *sickle cell disease* or SC anemia (i.e., genotype HbSS) and subsequent abortion of several affected fetuses (Grover et al., 1986). It is interesting to note that the parents of several AS newborns tested were found to have undiagnosed sickle cell disease, a point relevant to the issue of variation in severity of sickle cell disease (discussed below). Because the disease is usually severe, however, fetal diagnosis of sickle cell disease and counseling of parents to aid in their decision regarding abortion seem worthwhile. Sickle cell trait or HbAS is clinically benign, with no demonstrated effects on mortality, and occurs wherever the HbS gene is common—in U.S. blacks, in the Mediterranean and Near East, and in parts of the Far East (including India).

The *severity* of sickle cell anemia (HbSS) has been shown to vary considerably both within and among populations. Certain groups in India and Saudi Arabia, for example, have a less severe disorder (Perrine et al., 1978). One hypothesis advanced to explain population differences in severity involves intracellular polymerization of HbS, or formation of high-molecular-weight compounds (Brittenham et al., 1985). The clinical expression of sickle cell disease is a complex phenomenon. In vitro studies suggest that hemoglobin F or fetal hemoglobin (see later) is an inhibitor of polymerization of hemoglobin S, and cases with *low* HbF among western Saudi Arabians had infections and clinical severity comparable to African cases (Acquaye et al., 1985). The clinical (hematologic) mildness of sickle cell disease in persons with alpha thalassemia is well known (Higgs et al., 1982; Embury et al., 1982), although the extent of benefit is controversial.

A study in India confirms the apparent effect of alpha thalassemias and *high* fetal hemoglobin level on the clinical course of sickle cell disease. Higher hemoglobin levels and red cell counts in India versus Jamaican patients with HbSS are consistent with a lower rate of hemolysis and an inhibition of in vivo sickling (Kar et al., 1986). The HbS mutation, as noted earlier (Kan and Dozy, 1980), apparently arose independently in Asia and Africa, and this may also be involved in differences in clinical manifestations.

The issue of variation in clinical severity of sickle cell disease, along with various aspects of the distribution of abnormal hemoglobins in the world, has been reviewed extensively by Serjeant (1986). Finally, we note that pain associated with sickle cell disease has received renewed attention, and treatment programs used in Jamaica by Serjeant and associates may be applicable to other areas where the disease is common (Anon., 1986a), including the United States and Britain (Anon., 1986b).

The two-volume work edited by Winter (1986) includes more than 400 hemoglobin variants, some associated with particular racial/ethnic groups, and coverage includes China and the Soviet Union. A more recent survey of *abnormal* hemoglobins in China involved almost 1 million persons (Zeng and Huang, 1987). A newly discovered hemoglobin variant in China has been called hemoglobin (Hb) Shanghai. This variant cannot be identified by electrophoresis (see Chapter 3), because it is indistinguishable from normal hemoglobin (HbA). Investigation of a Chinese patient in Shanghai with chronic hemolytic anemia, however, disclosed an *unstable* mutant of the beta chain of hemoglobin that was synthesized at a normal rate but was rapidly degraded (Zeng et al., 1987).

Hemoglobin E will be discussed briefly. It is limited mainly to Southeast Asia (Mourant et al., 1976) and to refugees or migrants from that area, while it is rare in Japan, most of China, and the Pacific. A recent survey in China, however, reported a high frequency of HbE (i.e., 6.1 percent) in the Yunnan province of southern China (adjacent to Guangxi province) (Zeng and Huang, 1987). In the U.S. Southeast, Asian refugees have a high prevalence of HbE, and the gene frequency may be highest in the Khmer group than in Vietnamese, Hmong, and other ethnic groups (Monzon et al., 1986). Even in the homozygous state (HbEE), possession of this gene is not clinically important, except for microcytosis or reduced size of red cells (Lachant, 1987).

HbE is of clinical importance because of its common *co-occurrence* with thalassemias in the same person. In Thailand both thalassemias and HbE are common, and tens of thousands are estimated to have the two conditions simultaneously—for example, "hemoglobin E–beta thalassemias" (Table 5.1). The latter involves bone marrow expansion leading to spinal cord compression (Anon., 1982). Several independent origins of the HbE gene have occurred. An adaptation to malaria has been postulated for the maintenance of the HbE gene, as in the Semai Senoi of Malaysia (Fix, 1984); the latter group was mentioned in Chapter 3. However, evidence for this adaptation is inconclusive (Livingstone, 1984; Lachant, 1987).

Hemoglobin F and the genetic disease known as hereditary persistence of fetal hemoglobin (HPFH), probably represents another apparent malarial adaptation. HPFH, involving a gene on chromosome 11, is relatively frequent among blacks (Table 5.1) but is clinically benign; about 5–40 percent of the hemoglobin in adult heterozygotes for this gene is HbF. HPFH and another condition (i.e., delta beta thalassemia) involving continued expression of a fetal hemoglobin in adults are uncommon except in certain areas such as Sardinia, where a high carrier frequency has been recorded and the molecular basis elucidated (Ottolenghi et al., 1988). "Compound heterozygotes" with both beta thalassemia and either HPFH or delta beta thalassemia have a mild clinical condition or "thalassemia intermedia."

In normal adults without beta thalassemia or beta delta thalassemia, slightly elevated levels of fetal hemoglobin (i.e., 1–5 percent) occur in the "Swiss type" of HPFH, which was first described in the Swiss population. "Swiss-HPFH" has now been described in other countries including Yugoslavia, where the different molecular bases have been described by use of RFLPs (Efremov et al., 1987). Thus, as with other hemoglobins there is heterogeneity in the genetic basis of HPFH, because different amino acid substitutions have been identified in black populations and in Greeks (Huang et al., 1987). As noted above, HbF is involved in the amelioration of sickle cell disease, and understanding of HbF production could have clinical applications (McKusick, 1987). Prolonged elevation of HbF levels by pharmacologic treatment may be required to obtain clinical benefit in patients with sickle cell disease, and individuals may differ in their response to these drugs (Noguchi et al., 1988).

CONCLUSIONS

Although single-gene-related disorders are rare, they are clinically significant (e.g., cystic fibrosis and PKU) and reach relatively high frequency in certain racial/ethnic groups. DNA probes, along with RFLPs, are useful for diseases such as PKU and the thalassemias in which the basic gene defects have been characterized, and thus the nature of the defect can be compared in different populations. As McKusick (1988) has observed in some ethnic groups with a relatively high frequency of specific autosomal-recessive disorders, it is justified to assume that one or a few possible genic lesions are involved. The beta thalassemias in southern Chinese are an example, since the majority of cases can be detected by only four oligonucleotide probes. Thus prenatal diagnosis and genetic counseling, for prevention of the disorders, can be facilitated.

For cystic fibrosis, with an as yet unknown genic defect or defects, there is no strong evidence for genetic heterogeneity within or between the populations or racial/ethnic groups studied so far, and several tightly linked RFLPs have been identified for use in genetic counseling. Studies of CF using these RFLPs in specific racial/ethnic groups are continuing. A few other single-gene disorders are discussed later with reference to diseases of specific organ systems.

The great magnitude of the effects of malaria as a force of natural selection in human populations is evident in population differences in the frequencies of certain genes and diseases associated with these genes. Thus, some of the population differences in gene frequencies (Chapter 3) reflect the operation of these selective forces. Our discussion has emphasized abnormal hemoglobins and certain red cell disorders. Many genetic loci may be involved in malaria adaptation. In central Sudan, for example, adults resistant to malaria had a high frequency of the PGM^1 phenotype of the red cell enzyme phosphoglucomutase (Bayoumi et al., 1986) mentioned in Chapter 3.

Another influence of malaria is on susceptibility to other diseases. Expression of the AIDS virus may be promoted by underlying repeated infections with malaria, as discussed in the next chapter.

6

Infectious and Parasitic Diseases

Malaria, a parasitic disease, was mentioned in the last chapter as a major disease in human history and a force in natural selection. Human adaptation to this disease is reflected in genetic variation among populations. This is also true to some extent for other infectious diseases. Infectious diseases and their epidemic patterns have been of interest to epidemiologists since Hippocrates and in the early development of the discipline in the 19th and early 20th centuries (Lilienfeld, 1980; Lilienfeld and Lilienfeld, 1980).

Infectious and parasitic diseases account for about 40 percent of all deaths in the world, and more than 50% of all deaths due to these causes occur in developing countries, especially in Africa and South Asia (Hakulinen et al., 1986). Although ecologic and socioeconomic factors largely account for the distribution of infectious and parasitic diseases, sociocultural factors in specific populations also influence transmission in complex ways. Also, there is some role for genetic variation among populations, especially in HLA-associated diseases, as discussed later. All infectious diseases involve a complex interaction between host susceptibility and environmental factors, including individual and group behavior patterns.

DESCRIPTION OF RACIAL/ETHNIC DIFFERENCES

Our discussion of racial/ethnic differences in infectious diseases is selective, in view of the vast number of specific diseases encompassed. Emphasis is given to diseases for which there is some evidence for racial/ethnic differences, especially those involving sociocultural factors, independent of the predominant influences of environmental and socioeconomic factors. We shall begin with a few major bacterial diseases, and then discuss selected viral and parasitic diseases.

Tuberculosis

Tuberculosis is a chronic mycobacterial disease caused by *Mycobacterium tuberculosis*, or "Koch's bacillus." In active form, it is present in over 1 million persons worldwide and is endemic in Africa and Southeast Asia as well as among U.S. Indochinese refugees (Holdiness, 1985; McGlynn et al., 1985). In Thailand in 1977–82, for example, pulmonary tuberculosis was the second leading cause of death after age 44 years (Porapakkham and Prasartkul, 1985). In contrast in Hungary, due to mass X-ray surveys and drug prophylaxis in children since 1959, a rapid decline in incidence and mortality rates has occurred (Lugosi, 1985).

Racial/ethnic groups derived from parts of the Far East also have high rates. In two national surveys of tuberculosis notifications in England, rates for ethnic groups derived from the Indian subcontinent (i.e., Indians, Pakistanis, and Bangladeshis) were about 30 times higher than those for whites. Although crude rates suggested a rapid decline in the Asian population in recent years, direct standardization of rates for age, place of birth, and other characteristics showed a reduction occurring at the rate of 4–9% per year in the various ethnic subgroups (Nunn et al., 1986). The declining proportion of recent immigrants will result in a narrowing of the large gap between whites and Asians in tuberculosis incidence. Noteworthy was the similar rate of decline in annual incidence in whites and in Asians born in the United Kingdom.

Other evidence, however, suggests that "atypical" mycobacterial infections are increasing in prevalence among Asians in England and that these infections are life-threatening and difficult to treat (Yates et al., 1986). These atypical infections are due to strains of *M. tuberculosis* other than the classical human types and include bovine and "Asian" (or "South Indian") types. These differences in strains do not account for the higher prevalence of extrapulmonary (i.e., nonrespiratory) tuberculosis among Asians in England. These extrapulmonary forms include tuberculosis meningitis, or inflammation of the meninges (see later) due to tuberculosis. Extrapulmonary tuberculosis among Indochinese refugees in the United States (Powell et al., 1983) and among Southeast Asian immigrants in Australia (Dwyer et al., 1987) is important because of resistance to one or more drugs used in the treatment of tuberculosis. Tuberculosis is also common in some groups in the Solomon Islands of Melanesia (Friedlaender et al., 1987).

The incidence of tuberculosis in England among persons originating in the West Indies and other areas (including Africa) is also higher than that among whites (Nunn et al., 1986). Tuberculosis is endemic in Haiti, the poorest country in the Western hemisphere. Also prominent is the black–white disparity is South Africa, where mortality from pulmonary tuberculosis is especially high among rural Africans and "coloureds." Tuberculosis meningitis, one type of meningitis (see later), is frequent among both Asians and Africans in South Africa but rare among whites (WHO, 1983). The overwhelming importance of socioeconomic factors, including crowding and undernutrition, is undoubtedly evident from such comparisons. Tuberculosis may have been infrequent in South Africa before the arrival of whites and could be considered as a "virgin-soil" epidemic phenomenon. "Virgin soil" epidemics refer to the consequences of the introduction of a new microorganism, or more virulent strain of an existing form, in a population as a result of contact or acculturation. The possible role of genetic differences among populations is considered later.

Epidemics contributed to the decline in the American Native population between 1500 and 1900 A.D. Paleopathologic and historical evidence supports the conclusion that, although rare, tuberculosis was endemic in the pre-Columbian New World—perhaps as milder forms of the disease (Merbs and Miller, 1985). Changes in life style, health conditions, sanitation, crowding, and lack of medical care after European contact may have made native groups more prone to severe tuberculosis infections (El-Najjar, 1979; Pfeiffer, 1984). Research is planned among isolated South American tribes (e.g., the Yanomama of Brazil) undergoing rapid acculturation and already showing evidence of increases in tuberculosis (Salzano, 1985) and measles.

A survey of tuberculosis cases reported in 1969–73 in the United States, obtained by sampling 13 states, disclosed lower rates for whites than for blacks. Other races, mainly Orientals and Amerindians, had the highest rates for pulmonary and extrapulmonary cases per 10^5 population (Farer et al., 1979). In North Carolina in 1977–81, some 80% of childhood tuberculosis cases were in nonwhites, who had an incidence rate 10 times higher than that in whites. This underscores the opportunity for intervention in the transmission of this disease (Block and Snider, 1986; Norlan, 1986).

The disparity in tuberculosis death rates between U.S. blacks and other groups is still evident (Table 6.1). In the United States in 1981, some 27,373 new cases were reported with no substantial decline for the previous three years. In 1985 there was no decline in cases among blacks and an increase in Hispanics, American Indians, and Eskimos (Anon., 1986c) (Table 6.1). Among cases reported to the Centers for Disease Control (CDC) in 1985, age-specific rates of tuberculosis were from four to nine times higher, and mortality rates four to 16 times higher, among blacks than among whites (Anon., 1987c). Future CDC reports will focus on detailed information on tuberculosis in other groups such as Asians/Pacific Islanders, American Indians/Alaskan natives, and Hispanics.

The apparent predilection of tuberculosis infections for certain racial/ethnic groups such as blacks and American Indians has long been a subject of speculation and controversy, regarding the role of environmental factors and genetic susceptibility. As with malaria, genetic factors and environmental influences undoubtedly interact in explaining population differences (Livingstone, 1984).

Explanations for the apparently lower rates of tuberculosis in certain Jewish populations have long been a subject of speculation. Sawchuk and Herring (1984) have reviewed the evidence and presented data on Sephardic Jews of Gibraltar, showing an advantage in Gibraltarian Jews regarding respiratory disease mortal-

Table 6.1 Comparison of Change in Number of Tuberculosis Cases by Race and Ethnicity, United States, 1985 versus 1984

	Cases in 1984	Cases in 1985	Change in cases	Percent change
Race				
White	11,729	11,538	−191	−1.6
Black	7,678	7,734	+56	+0.7
Asian/Pacific Islander	2,473	2,532	+59	+2.4
American Indian/Alaskan native	375	397	+22	+5.9
Ethnicity				
Hispanic	2,750	3,134	+384	+14.0
Non-Hispanic	19,505	19,067	−438	−2.2

Abstracted from Anon. (1986c).

ity probably due to high standard of living, lower occupational risk, and possibly family size and degree of crowding.

The relationship between tuberculosis and the AIDS virus is a topic of current interest in the United States and other countries. The impaired cell immunity associated with tuberculosis appears to be both a result of and a factor contributing to susceptibility to infections caused by human immunodeficiency virus (HIV) (discussed below) and its sequelae such as AIDS and AIDS-related cancers. Thus in areas where tuberculosis is endemic, this disease contributes to the pattern of HIV-related diseases. Such interactions are complex, because not only ecologic and sociocultural factors but also genetic (HLA-related) factors contribute to the distribution of these diseases across geographic areas and racial/ethnic groups.

Leprosy and the Role of Crowding

Like tuberculosis, leprosy is a mycobacterial infection. The causal agent is the bacillus *Mycobacterium leprae*. In fact, most antigens of *M. leprae* are shared by *M. tuberculosis*, which leads to complications in the serologic testing for leprosy in many areas where both diseases are common. The World Health Organization periodically publishes data on the prevalence of infectious diseases such as leprosy (see Chapter 4). Some 1.6 billion people live in areas where leprosy is of some importance—that is, where the prevalence is more than one per 1,000 population (Nordeen and Bravo, 1986). In some developing countries prevalence remains as high as one per 100 despite the development of chemotherapy since the 1940s.

Now a tropical and subtropical disease, leprosy affects an unknown number of persons, estimated at about 5 million registered cases but 11 million or more. About 60 percent of known cases are in Asia, and less than half are regularly treated (Shepard, 1982; Nordeen and Bravo, 1986). Along with tuberculosis and certain sexually transmitted diseases, leprosy is common in sub-Saharan Africa. It is also frequent in other developing countries where crowded, unhygienic conditions, low socioeconomic status, poor nutrition, and inadequate medical care prevail. Leprosy is endemic in parts of the Americas, where it may have been introduced by colonists and emigrants from Europe (Anon., 1984c). Once common in the United States, especially Hawaii, small numbers of cases persist in eight countries of Europe, although the vast majority of cases are in tropical and subtropical regions.

In the United States the reported number of *indigenously acquired* cases per year (about 30) has remained constant since 1970, but a steady increase in *foreign-acquired* cases has occurred, and an increase in 1976–81 corresponded with an influx of Southeast Asian refugees (Anon., 1984d). The issue of foreign-acquired infections relates to many infectious diseases and is becoming even more important in view of the AIDS epidemic (see later).

Leprosy remains one of the most poorly understood major infections affecting humans, especially in terms of mode of transmission. Studies in mice, however, confirm the traditional view that overcrowding and intimate contact are involved in transmission (Chehl et al., 1985). The "contact hypothesis" is also supported by population studies in humans, showing a male excess in most societies (Fine, 1982) and the occurrence of multiple-case households in India

(DeVries and Perry, 1985) and other areas. Sociocultural factors involved in the spread of leprosy and other infections, and the role of genetic factors, especially HLA types, in leprosy susceptibility will be discussed later.

Bacterial Pneumonias and Acute Respiratory Infections

Although included in our discussion of infectious diseases, pneumonias are classified with diseases of the respiratory system in the International Classification of Diseases (WHO, 1977). Pneumonias are major infections in populations of many tropical, developing countries, especially among children in Africa and the Pacific (e.g., New Guinea). In fact, about 96 percent of the 15 million children under age 5 years who die each year are in the Third World, and about 30 percent of these die from pneumonia (Gwatkin, 1980; WHO, 1983).

Despite the reduction in streptococcal infections since the introduction of penicillin, streptococci are still major causes of infection, especially in underprivileged and developing countries. The evidence for the predominant role of only two bacteria, *Haemophilus influenzae* and *Streptococcus pneumoniae* (formerly pneumococcus), in pneumonias in developing countries is considerable. The apparent efficacy of penicillin (e.g., in India, Africa, and Papua New Guinea) is encouraging, although vaccines may also be needed (Shaun et al., 1984). Infections caused by these organisms are clinically similar, but gram-positive staining for microscopic analysis reveals pneumococci, whereas *Hemophilus* are gram-negative organisms. Vaccines against *Hemophilus* administered at 1 year of age may not be effective, because younger children who have lost maternal antibody protection are at risk, especially in populations without breast feeding (see below).

Other gram-negative bacilli (e.g., *E. coli*) also may be involved in pneumonia cases in some countries—for example, Costa Rica (Mohs, 1985). These infections may be acquired among hospitalized patients who are debilitated. The indirect effects of undernutrition and low SES may be reflected in the association between low birth weight and infant mortality (including deaths due to acute respiratory diseases) and the probable effects of improvements in birth weight on mortality (Mohs, 1985).

Children with sickle cell disease (HbSS) are at increased risk of pneumococcal pneumonia and have a poorer prognosis (DeCeulaer et al., 1985). Hence populations in which the abnormal hemoglobin (HbS) is common (see Chapter 5) are at increased risk.

Acute respiratory infections are a major worldwide public health problem, with great impact on the health of developing countries. Effective vaccines are not available for the major microorganisms involved, although rapid diagnosis of *Staph. aureus* is possible by immunofluorescence methods (Wafula and Onyango, 1986). The problem of drug-resistant strains is considered later.

Bacterial Meningitis

Cerebrospinal meningitis or inflammation of the meninges is caused by a variety of bacteria including *Haemophilus influenzae* and *Streptococcus pneumoniae*, mentioned earlier with reference to bacterial pneumonias. In addition to its role in pneumonia, *S. pneumoniae* bacteria are also a major contributor to (pneumococcal) meningitis among children under age 5 and among the elderly; the case fatality rate, or the chance of dying among those with the disease, is high. Pneumococcal meningitis (along with pneumonia) is frequent in Africa and in U.S. blacks, and the course of bacterial meningitis is especially severe in children with sickle cell disease (i.e., hemoglobin SS; see Chapter 5).

In the New World *H. influenzae* is a major factor in the high incidence of bacterial meningitis among Alaskan Eskimos (Ward et al., 1981).

Meningococcal infections, due to various strains of meningococci, are also involved in cerebrospinal meningitis. Meningococcal meningitis is common in temperate and tropical climates including sub-Saharan Africa. These infections are especially prominent in the semiarid areas north of the equator referred to as the "cerebrospinal meningitis belt," which extends from Benin and Burkina Fan in the west through Nigeria, southern Chad, the northern part of the Central African Republic, southern Sudan, and into Ethiopia. In this "belt" outbreaks of more than 25 cases per 100,000 population occur annually, and millions of cases have undoubtedly occurred in the past 30–40 years (Tikhomirov, 1987). Noteworthy have been epidemics of meningococcal meningitis in England and Wales and in northwestern Europe (Poolman et al., 1986) including an increase in 1986 in northwestern England and Wales (Guttride et al., 1986).

Underreporting of infectious diseases is a major problem worldwide (Chapter 4). The various strains of meningococci complicate the task of obtaining accurate data, but newer techniques (i.e., using monoclonal antibodies) offer the prospect of improved surveillance and eventual understanding of the causes of epidemics and the development of comprehensive vaccines.

Interestingly, immunization with meningococcal vaccine is now required for Moslem pilgrims going to Saudi Arabia for the hajj, or religious pilgrimage (Anon., 1988a).

In addition to the "meningitis belt" of Africa, *seasonal* outbreaks of meningococcal disease have recently been recognized and reported from parts of Asia— Mongolia, China, and Nepal (Cochi et al., 1987). Again, arid or semiarid conditions are important. In Africa, seasonal patterns are also prominent, and overcrowding may be a factor (Greenwood et al., 1984).

In Charleston County, South Carolina, the risks of both meningococcal and pneumococcal meningitis are greater for blacks than for whites (Fraser et al., 1973) as are rates for bacteremia. Differences appear to be independent of the SES factors measured (Filice et al., 1986). These apparent differences may be due to unidentified socioeconomic factors, sociocultural factors, or unknown genetic factors.

Extrapulmonary tuberculosis was mentioned earlier with reference to tuberculosis. Among certain Asian (i.e., Indian-origin) groups, *tuberculous meningitis* (TM) is relatively common. Thus, the importance of obtaining information on ethnic origin during clinical investigation of patients with fever has been emphasized (Damon, 1971). TM is also common among U.S. blacks and other groups at risk for tuberculosis (see earlier). In an urban (New York City) medical center the majority of TM patients were black and Hispanic. Despite treatment with antituberculosis drugs, mortality rates among TM cases were high, and one third of survivors had neurological sequelae (Ogawa et al., 1987).

Otitis Media

An increased incidence of middle-ear infections (otitis media) is well documented in North American Indians (including the Navajo) and Eskimos and in Australian aborigines, Maoris, and Melanesians. The early identification of persons at high risk for frequent attacks of acute otitis media, which begin to occur in the first year of life in most cases, is important in the prevention of hearing loss (Goodwin et al., 1980). Exposure to bacterial agents at an early age, related to crowding and low SES, is a major factor underlying this disease pattern (Hudson and Rockett, 1984). Similarly, for bacterial meningitis among Alaskan Eskimos (noted earlier), early exposure to the agent is involved, and vaccines need to be developed for use in children as young as 2 months of age (Ward et al., 1981).

Other Bacterial Diseases

Typhoid fever, caused by gram-negative coliform bacteria (*Salmonella typhi* with various disease manifestations), is now sporadic in the United States but still occurs among medically underserved populations worldwide. As a reportable disease (Chapter 4), numbers of reported cases are routinely recorded, with an average of 123 cases in the United States each year in 1983–87.

Also reportable is cholera, caused by the gram-negative *Vibrio cholerae*, transmitted by the fecal–oral route (i.e., contaminated water). Like tuberculosis it is still a major worldwide problem, with 54,000 cases reported worldwide to the WHO in 1983 (and underreporting occurs). Of great interest in the history of epidemiology because of the classic work of John Snow in mid-19th-century London, showing the association with water contamination, cholera is still endemic (i.e., uniformly frequent without epidemics) in the Ganges area, Bangladesh, Indonesia, and in parts of Africa and other developing areas. Mulitple-drug resistant strains of *V. cholerae* have been reported in East Africa (Finch et al., 1988), which further exacerbates the problem (see later). Importation of cases in developed countries due to worldwide travel is a problem, as with other diseases (see below), but a minor epidemic in the United States in 1978 was not traceable to an imported source. Large outbreaks occurred in Florida in 1973 and in Texas in 1981, and about half of the cases are acquired during foreign travel, others from chronic carriers, laboratory sources (Anon., 1984d), and raw shellfish.

The gram-negative spiral bacteria *Campylobacter jejuni* is an important cause of infant diarrhea and dysentery, apparently more common in males than females. It may be carried by dogs, but contaminated milk is a common source of epidemics. Epidemiologic study is complicated by wide variation in clinical expression, from subclinical or asymptomatic or mild to incapacitating abdominal pain and dysentery; hence reporting of disease varies considerably. *Campylobacter* species have been strongly implicated in the causation of gastritis and peptic ulcer (Chapter 9).

Last to be mentioned are infections due to clostridia, or enzyme- and toxin-producing gram-positive anaerobes of which *Clostridia perfringens* is the prototype. A severe "necrotizing" form (i.e., invasive or causing necrosis of the small intestine), which appeared in malnourished children during World War II, has been associated with pork ingestion in the highlands of Papua New Guinea, but a more severe form (often fatal) occurred in Khmer children at an evacuation site in Thailand in 1985–86 (Johnson et al., 1987). Lack of history of pork ingestion or other dietary factors suggested a pathogenesis different from the New Guinea variety, perhaps involving intestinal parasites (i.e., worms) as a cofactor. Cases have been reported in other parts of Melanesia (i.e., the Solomon Islands), other areas of the Far East including Malaysia, and other parts of Southeast Asia, India, Bangladesh, and Nepal, as well as East and West Africa.

In conclusion, the distribution of most of these bacterial diseases is related to ecologic factors and crowding, the latter reflecting mainly socioeconomic status. Sociocultural factors affecting crowding and spread of infection in different populations, along with genetic factors, are discussed later.

Hepatitis B and Poliomyelitis

Turning to the viral diseases worldwide, variation in incidence of hepatitis B virus (HBV) infection or infectivity is of major interest to epidemiologists and public health workers. This interest is due mainly to the long-term sequelae of chronic HBV infection, such as chronic liver disease and liver cancer (i.e., primary hepatocellular carcinoma or PHCC). The role of chronic HBV in PHCC has been confirmed in prospective studies of HBV carriers in Taiwan (Beasley et al., 1981; London and Blumberg, 1985) (see Chapter 8). HBV carriers are positive serologically for the HBV surface antigen and are designated as "HBsAg+."

Comparison of rates of HBV infection across countries and racial/ethnic groups is difficult because of noncomparability in surveys samples—that is, the varying representativeness of surveys which include blood donors, school and community groups, hospital patients, and various other sources. Also important are age differences in prevalence of HBsAg related to modes of transmission, aside from statistical issues regarding variability in estimated prevalence rates due to varying sample sizes.

Despite these limitations in the data, some generalizations can be made, using data on HBsAg as an indicator of chronic infection. HBV infection is particularly common in parts of Africa and the Far East, but numerous other populations have been studied (see Table 6.2). In Thailand, for example, by the age of 15–19 years, 50 percent of the populations surveyed had serologic evidence of previous experience with HBV—either antibody positivity or surface antigen positivity (Grossman et al., 1975). In other parts of the Far East, the prevalence of HBsAg positivity is lower—for example, about 8 percent among apparently healthy Chinese male blood donors in Singapore or 10 percent in samples from all sources (including hospital outpatients and nonhepatic patients), and 10–15 percent in Chinese adult males in Hong Kong and Taiwan (Phoon et al., 1987).

In Africa the infectious pool comprises 12–20 percent of adults but over 33 percent in hyperendemic areas of Kenya (Bowry et al., 1985). In rural communities of Senegal, 50 percent of the population is infected by age 7 years, and 80 percent by age 15 years. Intervillage variation in prevalence of surface antigen positivity (HBsAg+) may be related to degree of crowding (Feret et al., 1986).

Table 6.2 Prevalence of Hepatitis B Surface Antigen
in Various Populations

Population	Prevalence
Kenya, Turkana groups	29%
Taiwan, adult Chinese males	15%
Senegal, Tip villages	10–14%
Yupik Eskimos	13.9%
Alaskan Eskimo villages	0–20.1%
Papua New Guinea	10–13%
Fiji	11–12%
Thailand, Bangkok	8–10%
Singapore, adult Chinese males	8%
Shanghai, China	6.9%
New Zealand, all ages (whites)	6.6%
Maori, all ages	~25%
Israel	1.0%
Cochins	1.2%
Askenazi	3.4%
Yemenite	3.9%
Kurds	6.7%
Central Tunisia, children	3.3%
N. Africa, Middle East, S. Europe	2–5%
U.S., N. Europe	0–3%

Sources: Various studies, mostly adult males (see text). These estimates
are crude because of age differences in the populations compared and
variation in the prevalence of surface-antigen positivity with age.

Crowding was discussed earlier with reference to leprosy. In the nomadic Turkana
inhabitants of Kenya, a group of anthropological interest for their adaptations to
food scarcity, there is also interest in intrinsic host factors (i.e., cellular immunity)
in relation to HBV infection (Bowry et al., 1985). The growing body of seroepidemiologic studies on HBV infection is "highly informative and reveal numerous
inter-tribal and inter-racial differences which could provide an insight in genetic
and environmental factors involved in host immunity against HBV and its relation to chronic liver disease and PHC [primary hepatic cancer]" (Bowry et al.,
1985).

As always, comparisons of racial/ethnic groups within the same country are
informative. In a survey of 93 percent of all residents in a community in the North
Island of New Zealand, for example, the overall prevalence rate of HBsAg
positivity was 6.6 percent for all ages combined and highest at age 15–19 years,
but the rate, standardized for age and sex, was about four times higher in non-
Europeans (chiefly Maoris and Pacific Islanders) than in Europeans (Milne et al.,
1987). In children an important risk factor was the number of people in the
household, again suggesting the role of crowding; however, multivariate analysis
using multiple logistic regression showed that ethnicity (i.e., non-European vs.
European) was a significant predictor of HBsAg positivity independent of size of
household and number of siblings.

From surveillance reports there is evidence that HBV infection is more
common among U.S. blacks than whites, as also shown in military personnel, but

explanations are unknown (Dembert et al., 1987). Such factors as maternal transmission, crowding, and drug abuse should be considered.

Antigenic subtypes of HBsAg, involving several pairs of allelic determinants, have been found to vary geographically, but their significance to chronicity of HBV is uncertain. *Modes of transmission* of HBV also differ across populations. In Western developed countries, "horizontal" transmission in adults is a major source of infection, often related to intravenous drug use and sexual practices. The latter include both homosexual and heterosexual behaviors, especially experiences with multiple partners.

In developing countries the pattern of infection is more complex, involving both "vertical" (i.e., maternal–infant) and "horizontal" (e.g., sibling–sibling) spread. In tropical Africa nearly all children are infected during childhood, and about 20% become chronic carriers (i.e., HBsAg$^+$); perinatal transmission also occurs in Africa. In *some* Far Eastern countries the frequency of vertical versus horizontal transmission is apparently more important than in Africa and the United States (Arthur et al., 1984; Botha et al., 1984; London and Blumberg, 1985). In Taiwan the key role of perinatal mother-to-child transmission in maintaining HBsAg positivity has led to vaccination programs for infants of HBsAg-positive mothers (Chen et al., 1987). Similarly in Japan, mothers who are positive for the hepatitis B e antigen (HBeAg), which is indicative of infection, transmit the virus to their children, who become chronic carriers. Immunization programs initiated in Japan in 1986 for infants with HBsAg or HBeAg positivity may lead to a further reduction in the rate of HBeAg positivity among HBsAg carriers already shown in voluntary blood donors between 1977 and 1984 (Tsukuma et al., 1987).

In Okinawa, Japan, apparent sibling-to-sibling transmission of hepatitis B was more frequent than apparent maternal transmission, and children under 4 years of age seemed to become carriers more easily than older children (Kashiwagi et al., 1984). A comparison of family studies in the same area of Okinawa, however, suggested changing patterns of intrafamilial transmission over time (i.e., 1968–85), with the vertical mode becoming most important (Kashiwagi et al., 1988).

Elsewhere, such as in the People's Republic of China or among Eskimos in Alaska, transmission from family members (especially sibs) may be as important as or more important than maternal transmission. Also, in Singapore, both vertical and horizontal transmission occur, but infection in the majority of 1-year-old children must be acquired horizontally from other household members through sharing of utensils and personal items (Goh et al., 1987). Thus, generalizations about modes of transmission are difficult to make, and changes may occur over time. More work needs to be done on the modes of transmission in different populations and ethnic groups and on changes over time in order to plan effective preventive strategies.

For *poliomyelitis* (PM), another viral disease, there is also a contrast in mode of disease spread as well as in clinical picture in developed versus developing countries. In India 500 or more children per day become paralyzed from PM, although resistance to infection results from early exposure to wild virus in such poor countries and in certain groups in South Africa (Johnson et al., 1986).

Paralytic PM is a significant health problem in West Africa, where "lameness surveys" have found annual incidence rates of 28–53 per 100,000 children 5–11 years of age (Heymann et al., 1987) and an outbreak occurred in Senegal in 1986. The importance of immunization in these areas, even if *direct* coverage is incomplete, and the need for continuing surveys of paralytic PM in developing countries are evident from West African experiences.

In developed countries epidemics can result from new strains of PM viruses, due to genetic variation within these organisms. An outbreak of paralytic PM in Finland in 1984–85, with nine proven cases and an estimated 100,000 persons infected with a type of PM, was due to a strain of "type 3" PM that differed from strains in vaccines. The epidemic was controlled by a vigorous vaccination campaign (Hovi et al., 1986). In some countries partial immunization, through inefficient programs, may lead to the buildup of susceptibles and, hence, epidemics—as in the Netherlands and Taiwan. Continued surveillance is needed including testing for PM virus excretions in the community as part of vaccination programs.

Through lameness surveys in developing countries, some previous dogma about PM—regarding the rarity of *paralytic* disease in poor, crowded areas—has been disputed, although the importance of late age at exposure in predicting paralytic outcome is still evident. In any event, population differences in PM appear to be due mainly to socioeconomic factors, including availability of vaccines, which influence host immunity.

Acquired Immune Deficiency Syndrome

AIDS and AIDS-related illnesses are now recognized as epidemic and spreading in many parts of the world, through transmission of the causal agent, a retrovirus known as human immune deficiency virus type 1 or HIV-1 (formerly called HTLV-III). AIDS or AIDS-related clinical disease must be distinguished from *seropositivity* or detection of antibodies to the HIV-1 virus in serum, although the majority of seropositives may eventually manifest some form of clinical expression. Understanding of the epidemiology of AIDS-related diseases has been made difficult by the increasing numbers of viruses identified and by changes in the system of nomenclature for these viruses.

Table 6.3 summarizes data on AIDS cases reported as of the middle or end of 1987 versus March 1988 and shows the large recent increases worldwide and in selected countries. Comparability of data across areas is influenced by such factors as variations in criteria used to define AIDS and time lags in reporting as with other infectious diseases worldwide (Chapter 4). Definitions of AIDS may be based on "surveillance" criteria of the CDC/WHO, a WHO system based on clinical criteria, and physician's diagnosis. The major clinical features of AIDS include a variety of "opportunistic" infections, reflecting a host immunocompromised by the virus, and a cancer known as Kaposi's sarcoma. The history of the epidemiology of the AIDS epidemic will not be reviewed here, but key early observations (Friedman-Kien et al., 1981) involved increases in numbers of cases of previously rare opportunistic infections and Kaposi's sarcoma (see Chapter 8) in young males in the United States.

Table 6.3 Total Numbers of AIDS Cases Reported to the WHO as of 1987 and 1988

Continent	No. of Cases	No. of countries reporting (March 1988)
Africa	10,973	50
Americas	61,602	44
Asia	232	37
Europe	10,616	28
Oceania	834	14
Total	84,256	173

	No. of cases	
Selected countries	Mid-1987	Early 1988
Brazil	1,012	2,325
Haiti	851	912
Mexico	407	713
Trinidad and Tobago	134	206
Dominican Republic	127	352
Canada	1,000	1,517
U.S.	35,219	54,233[a]

Sources: Piot et al. (1988), Mann (1987), Chin et al. (1988).

Note: These numbers are increasing rapidly with time.

[a]56,212 by March 1988 (Chin et al., 1988) and 90,099 through March 1989 (CDC).

Worldwide Data

The number of countries reporting to the WHO Global Programme on AIDS has increased recently (Table 6.3), especially for Asia (see Piot et al., 1988; Chin et al., 1988). The majority of reported cases of AIDS are from the Americas, but most countries of Europe are now experiencing an epidemic of HIV infection (i.e., HIV seropositivity). In the Americas the United States accounts for the majority of AIDS cases, but the substantial numbers of cases from Brazil and Haiti are noteworthy, as are the recent increases in numbers for Brazil, Mexico, and the Dominican Republic. Only small numbers of AIDS cases and very small increases have been reported thus far from Asian countries, mainly related to exposure to persons (or blood products) of Western origin (Mann, 1987), but this situation is changing rapidly. In Asia the presence of male and female prostitutes in such areas as Hong Kong and Bangkok suggests the need for continued surveys.

Areas of low prevalence of AIDS are suggested from seroprevalence surveys for HIV-1. Only two of 1,124 persons in Jordan, mainly healthy rural and urban residents, were HIV antibody positive; one of the seropositives had received blood transfusion in another country, and the other had lived in West Germany and Lebanon (Toukan and Schable, 1987). Another case of AIDS in the Middle East due to imported blood has been reported (Kingston et al., 1985).

Africa

"Africa" has often been considered as a whole in discussions of the AIDS epidemic. The African continent includes 50 countries and a wide variety of ecosystems and racial/ethnic groups (Chapter 3). Konotey-Ahulu (1987) has decried this monolithic view of Africa and presented evidence for both the exaggeration of the present problem in most of Africa (see Table 6.3) and the variability in the frequency of AIDS in African countries. In some parts of rural Africa, except Uganda, prevalence of HIV-1 seropositivity has remained lower than in areas undergoing urbanization and social change (Piot et al., 1988), and many studies have been in small, selected urban populations (Mann, 1987).

Concerns are great, however, for the future impact of AIDS in Africa, including maternal-infant transmission and the appearance of other HIV viruses (i.e., type 2) with uncertain clinical effects. Although HIV-1 has been the major agent involved in AIDS and AIDS-related syndromes, HIV-2 was isolated in Africa in 1985 and apparently resembles HIV-1 in its mode of transmission in West Africa. The clinical expression of HIV-2 infection is less well known at present (Piot et al., 1988). In the Ivory Coast, where overt AIDS has been rare, seroprevalences of HIV-1 and HIV-2 were high among healthy female prostitutes. Thus the incidence of HIV-associated AIDS may increase in some areas of Africa in the future (Denis et al., 1987).

Central Africa exhibits a high prevalence of AIDS, and the disease is being spread to other African countries by travelers who frequent prostitutes. Studies in Africa show a high prevalence of AIDS virus infection in prostitutes, including those in East Africa (Nairoibi) (Kreiss et al., 1986) and Zaire (Mann et al., 1987). In the latter study, condom use by the sex partners of prostitutes was significantly associated with reduced prevalence of HIV positivity among prostitutes (see later).

The importance of host factors such as coexisiting parasitic diseases in AIDS in Africa has been noted (Pearce, 1986). The immune systems of African heterosexuals, similar to those of U. S. homosexuals, are chronically activated owing to the effects of other infections, and this activation may increase susceptibility to HIV infection and risk of disease progression (Quinn et al., 1987). In Africans this activation is presumably due not only to infections acquired by heterosexual practices but to the underlying burden of infectious diseases common in African countries—for example, malaria and trypanosomiasis (as discussed later) (Zagury et al., 1986). Thus, malaria, the great force of natural selection in Africa's history as evidenced by polymorphisms in various genetic loci, may have further impact on another epidemic.

United States

In the United States the reported cumulative incidence of AIDS, or total rates per million population based on all cases reported in 1981–87, in blacks and Hispanics is 3–13 times the rate for whites, and the highest ratios of rates are for females (Curran et al., 1988). The cumulative incidence rate in black adults reaches as high as 1,068 per million in males and 161 in females (for 1981–87) or slightly higher for 1981 to January 1988, especially for black females (Selik et al., 1988). Rates are not higher for other minority groups (i.e., American Indian/Eskimo-Aleut or Asian/Pacific Islanders).

Among all applicants for military service tested since October 1985, HIV *seroprevalence* rates also were 3–10 times higher in blacks and Hispanics than in whites. Underlying differences in socioeconomic and sociocultural factors, which in turn affect certain risk factors (especially intravenous drug use), may be the main explanation for these differences (Anon., 1984d) (see later). The estimated AIDS incidence "rates" are especially high in blacks and Hispanics versus whites for adult heterosexual IV drug abusers and for children whose mother (or mother's partner) used IV drugs (Curran et al., 1988). Denominators for these "rates" were all persons in the population, because numbers of persons in the specific risk categories (such as all black adult drug abusers) are unknown. Thus, the extent to which the "rates" reflect underlying differences in prevalence of drug abuse is uncertain but undoubtedly great.

Intravenous drug abuse is a risk factor of HIV antibody positivity in all racial/ethnic groups, including high-risk subgroups such as prostitutes. Seroprevalence surveys in the United States, however, indicate higher HIV-1 rates in black and "Hispanic" than "white" prostitutes independent of intravenous drug use (Cohen et al., 1987; Curran et al., 1988). Factors such as sharing of needles, SES, use of condoms (see later), and characteristics of sex partners need to be investigated.

As noted previously, "Hispanics" are a diverse group in terms of residence as well as country of origin and racial/ethnic background. In a surveillance system for western Palm Beach County, Florida, community samples living near reported AIDS cases showed *seroprevalence* rates for HIV-1 of 0 percent of 60 non-Hispanic whites, 0 percent of 42 Hispanics (undoubtedly mainly of Cuban origin), and 4.2 percent among 616 non-Hispanic blacks including 8.7 percent among 150 "blacks" born in Haiti) (Roberts et al., 1986). Haitian-Americans in the Miami area may be at risk for AIDS because of certain risk factors such as intravenous drug use (Pitchenik et al., 1983). In Haiti the appearance of certain sequelae of AIDS—chiefly, Kaposi's sarcoma (discussed earlier), which was unreported prior to 1978—in recent years may be related to contacts with HIV-infected persons from the United States, spread of HIV virus in the large prostitute population, and antecedent or concurrent infections of other types (Mitacek et al., 1986).

Pediatric AIDS

We have noted the higher risk of AIDS in U.S. children whose mother (or her sex partner) used IV drugs. In the United States incidence rates for children under 15 years of age are about 12 times higher in blacks and 6.6 times higher in Hispanics (versus white) (Selik et al., 1988). Infection with the AIDS virus may account for a substantial proportion of hospital pediatric admissions in some countries. The importance of maternal–infant transmission, along with medical injections in children, has been shown in Zaire, where a prevalence study of HIV virus was conducted among children under 2 years of age and their mothers (Mann et al., 1986). Although HIV-1 has been isolated from breast milk, breast feeding probably represents much less risk of vertical transmission than the in utero mode (Piot et al., 1987), but further studies are needed. Thus population patterns in breast feeding probably contribute little to variation in HIV-1 transmission. As with hepatitis B, prevention of this vertical transmission from mother to child is a major public health goal in some developing countries. In the United States the suggestion that black–white differences in pediatric AIDS incidence associated with blood transfusions reflects treatment for low birth weight, which is more common in blacks (Chapter 9), requires examination.

HTLV-I

"Tropical" areas endemic for another virus, called HTLV-I or adult T cell leuke-mia/lymphoma (ATL) virus, include the Caribbean (e.g., Trinidad), equatorial Africa, and southeastern Japan, but also southeastern Italy. HTLV-I was the first human retrovirus to be discovered, as reported in the United States (1980) and Japan (1981), but infection appears to have been rare in the United States. A case of adult ATL was reported in a U.S. black male in December 1986, and the seroprevalence of the virus appears to be increasing, especially among U.S. black IV drug abusers (Weinberg et al., 1987).

HTLV-I is less efficiently transmitted than HIV-1, but coinfection with both viruses may increase the clinical effects (Bartholomew et al., 1987). Race per se does not appear to be important in determining seropositivity in Trinidad or elsewhere; rather, certain sexual practices as well as coinfections with other diseases appear to be prominent risk factors. In Italy, both IV drug abuse and "sexual promiscuity" may influence HTLV-I seropositivity (Rezza et al., 1988), as discussed later.

Summary

An increasing number of immune deficiency-producing retroviruses have been associated with infection and varying clinical manifestations. Clinical infections with HIV-1 (formerly HTLV-III) include AIDS, which occurs worldwide, especially in the Americas, Europe, and Africa, while HIV-2 has uncertain clinical effects and has been reported in West Africa. HTLV-I occurs most frequently in certain tropical areas and southeastern Italy and is involved in a specific type of lymphoma. Modes of transmission and risk factors for infection with these viruses are similar, but the risk factors vary across populations and racial/ethnic groups, as discussed later.

Kawasaki Disease

Kawasaki disease (KD) is discussed after AIDS-related diseases, because a role for a retrovirus has been suggested. Outbreaks of KD or "mucocutaneous lymph node syndrome," first recognized in Japan by T. Kawasaki in 1967, have appeared in children in the continental United States and Hawaii since 1979. It is a major childhood disorder in Japan, where over 67,000 cases have been reported, involving fever and disorders of immune regulation but no known effects on cancer risk (Shulman and Rowley, 1986; Shulman, 1987). A major epidemic in Japan in 1985–86 suggested an unknown factor that was easily spread and produced immunity in those exposed (Yanagawa et al., 1986). The occurrence of another retrovirus (i.e., HTLV-I) in Japan, among other areas, is also noteworthy. The epidemic pattern of KD with waves in 2- to 3-year cycles in Hawaii, Los Angeles, and other areas, however, is quite dissimilar from the pattern shown by retro-virus-related diseases such as AIDS. The AIDS epidemic, as we have noted, is a steady progression of accumulated incident cases, suggesting spread by contact.

Herpes Viruses, Measles, and Other Viruses

Herpes viruses will be mentioned, because racial/ethnic differences in frequency are related not only to differences in socioeconomic status but to sociocultural factors. Various economically disadvantaged populations exhibit high prevalences of seropositivity for herpes simplex virus type 1, along with cytomegalovirus and Epstein-Barr virus, in children. Included are such diverse groups as the Navajo, Nigerians, and Amerindian tribes in Brazil (reviewed by Becker et al., 1988). In Navajo children seropositivity was associated with cultural practices of sleeping with parents in infancy and attendance at community events, presumably indicating modes of transmission. Overt symptomatic oral herpes type 1 infection was also common in Navajo children, in contrast to symptomatic Epstein-Barr virus infection (i.e., mononucleosis) (Becker et al., 1988). Herpes virus type 2 was not found in Navajo children, suggesting that nonsexual transmission is uncommon (Becker et al., 1988). In general, herpes type 2 (vs. type 1) involves sexual transmission.

Measles shares many epidemiologic features with poliomyelitis (discussed above), including a predilection for impoverished or developing areas such as parts of Africa. Worldwide it is estimated that more than 1 million deaths from measles occur annually, mostly in developing countries. Incomplete vaccination efforts, as with poliomyelitis, leave reservoirs of susceptible children which allow transmission of infection. Crowding and urbanization contribute to high risk of infection in young children, and immunization efforts in Africa have concentrated initially in cities where rates of transmission are high and vaccination programs can be effectively applied. In Kinshasa, Zaire, an estimated 87,600 measles cases occur each year, and annual incidence rates are about 24–35 per 10,000 population per year, with highest rates in children aged 6–11 months (i.e., 240 per 10,000 per year) (Taylor et al., 1988).

The fact that a significant proportion of measles cases in Africa occur in children under 9 months of age, which is the recommended age of vaccination, underscores the need for using newly developed vaccines for children 4–6 months of age. Current immunization programs result in a shift of the proportion of "nonpreventable" cases, defined as those occurring at less than 9 months of age (i.e., before available vaccines can be used). More than 50% of all children aged 9–23 months must be vaccinated in such areas as the Congo in order to show significant reduction in cases and death rates (Dabis et al., 1988). An epidemiologic study in Pointe-Noire, Congo, is noteworthy for its inclusion of measles surveillance through both hospital and community surveys, and for showing the beneficial effects of the WHO's Expanded Programme of Immunization in Africa (Dabis et al., 1988).

In 1988 in England and Wales, five of the six reported deaths from measles in children were preventable because the child was old enough for vaccination. In developed countries such as England and Wales, the advice to vaccinate is not being taken by physicians despite the well-known complications of measles (Anon., 1988b). Most children born in recent years in developed countries will not have been exposed to natural measles and are therefore at risk of infection. The accumulation of susceptible children, due to absence of "herd immunity," is a major problem that must be recognized by the medical community in developed countries.

Various eye diseases involve viruses and chlamydiae (i.e., intracellular organisms larger than viruses). We shall mention *acute hemorrhagic conjunctivitis* (AHC), or signs of inflammation and subconjunctival bleeding, which occurs in outbreaks in Africa, India, and Asia and is due to various viruses (e.g., enteroviruses, and adenovirus and Coxsackie virus variants). AHC is not serious and tends to resolve spontaneously in 7–10 days, except for rare neurologic complications. Crowding is again a factor, as with other infections, as shown in an outbreak of Coxsackie virus AHC in Taiwan, where large numbers of persons sharing a bathroom was a predictor of secondary spread of infection (Chou and Malison, 1988). Large numbers of cases per family have been reported in India (Srinivasa and D'Souza, 1987). *Epidemic keratoconjunctivitis*, usually caused by adenoviruses, is common in Asia and parts of Africa; corneal opacities usually resolve spontaneously but in rare instances become permanent (Ford et al., 1987). Again, overcrowded conditions and hygienic practices are important in transmission.

In urban, lower-SES areas of Nairobi, Kenya, and other parts of Africa, neonatal conjunctivitis is often due to maternal infection with sexually transmitted *Chlamydia trachomatis*, which may cause permanent damage due to corneal involvement (Laga et al., 1986). Trachoma, a chronic keratoconjunctivitis caused by chlamydiae, is a leading cause of blindness globally (see Chapter 9).

Smallpox, caused by variola virus, is mainly of historical interest as a previous force in natural selection, in view of successful worldwide eradication efforts that provide a model, as yet unequaled, for other infectious diseases. The last outbreak occurred in Somalia in 1977, and in 1980 the 33rd World Health Assembly declared the global eradication of smallpox, after which a system was established to maintain surveillance (Jezek et al., 1987). A bacterial disease (see above), *plague*, caused by the "zoonotic" (i.e., transmitted from animals via insect vectors) *Yersinia pestis* (formerly *Pasteurella pestis*), has also been largely controlled. Although global outbreaks no longer occur, individual cases continue to occur in areas where rats and other animals carry the insect vectors. The occurrence of a large proportion of reported cases in the United States among Amerindians in the Southwest is probably largely due to regional environmental factors (i.e., the presence of animals susceptible to plague, along with insect vectors), and perhaps in some cases to the handling of plague-infected animals (i.e., prairie dogs) used for food (Barnes et al., 1988).

Viral Fevers: Obscure and Not So Obscure

There is renewed interest in *yellow fever* in tropical Africa, where hundreds of thousands of people are affected and thousands die annually, as well as in the more publicized but less common viral fevers such as *Lassa fever* (Anon., 1986e). Many of these diseases have come to the attention of Westerners because of increased international travel. Lassa fever is endemic in West Africa, and new ELISA (enzyme-linked immunosorbent assay) techniques are being tested for early diagnosis (Jahrling et al., 1985). Early diagnosis is important to allow effective therapeutic intervention and reduce secondary spread.

Syphilis and Other Venereal Diseases

For *syphilis*, caused by the spirochete or spiral bacterium *Treponema pallidum*, mortality continued to be higher in U.S. blacks than whites in 1985 (Table 4.1). Rates had declined since 1980, but have shown increases in 1985–88 as high as 70% (in Connecticut), with larger proportions reporting illicit drug use and prostitution (Joachim et al., 1988). Black–white differences in sexually transmitted diseases, including *urethritis*, or urethral inflammation, appear to be largely explained by other risk factors. Recent increases in the incidence of early syphilis in a Florida county were accounted for by heterosexual transmission and female prostitution and were concentrated in low-income areas (Anon., 1987d), again suggesting that underlying socioeconomic differences that mediate other risk factors may explain racial differences (see later). This same pattern holds for the high prevalence of sexually transmitted diseases in Africa.

The history of worldwide efforts since 1948 in the control of STDs by WHO and UNICEF includes mass campaigns with penicillin injections, reaching some 43 million persons during the 1950s and early 1960s, followed by a resurgence of treponematoses in the 1970s and 1980s. Increases in STDs involved both the classical venereal diseases (e.g., syphilis and gonorrhea) and other STDs such as chlamydial infections, genital herpes (both mentioned earlier), and human papillomavirus infections (Causse and Meheus, 1988). In the United States, the incidence of reported cases of syphilis declined from 1950 to 1975, then leveled off (by 1984), while gonorrhea increased during the 1960s to a peak about 1975. The treponematoses include bejel, yaws, pinta (confined to Latin America and involving only the skin), and syphilis, and all are caused by spirochetes. Syphilis and yaws are endemic in Africa, while yaws is endemic in South America, the Caribbean, and Southeast Asia (though now only in Indonesia) and the Pacific Islands (i.e., Papua New Guinea and the Solomon Islands). It is estimated that about 2.5 million cases of yaws, bejel, and pinta still exist, mostly in children, and the WHO has revived active surveillance of the treponematoses and has mobilized resources for control.

Some Parasitic Diseases

Brief mention will be made of parasitic diseases with tremendous social and economic impact in some populations, especially in Africa and the Far East. The World Health Organization (WHO, 1986) has surveyed the major parasitic infections, including maps of estimated worldwide distributions and indications of inadequacies in data on prevalence.

Malaria is caused by four species of plasmodia which require suitable arthropod vectors (i.e., various species of female *Anopheles* mosquitos) and a mean temperature high enough for malarial parasite life cycle completion within the mosquito. This situation holds for much of Africa, where malnutrition may have a complex effect on parasite and host (Parry, 1984). *P. falciparum* malaria, for example, is endemic in coastal Madagascar, but the central highland plateau, with a cold dry season in May to October, presents an environment less favorable for transmission by *Anopheles*. The unexplained recent return of *P. falciparum* malaria to the highland plateau, near the main city of Madagascar, however, has been the cause of concern (Lepers et al., 1988). In the Solomon Islands malaria is also less frequent in groups inhabiting higher altitudes versus coastal areas (Friedlaender et al., 1987), as in New Guinea also (Chapter 5).

The disease continues to be a major public health problem in the 100 endemic countries or areas recognized by the World Health Organization, comprising perhaps half of the world population. Of *reported* malaria cases, the largest numbers are from Southeast Asia (i.e., about 2.5 million in 1985), followed by the Western Pacific (1.1 million), but the numbers are certainly larger for Africa. Unfortunately, reporting of malaria is very limited from most countries south of the Sahara, but the worldwide prevalence may be approximately 100 million clinical cases each year (WHO, 1987). The predominant species of parasite varies by region. *P. vivax* malaria is unusual in Africa but common in other tropical areas, as in Thailand, where *P. vivax* and *P. falciparum* are about equal in frequency. The death toll from malaria worldwide is often not appreciated by persons in developed countries. In Thailand, for example, malaria is the second leading cause of death among children and young adults (ages 15–24) (Porapakkham and Prasartkul, 1985). In children aged 1–4, the absolute death rate is higher, but the ranking is lower because of the prominence of upper respiratory tract infections and pneumonia (discussed earlier).

In Africa and Asia, mortality rates from malaria are highest in children under 4 years of age. Intensive studies of selected areas of Africa, in connection with malarial control efforts, provide better data on the public health importance of malaria. In a defined population of subsistence farmers in Gambia, comprised of three main ethnic groups, malaria accounts for about 4% of deaths in infants and 25% of deaths in children aged 1–4 years. A combination of treatment (with chloroquine) and chemoprophylaxis (using another drug) resulted in a significant reduction in mortality in children as well as a reduction in fever episodes associated with malaria parasitemia (i.e., parasite rates in blood) (Greenwood et al., 1988).

Genetic adaptations to malaria were discussed in Chapter 5, and issues of drug-resistant strains and vaccine development are discussed later.

Sleeping sickness or (more properly) *trypanosomiasis*, due to infection with various species of *Trypanosoma*, is another arthropod-borne disease. In this case the vector is the tsetse fly (*Glossina*), which exists only in Africa. It was one of the diseases that led Dr. Albert Schweitzer (1875–1965), the "jungle doctor," and his wife to Africa many years ago. Control of the disease is still of major interest, as in East Africa (Parry, 1984), where relapses after treatment with the trypanocidal drug suramin may be due to sequestration of the causal microorganism (*T. brucei*) in certain brain cells (Raseroka and Ormerod, 1985). The WHO reports that use of insecticides for tsetse fly control is increasing and that adverse effects on humans have not been reported. "American trypanosomiasis," or Chagas' disease, is carried by bugs. Although common in Central and South American countries, this disease will not be discussed here because the prevalence is uncertain (WHO, 1986).

Man-made sources of transmission, via new habitats for vectors, are important in *schistosomiasis* (or bilharziasis) (Parry, 1984). Schistosomiasis infects more than 200 million persons and is endemic in the tropics and subtropics wherever the snail vector carries the schistosome parasite, but different species occur in different populations throughout the world. In southwest Japan (i.e., Kyushu Island) *Schistosoma japonicum*, once highly prevalent, has been largely eradicated by intensive countermeasures. It now occurs only in China, Indonesia, and the Philippines. In the Philippines, *S. japonicum* infection may include cerebral involvement and be treated by a recently introduced drug (Watt et al., 1986). As with viral hemorrhagic fevers such as Lassa fever (see earlier), there is interest in schistosomiasis in travelers returning from the tropics (Harries et al., 1986).

Guinea worm infection or dracunculiasis is endemic in Africa and parts of the Far East (e.g., India and Pakistan), because of contaminated water supplies. Other worm infestations involve animal contact, as discussed later.

Examples of dietary factors, including the consumption of raw fish and dragonfly larvae in Thailand and the resultant infestation with *liver flukes* are discussed later. Indochinese immigrants to the United States may bring with them a variety of infections and parasitic diseases, but trichinosis or infection with *Trichinella spiralis* parasites from uncooked meat appears to develop after arrival (Stehr-Green and Schantz, 1986). Trichinosis outbreaks also occur in Thailand and other Southeast Asian countries, as well as among certain U.S. ethnic groups (e.g., those of German, Italian, or Polish descent) who consume raw or under-cooked pork.

EXPLANATIONS FOR DIFFERENCES

Socioeconomic Status, Sanitation, and Nutrition

Most of the burden of infectious disease, and the paramount importance of these diseases as contributors to mortality, is related to a combination of ecologic factors and low socioeconomic status which contributes to poor sanitation and lack of clean water. In such areas as rural Bangladesh, overall public health, and especially infant mortality rates, could be improved by use of low-cost latrines and tube-well water along with health education on the use of these technologies (Rahman et al., 1985) and on hygienic practices. Beneficial health impacts due to improved water quality and sanitation would occur worldwide, largely through the impact on infectious diseases and resulting diarrhea and their sequelae (Esrey and Habicht, 1986).

Poor nutrition contributes to susceptibility to infection and infectious diseases, such as those involved in diarrhea, and thus to poor growth and development and increased mortality in a vicious cycle of interrelated effects. This cycle has been shown convincingly for Bangladesh (Black et al., 1982a). The immunologic mechanisms, especially cell-mediated versus humoral immunity, whereby malnutrition affects the host's immune system and increases susceptibility to infection, are under close investigation (Hoffman-Goetz, 1986).

The importance of malnutrition has been demonstrated in a longitudinal (prospective) study of child health in Juba, southern Sudan, which may be representative of much of the indigent parts of the developing or Third World. Exceptionally high mortality during the second year of life in Juba was attributed to chronic undernutrition, either caused or complicated by repeated infections (Woodruff et al., 1984, 1986). Thus the oral rehydration program of WHO/ UNICEF may be expected to prevent some deaths from acute diarrhea but would not affect the huge, and worsening, problem of chronic undernutrition in that part of the Sudan (Woodruff et al., 1986) and other parts of Africa and the developing world.

Variation in the severity of certain infectious diseases among racial/ethnic groups may be due in large part to socioeconomic and sociocultural factors. The severity of measles in African children may reflect higher risk of early infection due to overcrowding and the co-occurrence of several susceptible children in the same polygynous or extended family (see sociocultural factors, next section), which appears to increase the severity of disease (Aaby et al., 1984, 1986). Death among children with measles, due to complications, within developing countries such as India and Bangladesh is related to low SES and lack of education, which lead to poor medical care (Bhuiya et al., 1987). Lack of immunization to various infections, including poliomyelitus, is due largely to socioeconomic status, although sociocultural and religious factors are sometimes involved.

Crowding, as we have noted, is associated with increased risk of spread of various infectious diseases. Degree of crowding may, of course, simply reflect socioeconomic level, which is the major factor underlying population differences and apparent racial/ethnic differences in the frequency of infectious diseases. In some instances, however, sociocultural factors may modulate the degree of crowding (see later).

In the United States, mortality from infectious-parasitic diseases, including pneumonia, is highest in lower socioeconomic areas that contain large proportions of blacks (e.g., in Philadelphia) (Dayal et al., 1986). In contrast to the general pattern of adverse effects of SES disparities, the rarity among U.S. blacks of paralytic poliomyelitis in the past, and of infectious mononucleosis at present, may be attributable to factors related to their lower SES. Scientific dogma has held that overcrowding and poor sanitation lead to earlier exposure to mild forms of infectious disease and subsequent immunity to paralysis due to infection. This dogma is being questioned, however, in view of data from poliomyelitis (or "lameness") surveys in developing countries, where paralysis is not rare despite low SES and poor sanitation (Raymond, 1986). Among Navajo children the rarity of overt Epstein-Barr virus infection (i.e., mononucleosis) may be due to the high proportion of antibody-positive children exposed to the virus prior to adulthood (Becker et al., 1988).

Among developing countries the high frequency of hepatitis B virus (HBV) infection and its sequelae, especially hepatocellular carcinoma, in certain populations in Southeast Asia, the Western Pacific, and Sub-Saharan Africa may be due largely to low socioeconomic status and associated sanitary conditions. Hepatitis B is but one example of the influence of SES on infectious diseases, as evidenced in the vicious cycle of malnutrition and infection. Unfortunately, the presently high cost of hepatitis B vaccine is prohibitive to large-scale programs in these areas, and new vaccines must be developed (Arthur et al., 1984). In high-risk areas such as Taiwan, because of the high costs of vaccines, mass HBV vaccination programs have begun by targeting infants of carrier mothers, with other groups to be screened in later phases of the program (Chen et al., 1987). Newer, very low dose HBV vaccines, however, may make control economically feasible for all infants in endemic areas (Moyes et al., 1987).

Thus, population differences in infectious diseases that coincide with racial/ethnic groups largely reflect ecologic and SES-related factors, although sociocultural factors may act independently of SES.

Sociocultural Factors

Sociocultural factors involved in population differences in parasitic diseases have already been noted, but other examples relevant to population differences in infectious and parasitic diseases will be discussed.

The role of sociocultural factors in *sexual behaviors* is an important issue which requires further investigation. Sexual behaviors differ among adolescent blacks and whites in southern U.S. cities (Smith and Urdy, 1985), but the role of SES versus ethnic or cultural factors is not clear and requires further study. The higher rates of sexually transmitted diseases, including syphilis and urethritis, in U.S. blacks may be due largely to SES-related factors including education. For both gonococcal and nongonococcal urethritis (GCU and NGCU) among men at a U.S. military post, the large black–white differences in rates almost disappeared after controlling for marital status, education, and number of sexual partners (Smith et al., 1987). Again, the role of sociocultural factors such as attitudes regarding number of sex partners and sex practices has not been explored. Although circumcision was less common in blacks than whites, it had a negative association with NGCU and no association with GCU risk.

The worldwide epidemic of AIDS-related diseases has increased interest in cross-cultural and international comparisons of sexual behavior, including homosexuality and specific sexual practices. The paucity of cross-cultural anthropological data on sexual behavior, especially homosexuality (Davis and Whitten, 1987), was noted in Chapter 2. Even in the United States, there is a paucity of survey data and controversy regarding the frequency of homosexual orientation (Cameron, 1988; Reinisch, 1988). Reliable data on the prevalence of bisexuality in U.S. blacks and whites are needed to interpret racial differences in incidence of AIDS (Selik et al., 1988). Specific homosexual practices, such as large number of partners and anal intercourse, are important risk factors for HIV seropositivity in studies of homosexual males in Holland (Van Griensven et al., 1987) and other Western countries. In Africa, however, a role for anal intercourse has not been shown, and number of sexual partners (vs. sexual orientation), especially prostitute contacts, appears important in AIDS (Piot et al., 1988).

The ratio of male to female cases of AIDS in Africa, which is near unity (about 1.1:1), has suggested that heterosexual spread of the disease is more prominent in Africa than in other countries, such as the United States. Although this conclusion has been questioned because of the unknown role of bisexual spread (Padian and Pickering, 1986), spread by prostitutes appears established.

Homosexual behavior is reportedly condoned in Afro-Brazilian possession cults (Davis and Whitten, 1987), and this could contribute to the prevalence of AIDS in Brazil. The increasing prevalence of AIDS in Brazil (Table 6.3) was predicted by Parker (1987) on the basis of surveys of sexual behavior in urban Brazil, where active and passive roles (rather than "homosexualidade" and "heterosexualidade") are recognized, and male–female anal intercourse is reportedly common. In contrast, male homosexuals are reportedly more "conservative" sexually and HIV positivity was infrequent in Panama, where the AIDS epidemic is only beginning (Reeves et al., 1988).

Hepatitis B, which shares some epidemiological features with AIDS, was common among older men in a Melanesian population owing to cultural factors related to traditional men's houses where homosexual encounters occurred; the gradual disappearance of traditional customs led to a lower prevalence among younger men (Langendorfer et al., 1984). In contrast, the rarity of seropositivity for HIV in one survey in Jordan has been ascribed to religious codes against communal homosexual practice and "sexual promiscuity" (Toukan and Schable, 1987).

Regarding AIDS, anthropological studies on variation in the social status of prostitutes and on changes in the institution of prostitution in such countries as Ethiopia (Davis and Whitten, 1987) would be useful. Also needed is more information on knowledge of AIDS, specific sex practices, and protective measures among prostitutes in different countries and cultures. In Singapore, for example, 100 transsexual prostitutes registered at Middle Road Hospital all practiced receptive anal intercourse, and only 53 percent used condoms; among the 100, only 48 percent of Malays, who comprised a larger than expected proportion, versus 67 percent of Chinese had ever heard of AIDS (Ratnam, 1986).

The importance of condom use by the sex partners of prostitutes in the spread of HIV infection has been established through studies in various countries including Zaire and the United States (Table 6.4). In a case-control study in Zaire (Mann et al., 1987), use of condoms by the sex partner was negatively and

Table 6.4 Association Between Positive Blood Test for HIV Virus in Prostitutes and Use of Condoms by Sex Partners: Studies in Zaire and in the U.S.

| | Use of Condoms by Sex Partners in: | | | | |
| | Zaire | | | U.S. | |
	Used condoms	Tended not to use condoms		Condoms always used	Condoms not always used
HIV test					
Positive	A = 0	B = 26	A+B = 26	0	60
Negative	C = 8	D = 51	C+D = 59	22	486
Total	A+C = 8	B+D = 77	N = 85	22	546

For Zaire, the probability (p) of observing this result, based on the hypergeometric distribution (Siegel, 1956), is

$$\frac{(A+C)! \ (B+D)! \ (A+B)! \ (C+D)!}{A! \ B! \ C! \ D! \ N!} = \frac{8! \ 77! \ 26! \ 59!}{0! \ 8! \ 26! \ 51! \ 85!} = .046.$$

This is the same p value as reported by Mann et al. (1986). For the U.S. study, after controlling for intravenous drug abuse, the reported p value was .10 (Cohen et al., 1987).

significantly associated with HIV seropositivity in female prostitutes. In U.S. surveys of larger samples of prostitutes in seven geographic areas, though not necessarily representative of all female prostitutes in these areas, surveyed through January 1987, similar results were obtained (Cohen et al., 1987); the statistical result quoted reportedly controlled for IV drug abuse. In 448 licensed female prostitutes in Nuremberg, West Germany, studied in 1986, none of the 89% tested were HIV antibody positive. Although only 50 percent completed an anonymous questionnaire, 97.5 percent of these respondents reported using condoms in vaginal sex, only one was an IV drug user, and 5 percent had rectal sex (55.5 percent of these with condoms) (Smith and Smith, 1986). Thus the zero HIV positivity rate probably reflected the low prevalence of these risk factors. The explanation for zero prevalence of HIV seropositivity among 183 female prostitutes in Panama City (Reeves et al., 1988) should be explored.

The importance of risk factors has also been shown in the transmission of HTLV-I in Italy, where stratified and multivariate analyses of 289 IV drug users at public assistance centers in Rome revealed an interaction between "promiscuity" (i.e., >10 partners in the past 5 years) and needle sharing. That is, the odds ratios for anti-HTLV-I positivity was highest when both exposures occurred together (Rezza et al., 1988). Thus both sexual behavior and specific practices involved in drug abuse may be important in predicting infection with retroviruses.

"Promiscuity" and premarital or extramarital sexual intercourse, of course, vary in frequency by time and place, associated with changing cultural norms and attitudes. In the cross-cultural summary of ethnographic data on 400 cultures in the Human Relations Area Files (Textor, 1967), 22 cultures were characterized by "restricted" sexual expression in youth, but 314 cultures were "unascertained"; 47 cultures had "insistence on virginity," and premarital sexual relations were "in fact rare" owing to prohibitions. Cross-cultural surveys, although limited, suggest that more "complex" societies tend to have more restrictions regarding premarital sexual practices (Davis and Whitten, 1987). Although such generalities may have some support, the importance of specific attitudes in specific cultures or urban versus rural areas within a region has become recognized with regard to their effects on risk of HIV infection.

Piot and Carael (1988) observed that in many societies in Central and East Africa, the norm is for female virginity at first marriage, except among matrilineal groups, which have somewhat more relaxed attitudes. Views regarding male chastity are generally more relaxed, and occasional sexual contacts of boys with prostitutes occur. In areas where chastity of girls is praised and premarital sex limited (as in Kinghala, Rwanda), sexual contacts with female prostitutes may be frequent (Piot and Carael, 1987). Complex interactions between marital stability and attitudes and practices regarding premarital sex in girls may be relevant to the spread of HIV.

As with other infectious diseases, the worldwide spread of AIDS has been influenced by travel. Among 17 Caucasian AIDS patients in France who developed the disease after long visits to Central Africa, none were IV drug abusers or hemophiliacs, but 12 of the 14 men had had occasional or frequent contacts with prostitutes, and some had not used condoms (Vittecoq et al., 1987). The importance of public health education programs regarding sexual contacts with prostitutes and use of condoms is evident. The effectiveness of education programs in increasing condom use among prostitutes has been shown in Nairobi, Kenya (Ngugi et al., 1988).

Religious beliefs and norms may influence the spread of infectious diseases in various ways. In the Netherlands a religious sect opposed to immunization and maintained as a distinct subpopulation provided a reservoir against "herd immunity" and permitted an outbreak of poliomyelitis in this group (Schaap et al., 1984).

Degree of *crowding* has been mentioned as an imporant risk factor for many infectious diseases such as leprosy, tuberculosis, and hepatitis B. Crowding or family size, along with malnutrition, may be important in measles mortality in Africa and other developing countries (Anon., 1983c; Aaby et al., 1984, 1986), and postnatal mortality in Bangladesh (Rahman et al., 1985) and other areas. Along with the overwhelming influence of socioeconomic factors affecting crowding, family structure and marriage patterns (e.g., polygyny) are related to crowding and may also influence rates of infectious disease in different geographic/ ethnic groups. In an outbreak of paralytic poliomyelitis in Taiwan, the county with the highest rates had a larger proportion of families sharing toilets despite the higher proportion of fathers with a professional occupation (Kim-Farlet et al., 1984). In New Zealand crowding was related to HBsAg positivity, but the higher prevalence of HBsAg among non-Europeans versus Europeans persisted after controlling for household size and number of siblings (Milne et al., 1987). Other aspects of crowding, including available space, should be explored.

Hygienic practices may reflect both SES and sociocultural factors. In urban Bangladesh, children with diarrhea and a control group differed in various practices such as washing of hands before food preparation and hygienic practices. These findings suggest that educational programs to influence these practices could influence disease patterns (Clemens and Stanton, 1987).

Cultural influences may be subtle or esoteric, and a few examples will be cited. In Ethiopia horizontal transmission of hepatitis B, especially in females, may occur by local customs of tattooing, tonsilectomy, circumcision, and ear piercing (Tsega et al., 1986). Tattooing also has been responsible for transmission of hepatitis B in Westernized countries. In New Zealand tattooing was associated with presence of HBs antibody (anti-HBs) but not with HBsAG positivity (i.e., chronic carrier state) (Milne et al., 1987). In Africa the practice of surgical removal of the uvula of the soft palate by "native doctors," owing to erroneous beliefs, leads to many serious medical consequences including infections as well as hemorrhage; public health education in collaboration with local chiefs and traditional rulers is needed (Adekeye et al., 1984). In contrast, lack of circumcision in African males has been associated with HIV-1 (i.e., AIDS virus) seropositivity, independent of the occurrence of genital ulcers, perhaps indicating viral survival under the foreskin (Piot et al., 1987). Further studies are needed on the role of circumcision in HIV virus infection, independent of other risk factors.

While various "life-style" factors in Westernized countries may vary across ethnic groups owing to cultural factors, in tropical diseases in developing countries the behavior of pathogens and "hosts other than man" have been studied in greater detail than the sociocultural behavior of man himself (Gillett, 1985).

Gillett cites many examples of the importance of human behavioral variation, such as the custom in Thailand of eating fresh dragonfly larvae which harbor liver flukes, and raw crabs or fish which carry other parasites (as noted earlier). Various breeding grounds for *Anopheles gambiae* mosquitoes are man-made in Africa, urban India and Pakistan, and Bangkok. The effects of agricultural practices in Africa on mosquito breeding grounds (i.e., stagnant pools) and hence on the spread of malaria are well known. The planting of mango trees provides shade conducive for the sleeping sickness vector in West Africa. Other cultural factors include local attitudes regarding the source of infection. Witchcraft rather than insects, for example, may be viewed as vector; also insects may feed on pigs kept in nearby compounds (Parry, 1984). Sleeping sickness would be rare in Africa without the intervening domesticated animal hosts, because wild animals do not appear to be a major vector.

The transmission of dracunculiasis, or guinea worm infection, in Africa involves a complex web related to drinking water contamination, but including the practice of immersion of body limbs with worm lesions into drinking water sources, that must be understood and modified (Watts, 1986). In Africa health education programs, involving filtration of drinking water through a nylon cloth, have virtually eliminated dracunculiasis in certain villages (Hopkins, 1988). Among the Turkana people of Kenya, parasites (i.e., tapeworms) responsible for the parasitic cysts or hydatid disease in the liver and other organs, are transmitted by close contact with dogs. Again, control of this disease will require education programs and administration of drugs to the dogs, or sheep in other countries where the disease is common. In Southern Morocco hydatidosis in humans is also related to exposure to dogs with hydatid cysts derived from eating infected animals slaughtered, especially during religious festivals; the human population is unaware of the mode of spread of the worm (Pandey et al., 1988). In southwest France, high rates of visceral larva migrans, a syndrome involving rash and difficulty in breathing, are due to the larva of *Toxocara canis*, the common dog roundworm; suggestive associations have been found with owning two or more dogs and with hunting (Glickman et al., 1987). Antibodies to *T. canis* are also reportedly common in U.S. children, especially among blacks in rural areas, but further studies are needed on the explanations.

Genetic Factors

Infectious diseases have long been a major factor in natural selection among human populations (Livingstone, 1980, 1984) as well as a significant influence on world history (McNeill, 1976). As a force in natural selection infectious diseases have been involved in the maintenance of certain genes, as witnessed by the effects of malaria on the population genetics of a number of gene loci. The demonstration of malarial selection for hemoglobin S led to investigation and establishment of associations between malaria and other red cell polymorphisms (Chapter 5). Evidence for associations between malaria and blood groups, however, is equivocal (Mourant et al., 1976), except for the protection afforded by Duffy-negative blood groups against vivax malaria in some studies (Livingstone, 1984) but not in others (Bayoumi et al., 1986).

Blood group O is apparently involved in *susceptibility* to cholera. In the Gangetic delta (Bangladesh), constant selective pressure, due to endemic cholera, against group O persons may account for the low prevalence of O genes and the high prevalence of B genes (Glass et al., 1985). Blood group O may be related to *resistance* against smallpox, and selection against A and AB phenotypes may have occurred in parts of India and in Iceland (Adalsteinsson, 1985). In contrast group O hosts were *favored* in choice for blood meals by mosquito vectors (*Aedes aegypti*) for yellow fever (Wood, 1976).

In general, natural selection via disease may have operated on fortuitous variation in phenotype (and hence genotype) frequencies in populations, leading to unusual gene frequencies in these populations (Livingstone, 1980, 1984). That is, present gene frequencies in different populations represent in part the operation of natural selection, for or against certain genes, of unknown or uncertain duration. Without knowledge of the history of genetic structure and disease in populations, the role of present-day variation in gene frequencies in explaining population differences in infectious disease frequency is especially difficult to unravel.

HLA and HLA-linked genes are involved in susceptibility of the host to the "tuberculoid" (or localized lesion) form of leprosy and to tuberculosis (Fine, 1981, 1982). Class II HLA antigens have been associated with these diseases, suggesting the possible role of immune responses in their pathogenesis. In tuberculoid leprosy, HLA-DR2 and HLA-DRw2, as well as DQw1 have been associated in some populations (DeVries et al., 1980; Schauf et al., 1985), but further studies are needed on other groups. Interestingly, DR2 is common in Thailand, and the origin of that population is mainly from southern China (see Chapter 3), where DR2 is also common. Thus the high frequency of DR2 despite its association with leprosy suggests that DR2 genes may have had some other survival advantage (Schauf et al., 1985). The assumption is that without such selective advantage the HLA-DR2 gene would not be as common. We must recall, however, that the historical background of infectious diseases in populations and hence the opportunity for the operation of selection are largely unknown but influence the present frequency of genes. This principle has been discussed by Livingstone (1980, 1984) with respect to malarial adaptations.

HLA-DR4 has been associated with skin test responsiveness to antigens of *M. tuberculosis* but not to antigens shared with other mycobacteria such as *M. leprae* among Caucasian leprosy patients in Spain (Ottenhoff et al., 1986). Methodologically, it is noteworthy that the finding of a statistical association remained after correction for the number of comparisons made (i.e., 40). The biological mechanism may involve the immune response genes in the class II region of the HLA gene complex, which control T cell (lymphocyte) responses to foreign antigens. In tuberculosis hypersensitivity to the tubercle bacillus results from cell-mediated responses, and the inflammatory reaction produces granulomas, which form the typical tubercules of tuberculosis. Thus, if HLA-DR4 is a marker for a gene conferring skin hyperresponsiveness to *M. tuberculosis*-specific antigens (Ottenhoff et al., 1986), persons of HLA-DR4 phenotyope may be at increased risk of the disease. Although frequency of the DR4 phenotype varies considerably by racial/ethnic group (Table 3.4), the data (i.e., highest frequency in "Amerindians" and lowest in certain black populations) are not immediately useful in interpreting racial/ethnic differences in tuberculosis. Further studies are needed on the role of HLA genes, along with environmental factors such as degree of crowding, in tuberculosis in specific racial/ethnic groups.

The high frequency of pneumococcal meningitis in Africa (Davies, 1977) and the high prevalence in U.S. blacks, even after controlling for income level and the presence of sickle cell disease, have led to speculation that a genetic factor may predispose to the disease (Henneberger et al., 1983). Control for the presence of sickle cell disease (HbSS) is necessary because of the well-known increased prevalence of pneumococcal septicemia and bacterial meningitis and the severe course of pneumonia in these children (DeCeulaer et al., 1985). Further studies are needed to explore the hypothesis of genetic factors in black–white differences in meningitis, perhaps using degree of admixture as a variable (Chapter 3).

The growing body of data from seroepidemiologic studies of hepatitis B among various racial/ethnic groups should provide a basis for more detailed studies of both environmental and genetic factors influencing host immunity. In New Zealand the independent effect of non-European versus European ethnicity, controlling for other factors including size of household through multiple logistic regression, suggested that "immunogenetic" factors might be involved. The earlier age of infection in non-Europeans, however, in the cross-sectional data (Milne et al., 1987) requires further study. Earlier acquisition of infection could result from environmental factors not controlled for in the analysis, including other aspects of crowding or sociocultural differences.

It will be difficult to separate the effects of nutrition and concomitant infections from genetic factors in studies of susceptibility of racial/ethnic groups to hepatitis B. The same situation holds for AIDS, where evidence for the role of genetic factors in mediating susceptibility has been regarded as inconclusive (Piot et al., 1988), although some rather consistent HLA association have been reported for Kaposi's sarcoma (see Chapter 8).

One recent study of HLA associations with outcome after exposure to HIV virus merits some discussion. In cohort of 32 hemophilia patients in Edinburgh exposed to HIV-contaminated blood products (i.e., factor VIII, discussed in Chapter 5) in March to May 1984 and followed to 1988, a "strong association" was found between the HLA haplotype A1 B8 DR3 and development of HIV-related symptoms (without Kaposi's sarcoma) after seroconversion (Steel et al., 1988). The data were analyzed in a case-control fashion, with various outcomes including seroconversion and symptoms among those who seroconverted. Although the "relative risk" (i.e., odds ratio or estimate of the relative risk) for seroconversion associated with the HLA A1 B8 DR3 haplotype was 2.9, a confounding factor was evident regarding the outcome of seroconversion. That is, the HLA A1 B8 DR3 group had received a larger average number of bottles of contaminated fluid. This confounding was considered less likely to have affected the odds ratio for symptomatic infection (excluding persistent generalized lymphadenopathy) among those who had seroconverted (i.e., seven of nine with HLA A1 B8 DR3 vs. one of nine without this HLA haplotype). One cannot be certain, however, that the amount of initial exposure to contaminated factor VIII could not influence subsequent risk of symptoms.

As noted in Chapter 3, A1 B8 DR3 is the most frequent HLA haplotype among Europeans, especially northern Europeans (Bodmer et al., 1987). The Edinburgh study needs to be replicated in other populations, with consideration of potential confounders in the statistical analysis. Meanwhile Steel et al. (1988) have raised several interesting and important issues. *First* the different ethnic compositions of other groups studied for HLA associations, with less frequent occurrence of the A1 B8 DR3 haplotype, were pointed out. We have noted the importance of statistical issues in the interpretation of findings from epidemiologic studies in different populations (Chapter 1). The higher expected frequency of the specific HLA haplotype in the total cohort studied in Edinburgh increased the chances of detecting an association, if in fact one existed. Reports on non-hemophiliac blood donors in France (Halle et al., 1988) and hemophiliacs in Vienna (Pabinger et al., 1988) have not confirmed the association. Additional studies are needed in northern European cohorts at high risk for HIV infection and its sequelae. *Second*, the immune hyperresponsiveness associated with the A1 B8 DR3 haplotype and the observation that HIV virus replicates preferentially in activated lymphocytes (i.e., T4 cells), suggested to Steel et al. (1988) a possible biological explanation for the association observed with HIV progression, but further studies are needed.

The number of studies on associations between HIV-related diseases and genetic factors has increased in recent years. A case-control comparison of the serum protein known as group-specific component (Gc) (see Chapter 3) in London, "Gc-1 fast," or Gc-1F, was associated with susceptibility to infection and severity of illness (including risk of AIDS) (Eales et al., 1987). It was also observed that the gene frequency of Gc-1F is apparently higher in central Africa, where HIV infection prevalence is relatively high, than in Europe (see Chapter 3). High frequencies of Gc-1F have been reported in Asiatic populations, Lapps (Beckman et al., 1988), and some groups in India (Papiha et al., 1987), but the relevance of these data to AIDS prevalence is uncertain. As the number of reported AIDS cases increases in the Far East, including Thailand with its large population of prostitutes, further studies of Gc and other polymorphisms may be rewarding.

KEY PROBLEMS: VACCINES, DRUG RESISTANCE, AND ADVERSE EFFECTS OF DRUGS

We have noted the prominence of infectious diseases as the greatest causes of worldwide mortality and morbidity, especially in developing countries. Disease *prevention* involves the development and dissemination of vaccines, while improvements in *therapy* can lead to increased survival and improved quality of life among patients with the disease. Hepatitis B virus (HBV) is a major cause of chronic liver disease and primary liver cancer worldwide, especially in Africa and Asia (see Chapter 8). The World Health Organization, keenly aware of this situation, has launched a number of programs including a global effort for control of HBV (Anon., 1983c; Arthur et al., 1984). Developments in genetic engineering have reduced dependence on human plasma as a source of hepatitis B vaccine (Grady, 1986). A recombinant HBV vaccine produced by a common bread yeast has been shown to be effective in prevention of perinatal transmission of HBV (Stevens et al., 1987). Poor responders to vaccine are still a problem, and genetic factors may be involved. Also recently noted is the need for booster vaccination in children in endemic areas such as Senegal (Coursaget et al., 1986).

For cholera, the WHO has collaborated in a field trial of oral vaccines in Bangladesh which demonstrated protection of both children (the highest risk group) and adults, but longer-term follow-up is required (Clemens et al., 1986). For leprosy, another major worldwide problem (discussed earlier), WHO has also sponsored human trials of vaccines developed, interestingly, from killed armadillo-derived *Mycobacterium leprae*. The vaccine appears to be safe (Millikan et al., 1985). Pneumococcal vaccine has been recommended for persons with sickle cell disease, although it is ineffective in children under 2 years of age (Noah, 1988).

Multiple vaccines may be needed for control of malaria, because of antigenically distinct stages in the life cycle of the parasites, and complete protection by vaccination may require further advances in knowledge of T and B cell responses to infection (Miller et al., 1986). Prospects for development of a vaccine to prevent infection with Epstein-Barr virus, responsible for endemic Burkitt's lymphoma and probably other cancers (nasopharyngeal carcinoma), have been discussed by Epstein (1986).

The development of vaccines against HIV viruses is a current issue of major importance, not only for the developed countries but for Africa and probably Asia, where AIDS and AIDS-related cancers are expected to increase.

In the area of therapy, the evolution of strains of microorganisms resistant to various agents has posed a major worldwide problem, to indigenous groups and to travelers from other countries (Anon., 1986f). Multiple-drug-resistant strains of cholera bacteria in Africa emphasize the need for alternate therapy (i.e., rehydration) and eventual primary prevention through vaccines. The presence of chloroquine-resistant malarial organisms (i.e., *Plasmodium falciparum*) was described in 1978 in travelers to Kenya and Tanzania, and such resistance has spread to most East African countries including Ethiopia (Teklehaimanot, 1986). Resistant strains have occurred in South and Central America since 1959, in Southeast Asia since 1962, and recently in the Pakistani Punjab (Fox et al., 1985). This phenomenon of failure of once successful treatment has been described by Bruce-Chwatt as "a spent 'magic bullet.'"

The human (i.e., medical) response to drug-resistant strains has been the development of new drugs. Mefloquine is a new single-dose antimalarial agent that is effective in the treatment of chloroquine-resistant *P. falciparum* malaria (Harinasuta et al., 1985). Noteworthy was the good tolerance by patients with G6PD deficiency (G6PDD) or heterozygous hemoglobin E. We have noted the well-known associations between abnormal hemoglobin and X-linked G6PDD genes and malarial frequency in human populations (Chapter 5). Kalow et al. (1986) have reviewed ethnic differences in reactions to drugs, including the antimalarial primaquine. Racial differences have been reported in metabolism of drugs used against chloroquine-resistant strains of *Plasmodium* in Papua New Guinea; the slower drug clearance in Papuans may be related in part to effects of their low-protein, high-carbohydrate diet (Cook et al., 1986).

Penicillin-resistant strains of pneumococci were first found in Australia in 1967 and subsequently in such areas as Papua New Guinea and South Africa as well as Europe and North America. In Papua New Guinea one third of 57 strains of pneumococci from infections were penicillin insensitive (Gratten et al., 1980). Thus, there is threat of epidemics of pneumococcal penumonia. As we have noted, pneumococcal pneumonia and meningitis are major problems in Africa and other areas. Guidelines for pneumococcal vaccine use are rather controversial except for selected groups such as sickle cell disease patients (mentioned earlier).

In addition to the evolution of drug-resistant strains of microorganisms, the side effects of therapeutic agents must be considered. One example is the development of severe neutropenia or reduced white cell counts with amodaquine which has been used for prophylaxis against malaria for over 40 years (Hatton et al., 1986). Other antimalarials are associated with severe skin reactions. Another example involves skin reactions, sometimes serious, to antituberculosis drugs (Holdiness, 1985). It is important to determine the reasons for these reactions in particular patients or groups.

CONCLUSIONS

Our review has emphasized the importance of ecologic factors (especially climate) and socioeconomic differences among populations, including racial/ethnic groups, in explaining population differences in frequency of infectious and parasitic diseases. Socioeconomic differences may operate through nutritional factors, sanitation, and crowding. Sociocultural factors are also important, however— especially those involving various sexual behaviors. Additional cross-cultural comparisons of sexual behaviors are needed to increase understanding of differences in disease risk and modes of transmission.

Genetic factors have operated in the past, and continue to operate, in influencing susceptibility or resistance to infectious diseases, which are still the major contributors to death worldwide. It is difficult to correlate worldwide variation in specific genetic markers such as HLA phenotype or genotype frequencies with variation in disease prevalence because of the unknown history of the disease in specific populations and factors that influence population genetics other than natural selection due to disease. Also, susceptibility to several infectious diseases (as well as chronic diseases) may involve the same gene locus, and a balance in selective forces may exist.

Reported associations between specific markers such as HLA and Gc types and specific infectious diseases, such as leprosy, tuberculosis, and AIDS, however, should lead to further studies of these associations in different racial/ethnic groups. In these studies the role of genetic factors, along with specific environmental influences, can be studied and the results compared across populations. With the expansion of population genetics and the emergence of new genetic markers or polymorphisms in genes and their products (Chapter 3) and the increasing importance of AIDS, further studies of genetic host factors in different populations can be expected.

Comparisons of the results of studies in different populations, including racial/ethnic groups, suggest similar environmental risk factors for many infectious diseases including AIDS. These risk factors include individual and group behavior patterns. The prevalence of these risk factors may vary across populations and racial/ethnic groups. The underlying explanations, however, are unclear, and the independent role of sociocultural versus socioeconomic factors is rarely studied. Evidence is increasing for the importance of sexual practices reflecting, in part, cultural norms, and further cross-cultural studies of these practices are needed.

Whatever the mechanisms underlying the influence of SES on infectious diseases, there is increased recognition by the World Health Organization (WHO) of the importance of their control through vaccination programs in developing countries. The year 2000 goals of the WHO include specific programs for vaccination development and administration. For parasitic diseases control involves both improved treatment and prevention, the latter including measures to increase host resistance (through drugs) and to interfere with the vectors. In developed countries, such as the United States, targeted programs for prevention of AIDS are needed for racial/ethnic groups such as blacks and Hispanics, who are at high risk because of socioeconomic and sociocultural factors related to drug abuse and maternal–infant transmission.

Evans (1985) has projected that around the years 2000 to 2025 the large proportion of the total population living in developing or Third World countries will perpetuate the problems of poverty, malnutrition, and infectious diseases. Many of the "old diseases" such as malaria, schistosomiasis, hepatitis, and arboviral infections may still be prominent in developing areas, whereas in developed countries diseases related to behavioral and sexual activity and to travel would head the list of infectious disease articles in prominent medical journals. We have noted the growing AIDS epidemic, its relationships to sexual and other behaviors, and the role of increased travel in the spread of many infectious diseases. Another trend worldwide is increased crowding, which could also affect the spread of various infectious diseases, especially in developing countries, where other risk factors are omnipresent.

Evans (1985) also predicted that journal articles would consider vaccine trials for malaria and various viruses as well as the elimination of poliomyelitis, measles, and hepatitis B in developed countries. Some of these trends in infectious disease control and in discussions in the literature are already evident. Examples are the intensified discussion of the worldwide eradication of poliomyelitis and the development of malarial vaccines and control of hepatitis B in both developed and developing countries. Mass vaccination programs for HBV are under way in Africa, Asia (including Japan and Taiwan), and other areas.

The continuing burden of chronic diseases related to infectious diseases, including hepatitis B, is also reflected in the worldwide distribution of certain cancers, including liver cancer (as discussed in Chapter 8).

7

Cardiovascular Diseases

While infectious diseases still account for the largest proportion of deaths world-wide, the predominance of cardiovascular diseases in mortality in developed countries is also apparent. As urbanization and Westernization increase in developing countries, rates of cardiovascular diseases are also increasing. Indeed these changes provide an opportunity to study the effects of the processes of urbanization, Westernization, and acculturation—and their specific components such as diet, exercise, smoking, alcohol use, and stress—on specific cardiovascular diseases. Also apparent is the need for multidisciplinary approaches involving understanding of cultural, social, and biological phenomena, as well as appropriate epidemiologic methods.

The problem of comparability of epidemiologic data across different countries or racial/ethnic groups is evident for cardiovascular diseases. Using the best available data worldwide, diseases of the circulatory system accounted for 26.2 percent of all deaths around 1980, with striking differences in this proportion and in age-adjusted death rates for regions by level of development. In Europe and North America, for example, more than half of all deaths were attributed to this category, while proportions of deaths and age-adjusted death rates were much lower in all other regions except Oceania (Hakulinen et al., 1986). This international group of authors recognized the limitations of the statistics and saw their work as a step toward the ongoing monitoring and evaluation process needed for formulating health policies in the developing world. One major problem, even with statistics on such gross categories as diseases of the circulatory system, is the large proportion of deaths due to "other and unknown causes" in developing countries (see Chapter 2).

The WHO's MONICA Project (Chapter 4) on cardiovascular diseases and the Seven Countries Study are examples of the recognition of the need for better worldwide data on mortality and morbidity from cardiovascular diseases. The MONICA Project will also permit regional comparisons within the cities/countries involved. In general there is a need for more data on racial/ethnic groups within broad regions or countries. Although some countries such as Japan and China include only a few major racial groups, data on regional differences in disease must be obtained to explore ethnic and cultural influences within these countries.

DESCRIPTION OF RACIAL/ETHNIC DIFFERENCES

United States

Hypertension

For blacks and whites the earlier literature on hypertension has been reviewed extensively by Phillips and Burch (1960) and by others (see Moriyama et al., 1971). The persistent black excess in mortality rates for hypertension and hypertensive heart disease, as well as cerebrovascular diseases, is evident in Table 4.1. The higher frequency of essential hypertension and its sequelae in blacks versus whites is now well documented (Frisancho et al., 1984; Prineas and Gillum, 1985).

Longitudinal studies in childhood and early adulthood do not indicate major ethnic differences in blood pressure in U.S. blacks, whites, and Hispanics prior to 20 years of age (Schachter et al., 1984; Baron et al., 1986). Resurveys of the eighth-grade population in Dallas, Texas, 2 and 4 years after initial survey showed no substantial differences in blood pressure among blacks, whites, and Mexican-Americans before age 20 years (Baron et al., 1986). Regional variation may exist, however, in the development of black–white differences in blood pressure in childhood. In the Bogalusa, Louisiana, Heart Study, no black–white differences in blood pressure were evident in children followed longitudinally from age 2 to 7 years, but slightly higher blood pressures were evident in black than in white children, especially with regard to the proportions at the higher percentiles of blood pressure after age 12 years (Berenson et al., 1984; Burke et al., 1987). Cross-sectional studies in urban areas suggest higher blood pressure levels in black teenagers (Prineas and Gillum, 1985).

Table 7.1 shows cross-sectional data on the 50th percentile levels of blood pressure in U.S. white and black adults in 1976–80 by sex and age group, according to the National Health Survey (Drizd et al., 1986). Black–white differences in blood pressure were small before age 35 years but increased thereafter and then diminished or disappeared by age 65 to 74. It should be emphasized that cross-sectional data may be misleading, due mainly to selective mortality (of persons with higher pressures). The small black–white differences in pressures prior to age 35 years in samples representative of the entire United States may obscure black–white differences in children and young adults in specific regions, as suggested for certain urban areas (noted above).

"Hypertension" is defined by various cutoff points in the distribution of blood pressures. Major sources of data on hypertension prevalence in blacks and whites include the mass screening programs of the 1970s—for example, the Hypertension Detection and Follow-up Program (HDFP) and the Community Hypertension Evaluation Clinic Program (CHEC) (Stamler, 1981). More recent data are available from the periodic U.S. National Health Survey (described in Chapter 4) (Table 7.1).

All of these surveys indicate higher prevalences of hypertension in black than in white adults, with black–white ratios of about 2 to 4 for diastolic pressure > 95 mm Hg, depending on the age and sex groups compared. In the U.S.

Table 7.1 Blood Pressure Levels (50th Percentile) and Prevalence of Definite Hypertension[a] by Age and Sex for Blacks and Whites in the U.S. National Health Examination Survey

	Age (years)						
	18–24	25–34	35–44	45–54	55–64	65–74	Total
Blood Pressure (50th Percentile, in mm Hg)							
Systolic							
Males, black	119	123	130	135	140	140	127
Males, white	123	124	125	129	135	140	127
Females, black	111	114	124	137	139	146	121
Females, white	110	111	115	125	134	143	119
Diastolic							
Males, black	75	79	87	89	88	83	81
Males, white	75	79	81	84	83	81	80
Females, black	71	73	82	87	87	84	79
Females, white	70	71	76	80	81	81	75
Hypertension prevalence (Percentage of Population)							
Males, black	(2.4)[b]	(13.3)	(23.8)	26.0	44.4	42.9	21.1
Males, white	(2.9)	8.9	12.1	26.2	31.3	37.5	17.1
Ratio, B/W	0.8	1.5	2.0	1.0	1.4	1.1	1.2
Females, black	(3.2)	(7.3)	(26.9)	58.3	60.1	72.8	29.5
Females, white	(0.9)	3.7	8.9	21.6	34.4	48.3	16.6
Ratio, B/W	3.6	2.0	3.0	2.7	1.7	1.5	1.8

Source: Drizd et al. (1986).

[a]Systolic pressure 160+ and/or diastolic 95+, and/or taking antihypertensive medication. This is defined as "definite" hypertension.

[b]Prevalence rates in parentheses are based on small numbers and have large standard errors.

National Health Survey, *"elevated blood pressure"* defined as a systolic pressure of 140+ or a diastolic pressure of 90+, was more prevalent among black than white adults in all age groups except males aged 18 to 24 years. By age 65 to 74 years, however, the prevalence rates in whites approached those in blacks (Drizd et al., 1986), as also shown for average blood pressure. The prevalence of *"definite hypertension,"* defined as systolic pressure of 160+ and/or diastolic of 95+ and/or use of antihypertensive medication, was consistently higher in blacks than whites after age 24 years (Table 7.1). The largest black/white ratio for prevalence of definite hypertension was among females 35 to 54 years of age, with small ratios for males after age 44 (Table 7.1).

A subgroup of blacks apparently at especially high risk for hypertension has been identified. A long-term cohort study of black physicians (mostly males) educated in Tennessee and initially free of hypertension has shown a very high risk of hypertension (i.e., 44% after an average of 23 years of follow-up) apparently strongly related to the development of obesity (Neser et al., 1986).

In some surveys, isolated systolic hypertension—or elevated systolic pressure without concomitant elevation of diastolic pressure—is more common among black than white women in older age groups (i.e., 55–64 and 65–74 years). This pattern may be related to the higher prevalence of obesity and diabetes among black female adults (McClellan et al., 1987), as discussed later.

Thus, higher prevalences of hypertension among adult blacks are noteworthy despite increased awareness of and treatment for hypertension among blacks (e.g., in Georgia). Black–white differences in prevalence and mortality from hypertension persist, although an analysis of time trends in U.S. blacks and whites indicates a decrease in racial differences in recent years due in part to improvements in hypertension control in blacks (Persky et al., 1986). Additional studies are needed on time changes in hypertension prevalence in blacks, which have important implications for planning for such conditions as *end-stage renal disease* or renal failure evidenced by uremia. The latter had been a more common sequela of hypertension among blacks before the use of modern antihypertensive drugs (Relman, 1982), and black–white differences in mortality rates for renal failure, though declining, still persist (Table 4.1). The poorer prognosis of blacks versus whites with hypertension has been confirmed by the U.S. Hypertension Detection and Follow-up Study (Tyroler, 1983).

In contrast to essential hypertension, *renovascular hypertension* (RH) or renal artery stenosis is less frequent in blacks than in whites, with a 1:3 ratio for surgically cured RH in the U.S. Cooperative Study of Renovascular Hypertension (Hall, 1985). Clinically the hypertension of RH resembles that of essential hypertension. The diagnosis of RH requires evidence of renal artery stenosis or narrowing, through special tests (i.e., renal arteriograms). Unilateral renal artery stenosis is an uncommon cause of hypertension, and hence the lower prevalence in blacks has little effect on the black–white difference in overall prevalence of hypertension. The pathogenesis of RH is probably different from that in essential hypertension, since renal stenosis often involves atheromatous occlusion of the renal artery at its origin; thus the pathogenesis may resemble coronary heart disease (discussed later). Parenthetically, we note that other renal diseases not related to hypertension include glomerulonephritis, which is classified with renal diseases in the ICD (WHO, 1977); this disease has an infectious etiology in some cases and shows higher mortality rates in U.S. blacks than whites (see Hall, 1985, and Table 4.1).

Turning to other U.S. racial/ethnic groups, Filipinos in California have rates of essential hypertension nearly equal to those of American blacks, especially among males aged 18 to 49 years and 50+ years and females aged 50+ years (Stavig et al., 1984).

Data on hypertension in U.S. Hispanic groups are limited, but analyses of the Hispanic Health and Nutrition Examination Survey (HHANES) data (Chapter 4) are in progress. In Mexican-Americans in Texas, the true prevalence of "hypertension" is debated, because of the uncertain prevalence of treatment for hypertension, which affects current levels of blood pressure (Stern, 1985). In San Antonio, hypertension defined as a diastolic pressure of 95 mm Hg or higher *or* current use of antihypertensive medication was not more frequent in random samples of Mexican-Americans than among Anglos, especially after adjustment for obesity level and SES (Franco et al., 1985). At the same SES, however, the lower proportion of Mexican-American hypertensives *under medication* suggested possible sociocultural barriers to medical care. This same situation appears to hold for control of diabetes mellitus and its consequences, including a proportion of cases of end-stage renal disease in Mexican-Americans (see Chapter 9).

Among Hispanics in a semi-rural area near Albuquerque, New Mexico, a survey in 1984–85 disclosed a lower prevalence of "definite" and "borderline" hypertension in males in comparison with U.S. data (i.e., Drizd et al., 1986, as shown in Table 7.1) and comparable rates for Hispanic vs. U.S. females (Samet et al., 1988). Borderline hypertension is defined as excluding persons taking antihypertensive medication (not shown in Table 7.1).

Data on prevalence of treatment for hypertension recorded in the NHANES, as reported for blacks and whites (Drizd et al., 1986), will be reported for Hispanics in the HHANES. Meanwhile, there is some evidence that major cardiovascular diseases for which hypertension is an important risk factor are not more frequent in various U.S. Hispanic groups than among Anglos (reviewed by Frerichs et al., 1984).

Hypertensive emergency is a heterogeneous, poorly defined clinical entity characterized by sudden severe hypertension and its complications. Included is *malignant hypertension*, or malignant nephrosclerosis, a renal disease associated with accelerated hypertension, previously recognized as more common among black males. In a case series of hypertensive emergency in a New York City hospital, both black and Hispanic young males of low SES predominated (Bennet and Shea, 1988). Absence of denominator data in such hospital case series precludes calculation of disease rates (see Chapter 2), but this study emphasizes the need for better data on this condition (especially among Hispanic groups). The often-mentioned problem of diagnostic uncertainty is evident in studies of conditions related to severe hypertension, as well as the importance of lack of proper treatment of hypertension. The majority of cases of hypertensive emergency reported by Bennet and Shea (1988) were not adherent to pharmacologic treatment and had no identifiable source of regular medical care.

In conclusion, despite some reduction in mortality from hypertension and hypertension-related diseases and increased treatment in U.S. blacks, their excess prevalence and mortality continue.

Cerebrovascular Diseases

Elevated blood pressure is a major risk factor for cerebrovascular disease as well as for other cardiovascular diseases. Although both U.S. blacks and whites experienced considerable declines in mortality rates for cerebrovascular diseases or "strokes" in the late 1960s through the 1970s, the persistent black–white differential in mortality (Table 4.1) is due in large part to differences in hypertension prevalence. Not all recognized pathologic subcategories of cerebrovascular diseases involve hypertension, however, and specialized diagnostic procedures are required to differentiate these subcategories. This complicates epidemiologic studies of populations within a country and across different countries (as discussed later).

U.S. mortality data for 1985 show higher death rates for both "intracerebral or other intracranial hemorrhage" and "thrombosis" in blacks than whites (Table 4.1), but before age 55 years, the black/white ratio is higher for the former category. Disregarding the formidable problem of diagnostic accuracy of subgroups of stroke, this pattern might be expected in view of the association between cerebral hemorrhage and hypertension.

Data on incidence rates of cerebrovascular disease in U.S. blacks appear to be limited. In the Evans County (Georgia) study, an early report (Heyman et al., 1971) showed a higher age-adjusted incidence of first cerebrovascular event in black versus white women, especially at 55 to 64 years of age. A later report of higher cardiovascular disease *mortality*, largely due to cerebrovascular diseases and explained by hypertension and other risk factors, among black versus white women in Evans County (Johnson et al., 1986) is discussed below.

In Los Angeles age- and sex-adjusted mortality rates from cerebrovascular diseases estimated for Hispanics, by using census tracts in which 75 percent or more of the population was Hispanic, were slightly lower (i.e., by about 15 percent) than those for Anglos in 1980 (Frerichs et al., 1984). Lower death rates from all cardiovascular diseases and from "cerebrovascular diseases" considered separately were also reported in Chinese and Koreans versus Anglos in Los Angeles. Despite high rates of hypertension, Filipinos in Los Angeles had much lower death rates for "cerebrovascular diseases" and "heart diseases" than Anglos (Frerichs et al., 1984); as noted above, hypertension is not involved in all subcategories of stroke. Further studies are needed on these subcategories of cerebrovascular diseases and their risk factors in Filipinos in the United States. Noteworthy was the nearly equal mortality rate for stroke in Japanese and whites in Los Angeles (Frerichs et al., 1984) in contrast to the higher death rates in Japan.

Studies of cardiovascular diseases among Japanese migrants to the United States have been illuminating. In these migrants there has been a rapid transition of cerebrovascular disease mortality, from the high rates characteristic of Japan to lower rates associated with U.S. whites (Haenszel et al., 1972). The "Ni-Hon-San" study involves three groups of Japanese men living in southern Japan, Honolulu, and San Francisco, who were 45–69 years old in 1965 (Kagan et al., 1974; Yano et al., 1979). Environmental changes related to diet are implicated—that is, increased fat and lower salt intake (as discussed below).

Temporal (giant cell) arteritis or inflammation of the temporal artery is an arterial disease, not classified with cerebrovascular diseases in the ICD, reportedly less common in U.S. blacks than whites. Apparently no data are available on other racial/ethnic groups. Since the disease is especially common after age 70, there may be increasing interest in its distribution in developed countries.

Ischemic (Coronary) Heart Disease

Definitions. Complicating epidemiologic studies of ischemic heart disease (IHD), also known as coronary heart disease (CHD), are the various *specific clinical manifestations* of this disease category and the different risk factors involved. This problem is similar to that encountered in the epidemiology of cerebrovascular diseases. The internationally recognized categories of IHD (Fraser, 1986) are *primary cardiac arrest* presumably reflecting electrical instability of the heart; *angina pectoris* or chest pain (with several subcategories); acute *myocardial infarction* (AMI) (both "definite" and "possible"), diagnosed by medical history (i.e., chest pain), electrocardiogram, and blood serum enzyme changes (i.e., in specific enzymes indicative of injury to the myocardium); *heart failure*; and *arrhythmias* resulting from IHD. Not included in this classification is *sudden cardiac death*, which includes "primary cardiac arrest" and part of "myocardial infarction," and involves death within a defined period (e.g., 1 hour, or 24 hours) after onset of symptoms. *Uncomplicated angina pectoris* involves only angina or pain, without other manifestations of CHD such as myocardial infarction, which involves a significant obstruction of blood flow in one or more of the coronary arteries.

It should be apparent that population comparisons of IHD frequency are influenced by quality of diagnostic information, including available technology for electrocardiograms and blood tests. Epidemiologic studies of angina have been facilitated by widespread use of the London School of Hygiene questionnaire developed by G. Rose (see Fraser, 1986). Since the "Rose questionnaire" has not been validated for use in black populations, however, data on angina pectoris in blacks and whites are of uncertain value.

There is increased interest in epidemiologic studies of risk factors involved in *arteriographically defined* coronary artery disease, or the extent of atherosclerois in terms of degree of stenosis or narrowing of coronary arteries (Fried and Pearson, 1987). As these arteriographic methods become used more widely, racial and ethnic differences in extent of disease and in the strength of associations with risk factors should be examined.

Risk factors. It is difficult to discuss racial/ethnic differences in frequency of IHD without considering differences in the risk factors associated with the disease. A brief review of important risk factors in IHD may be useful. Although devised in 1961, a "thumbnail sketch" of the man least likely to have "coronary heart disease" is still largely valid. This sketch depicted the following type of man.

> An effeminate municipal worker or embalmer in a mountain city with hard water. Completely lacking in . . . drive, ambition or competitive spirit who has never attempted to meet a deadline of any kind. A man with poor appetite, subsisting on fruit and vegetables laced with corn and fish oils. Detesting tobacco . . . scrawny and unathletic in appearance, yet constantly straining his puny muscles by exercise. Low in income, b.p. [blood pressure], blood sugar, uric acid and cholesterol, who has been taking nicotinic acid [niacin or vitamin B, a vasodilator], . . . and long term anticoagulant therapy ever since his prophylactic castration (cited by Dubos, 1965).

Further studies including use of newer technologies have modified this risk profile somewhat. The following is a brief summary of findings on various risk factors in IHD.

In most studies the excess risk of IHD is about equal for elevated blood pressure and serum cholesterol. In the prospective (U.S.) Western Collaborative Group Study of over 3,000 healthy middle-aged men followed from 1960–61 to 1982–83, for example, the relative risks of death from IHD were 1.49 for systolic blood pressure and 1.51 for serum cholesterol. These risks represent the excess hazard of dying from IHD associated with an increase of 1 standard deviation in the risk factor—in this study, 15 mm Hg for systolic blood pressure and 43 mg/100 ml for serum cholesterol (Ragland and Brand, 1988).

Technological advances have permitted more detailed studies of "cholesterol" in terms of dietary sources, including characterization of various types of fat (especially saturated vs. unsaturated fatty acids), and blood parameters. Cholesterol is carried in the blood as *lipoprotein* particles comprised of cholesterol and triglyceride, along with *apolipoproteins*, which make the particles soluble in the blood. Lipoproteins include low- and high-density fractions, or LDL and HDL, and their genetic–environmental bases are under study. Clinicopathologic and animal experimental studies indicate that levels of LDL cholesterol are directly associated, and levels of HDL are inversely associated with IHD risk. Apo-AI and apo-AII, the major apoproteins of HDL, are negatively associated with IHD in most studies, while apo-B, the major apoprotein of LDL, is positively associated with IHD.

Anthropometrically, the idea of a low-IHD-risk "unathletic" or nonmuscular (nonmesomorphic) body build has been modified by studies of weight/height indices and anatomical distribution of body fat (i.e., upper-body or abdominal vs. lower-body or hip measurements) (reviewed by Bailey, 1986; Polednak, 1987c). Additional epidemiologic studies have confirmed the roles of smoking, exercise, blood sugar, and serum uric acid and suggested the importance of dietary fish oils and fiber—including fiber from "fruit and vegetables" in the thumbnail sketch (see earlier). Blood factors (e.g., fibrinogen levels) influencing coagulation and thrombosis or blood clot formation have also been suggested as important. The role of the hard-driving, impatient or "type A" behavior pattern with regard to IHD mortality (Ragland and Brand, 1988), however, has not been confirmed, although there is agreement that psychological factors are involved in the risk of IHD. The relative resistance of women to atherosclerotic changes (except among diabetics), possibly involving sex hormone effects (see thumbnail sketch) on lipoproteins, is poorly understood.

Some further details on these risk factors and their distribution in racial/ ethnic groups will be provided below.

Findings in U.S. racial/ethnic groups. In IHD mortality rates the United States ranks 36th (from the bottom) among the 52 countries listed in Table 4.5, resembling other Westernized countries except for Japan, with low IHD rates (as discussed later). The decline in IHD mortality in the United States since around 1963–64 has been extensively reviewed (see Kuller et al., 1986). Most prominent in 35- to 44-year-olds, the decline is apparently limited to sudden deaths (vs. myocardial infarction, defined earlier).

U.S. blacks and whites. Although blacks have shared in the recent declines in IHD mortality rates, a rapid increase of IHD among U.S. blacks during the 1950s and 1960s resulted in similar rates for black and white males and higher rates for black than white females by the 1970s (Gillum et al., 1984). Since 1976 IHD mortality rates have continued to decline in white males at a constant rate, but a leveling off has occurred in black males and females (Sempos et al., 1988). Table 4.1 shows that death rates for CHD in 1985 were higher in blacks until age 65. Thus the commonly held belief or myth (Gillum et al., 1984), including "clinical impression," that CHD is still less frequent in U.S. blacks than in whites has been contradicted, as summarized by the proceedings of two meetings on CHD (Anon., 1985b). The factor of time (Chapter 1) must be considered in discussions of the epidemiology of IHD in U.S. blacks and whites.

Not shown in Table 4.1 are sex- and age-specific mortality rates for blacks and whites in 1985. The black/white ratio declined with age for males as well as females, but the ratios were lower for males—1.9 (males) versus 2.8 (females) at age 25–34, 1.6 versus 2.5 at age 35–44, and 1.2 versus 2.1 at age 45–54. By age 65–74, death rates were lower in black than white males, but this did not occur in females until age 75–84 years. Total age-adjusted death rates became higher in black than white males around 1978, but have been consistently higher in black than white females for a few decades (Sempos et al., 1988).

Mortality studies of blacks and whites in specific areas of the United States have been most informative. In the Evans County, Georgia, prospective study, mortality analyses have been reported separately for males and females. In *males* 40–64 years old at entry into the study, the age-adjusted 20-year mortality rates (to 1980) per 1,000 person-years of follow-up for IHD were 8.1 in blacks, 9.4 in all whites, 10.2 in low-social-status whites, and 9.1 in high-social-status whites (Tyroler et al., 1984). Thus, the rates were slightly lower in blacks, especially in comparison with low-social-status whites. In *females* 40–64 years old at entry the 20-year mortality for total cardiovascular diseases was higher in blacks than whites (especially blacks vs. high-social-status whites) (Johnson et al., 1986). The excess total mortality from cardiovascular diseases among blacks was due to cerebrovascular diseases and "other" cardiovascular diseases, explained by the higher prevalence of hypertension among blacks. Numbers of deaths from IHD in women were too small for multivariate analyses, but crude percent probabilities of dying from IHD were 8.2, 10.6, and 7.1 among blacks, low-social-status whites, and high-social-status whites, respectively. Thus, in this study there was no evidence for higher IHD death rates among black than white females. The mortality experience of Evans County blacks, however, is not representative of urban groups.

While Evans County is a predominantly rural, relatively poor area, blacks in the Charleston (South Carolina) study are mostly from urban areas. In the Charleston prospective study of randomly selected adults (age 35+ at entry) from 1960–61 to 1974–75, age-adjusted IHD death rates per 1,000 were 79.8 in 322 black males, 93.8 in 601 white males, 62.2 in 440 black females, and 46.3 in 718 white females (Keil et al., 1984). Thus, the higher IHD death rate in black females evident in the United States as a whole (Table 4.1) was also shown in Charleston.

Another population showing large black–white differences in mortality among young female adults is in a high-income area of New York State (Table 7.2), with black/white ratios as high as (or higher than) those for the United States (Polednak, 1988).

In contrast to mortality trends, *morbidity* from IHD may not have declined in the United States (Kuller et al., 1986). The patterns for incidence and prevalence in Southern blacks and whites, while resembling the mortality pattern, vary by manifestation of IHD. In the Charleston prospective study, *incidence* rates were calculated on the basis of all participants who died of IHD during the 1960–75 period or who were diagnosed as having IHD on reexamination in 1974–75. IHD diagnosis was based primarily on validated history, ECG findings, serum enzymes, and the Rose questionnaire for angina pectoris. Angina has been excluded from Table 7.3 because of uncertainties regarding the validity of the Rose

Table 7.2 Mortality Rates for Ischemic Heart Disease (IHD) in Young Adult Black and White Females in the U.S. and in Suffolk County (New York), 1979–83 (Total Deaths and Average Annual Rates per 100,000 Population)

Age (years)	Area	White No.	White Rate	Black No.	Black Rate	Black/White Ratio	Black/White (95% CL)[a]
35–44	Suffolk	36	8.9	9	33.7	3.79	(1.74–7.20)
	U.S.	4,958	8.4	1,788	23.0	2.74	(2.61–2.87)
45–54	Suffolk	155	46.5	18	101.5	2.18	(1.29–3.44)
	U.S.	23,036	45.4	6,447	102.4	2.26	(2.20–2.32)
55–64	Suffolk	545	208.9	45	363.5	1.74	(1.27–2.33)
	U.S.	89,913	174.2	16,270	303.5	1.74	(1.71–1.77)

Sources: U.S. Vital Statistics Reports, and Polednak (1988b).

[a]Confidence limits (95%) on the ratio (see Chapter 1). The lower limits do not include 1.00, indicating that the ratio is statistically significantly different from unity.

questionnaire in black populations (as noted earlier). Incidence rates for total IHD were higher in white than black males and higher in black than white females. Acute myocardial infarction (AMI) rates were much higher in white than black males but equal in females, while the sudden (i.e., within 1 hour) death rate was especially high in black males.

In conclusion there is some consistency in the findings for females, with higher total IHD mortality and morbidity in blacks than whites, while incidence and mortality rates (except for sudden death) in black versus white males are lower in some areas but not for mortality rates before age 65 years in the United States as a whole. Urban–rural differences may exist in the black–white ratio of IHD morbidity and mortality, with higher ratios among females in urban areas, but further studies are needed. Risk factor profiles for IHD in blacks versus whites, and the interpretation of black–white differences in IHD rates, are discussed later.

U.S. Japanese and other Asian migrants. The increase in rates of coronary (ischemic) heart disease (IHD) among Japanese migrants relative to those in Japan was noted by Haenszel et al. (1972). Although follow-up methods for

Table 7.3 Ischemic Heart Disease in Charleston, South Carolina, Study

Group	IHD prevalence in 1960–61	All types of IHD	AMI	Sudden death[a]
White males	75.8	188.4	80.5	10.2
Black males	32.7	131.7	28.5	32.2
White females	26.6	113.8	36.3	8.2
Black females	26.6	161.0	36.3	13.0
Black males high SES (N = 101)		61.2	26.4	0.0

(Age-adjusted incidence rates per 1,000 during follow-up 1960–61 to 1974–75)

Source: Keil et al. (1984).

[a]Death within 1 hour of symptoms.

Incidence rates include all deaths and all diagnosed with IHD on reexamination in 1974–75.

assessing IHD differed among the cohorts in the *Ni-Hon-San Study*, there was a trend toward increased prevalence and mortality among the Hawaiian and Californian groups versus those in Japan. All men were initially free of IHD, so this was a cohort (prospective) study design (see Chapter 1).

The Ni-Hon-San Study raised an important issue common to all migrant studies, whether in physical anthropology or epidemiology. This issue concerns selective migration or the comparability of migrant groups with their original ancestral groups in terms of genetic and other characteristics, including health status prior to migration. The demonstration of nearly identical ABO blood group frequencies in the Ni-Hon-San groups (Kagan et al., 1974) suggests that the southern Japanese population was indeed ancestral for most of the migrants (as discussed by Fraser, 1985). In the Honolulu Heart Program, a prospective cohort study that is part of the Ni-Hon-San study, analyses of coronary heart disease and cerebrovascular disease rates indicated that region of ancestral origin was unlikely to have greatly influenced changes in these disease rates after immigration to Hawaii (Carter et al., 1984).

Among Japanese in Los Angeles County the age-standardized death rate for "diseases of the heart" (including hypertensive heart disease as well as IHD) in 1980 was still only about half that in whites, and Filipinos, Chinese, and Koreans had even lower rates (Frerichs et al., 1984). More recent studies have compared the relative importance of specific risk factors in IHD mortality among Japanese in Hawaii versus Japan, as discussed later.

Other U.S. groups. For *Hispanics*, data on IHD incidence, prevalence, and mortality are limited. Studies of Spanish-surnamed (i.e., Mexican-American) populations in Texas do not indicate higher mortality from IHD than in Anglos, although obesity-related cardiovascular risk factors are higher than in Anglos of similar socioeconomic status (Stern and Gaskill, 1978; Stern et al., 1984). These Mexican-Americans also shared equally with Anglos in the national decline in coronary heart disease in the 1970s (Hazuda et al., 1983). Hispanics in Los Angeles, who are mainly of Mexican origin, had estimated death rates for "diseases of the heart" in 1980 that were similar to or slightly lower than those for Anglos (Frerichs et al., 1984).

Southwestern Amerindians have had low prevalence rates for IHD, according to various studies, but increases over time have been suspected (Sievers and Fisher, 1979, 1981). The quality of data is surprisingly poor for a developed country, indicating in part the situation for health care statistics in a disadvantaged subpopulation. Data on hospital admissions rates for about 150,000 Navajo in a relatively well defined area for 1956–83 suggested lower hospitalization rates than those for the United States as a whole for acute myocardial infarction and "other IHD." Thus, a large increase in IHD risk apparently has not yet occurred among the Navajo (Coulehan et al., 1986). A similar conclusion can be drawn from an analysis of *mortality* data for "American Indians" (i.e., Amerindians, Aleuts, and Eskimos), which showed a slightly lower death rate for IHD in 1979–81 than 1969–71 and a similar proportional mortality ratio for these time periods (Gillum, 1988). As with U.S. "Hispanic" populations, less frequent reporting of American Indian "race" on death certificates (than in the census) may lead to underestimation of death rates while undercounting in the census would have the opposite effect. *Incidence* data based on hospital admissions, however, show an increase among Navajo Indians in recent years (i.e., 1984–86 versus 1976–83) for confirmed acute myocardial infarction in both men and women (Klain et al., 1988). Thus, mortality rates may increase in the near future.

A survey of *gypsies* in Boston suggested very high prevalences of hypertension and cardiovascular (occlusive) disease, along with CHD risk factors such as hypercholesterolemia, obesity, smoking, and physical inactivity.

In contrast to gypsies, the religious–cultural group of *Seventh-Day Adventists* (SDA) in California (and in Europe) show a 50 percent lower mortality from IHD and lower prevalences of various risk factors (e.g., smoking, dietary fat, physical inactivity, and hypercholesterolemia) in comparison with other white groups. *Mormons* have IHD death rates about 35 percent lower than that expected on the basis of U.S. death rates, again due in part to the low prevalence of smoking (Lyon et al., 1978) as discussed later.

International Comparisons

Sources of data for international comparisons of cardiovascular diseases were discussed in Chapter 4. Variation in cardiovascular disease mortality in 52 countries is shown in Table 4.1, and Table 7.4 shows the highest and lowest rates for the selected countries involved in the MONICA Project. The major subcategories of cardiovascular diseases, although themselves comprised of subcategories (as noted above), must be considered in interpreting rates for total cardiovascular diseases. A few examples should suffice. While relatively high death rates for total cardiovascular diseases in Siberia are due to high rates for both IHD and stroke,

Table 7.4 Age-Standardized Annual Mortality Rates (with 95% Confidence Limits) per 100,000 for Cardiovascular Diseases in Selected Countries of the World Health Organization's MONICA Project (Males, Age 35–64)

All Cardiovascular (ICD 390–459)[a]		IHD (410–414)		"Stroke" (430–438)	
Top five countries or areas					
Siberia, USSR	560 (55)	Siberia	401 (46)	Siberia	119 (26)
Novi Sad, Yug	514 (77)	Finland	374 (37)	Beijing	98 (19)
Finland	495 (42)	Belfast	368 (41)	Novi Sad	96 (34)
Glasgow, Scot	486 (50)	Glasgow	365 (44)	Belgrade	80 (13)
Belfast, NI	453 (46)	Novi Sad	290 (57)	Czech	78 (16)
Lowest five countries or areas					
Catalonia, Spa	135 (17)	Beijing	40 (11)	Halifax	18 (13)
Toulouse, Fra	148 (20)	Friuli	64 (1)	Switz	21 (7)
Beijing	177 (25)	Catalonia	66 (12)	Denmark	25 (13)
Switz	195 (20)	Toulouse	72 (14)	Krakow, Pol	29 (11)
Friuli, Ita	201 (20)	Lille, Fra	90 (15)	Goteborg, Swe	30 (12)

Source: Tuomilehto et al. (1987).

In parentheses are standard errors of rates.

[a]ICD: International Classification of Diseases, code numbers (WHO, 1977).

Finland and Northern Ireland have high death rates for IHD but intermediate rates for stroke (Tables 4.5 and 7.4). In Beijing China, death rates for all cardiovascular diseases combined are relatively low, despite rather high rates for stroke among the MONICA countries (Table 7.4) (though not worldwide; see below).

Rheumatic Heart Disease

Brief mention will be made of rheumatic heart disease, which is important in developing countries. Severe heart failure in Africa and other developing areas is often due to *rheumatic* or *valvular heart disease* (RHD) of an infectious origin, but it may also involve immunological disorders. The epidemiology of rheumatic heart disease is influenced by the prevalence of primary and recurrent acute rheumatic fever (ARF), an infectious (i.e., streptococcal) disease. Although ARF has declined in incidence and severity in the United States and Europe, such a decline has not been reported from areas of the tropics where ARF is reportedly aggressive (i.e., involving severe carditis and congestive heart failure). Studies of initial ARF in children followed prospectively for 6 years in Kuwait showed that carditis in the initial attack predicted the occurrence of RHD and that recurrence rates and RHD were reduced by regular treatment. The previous reports of an aggressive form of ARF with severe involvement of the heart valves probably represented the selective reporting of hospitalized cases and the effects of recurrence of disease due to lack of regular treatment (Majeed et al., 1986).

Thus, regular treatment and adequate follow-up of children with initial ARF should reduce the prevalence and mortality from RHD in tropical and subtropical countries. One group in need of such intervention would be the Australian aborigines, among whom chronic rheumatic heart disease in the Northern Territories in 1975–78 caused an average annual hospital admission rate of 130 per 100,000 (vs. 10 per 100,000 in nonaboriginals) (Thomson, 1984). A WHO study group has summarized (in 1988) the available worldwide data on the prevalence of RHD and ARF, as well as carrier rates for the beta-hemolytic streptococci (Group A) responsible for these diseases. Prevalence rates for RHD in school-age children are high among Polynesians (i.e., New Zealand, Maoris, Rarotongans, and French Polynesians, about 8 to 19 per 1,000 children) and in Egypt and North Africa, parts of Latin America (including Bolivia and Mexico City), and the Far East (India, Pakistan, and Thailand). Improved diagnostic facilities including the use of ultrasound are needed in the clinical assessment of RHD. Maternal RHD is discussed in Chapter 9.

Hypertension

International and racial/ethnic comparisons of hypertension depend on adequate surveys involving blood pressure measurement. Inferences regarding hypertension can also be drawn from mortality patterns for diseases related to hypertension—especially cerebrovascular diseases (or its subcategories).

Blood pressure surveys in Africa show wide variation in the prevalence of higher pressures and in the pattern of change with age (Akinkugbe, 1985). In many but not all studies, the more settled or urban groups have higher pressures and greater increases with age than do nomadic or rural groups. In Africa, small pockets of populations, usually tribal and rural versus urban groups, have low blood pressure and no increase with advancing age (Mugambi, 1983; Akinkugbe, 1985).

Other populations with a similar pattern of little change in blood pressure levels with age and low prevalence of higher pressures are such diverse groups as Polynesians and Melanesians, including Solomon Island groups (Page et al., 1974; Friedlaender et al., 1987), and Brazilian and Guatemalan Indians. In an extensive review Marmot (1984) observed that the lack of age increases in blood pressure in such diverse groups indicated that "racial/genetic characteristics alone are not responsible."

A cross-sectional survey of an entire tribal community in the western highlands of New Guinea in 1966–67 (Sinnett and Whyte, 1973) showed no increase average (i.e., 50th percentile) blood pressure with age (Table 7.5). These data may be compared with data from the U.S. National Health Survey (Table 7.1); the 50th percentile was used here for the purposes of this comparison. Although absolute blood pressure levels are somewhat lower at younger ages in the United States, the higher levels at older ages in the United States as opposed to New Guinea are due to cross-sectional increases with age in the United States (Tables 7.1 and 7.5). A more recent survey in Papua New Guinea has confirmed the lack of increase in blood pressure with age (Table 7.5) and the virtual absence of hypertension (King et al., 1985a). In the latter study, however, higher pressures were found in the more traditional of the two villages, a difference not explained by differences in obesity; salt intake was not examined.

Interestingly, King et al. (1985) noted the possible role of genetic heterogeneity among the small isolated groups in the highlands of New Guinea, as well as social and environmental differences. We have noted (Chapter 3) the considerable degree of genetic heterogeneity among these Melanesian populations. Such genetic heterogeneity also holds for the Solomon Islands in Melanesia. In the Solomon Islands clinical hypertension and mean blood pressure levels remained low in a longitudinal survey of samples of persons in various ethnic groups in 1966–72 and 1978–80, and some groups retained low average levels of blood pressure and an absence of increases with age (Table 7.5) (Friedlaender et al., 1987). The effects of modernization were evident (see also later) in some groups, but the pattern was complex, and the clustering of blood pressures along ethnic lines suggested the possibility that genetic differences among the groups might be a factor.

Males in an isolated traditional island (i.e., Puka-Puka) in Polynesia (Fig. 3.2) had low average blood pressures and no age increase in pressure, in contrast with more urbanized and Westernized groups of Polynesians such as Samoans, Rarotongans, and the Maupiti of Society Islands (Harburg et al., 1982). Although an apparent lack of increase in blood pressure with age in cross-sectional or prevalence surveys could be due in part to selective removal of hypertensives from the population by death or migration, studies of level of urbanization and acculturation (see later) indicate the importance of environmental factors in explaining population differences in blood pressure levels and patterns with age.

There is some consistency in finding regarding increases in blood pressure with acculturation and/or modernization in traditional or tribal groups of varied racial/ethnic origin. Acculturation and urbanization may occur with migration,

Table 7.5 Cross-Sectional Blood Pressure Survey in an Entire Tribal Community (N = 1487) in the Western Highlands of New Guinea,[a] in the Asaro Valley of Papua New Guinea[b] and in a Solomon Islands Group[c] (Average Pressures in mm Hg)

Years	New Guinea, Western Highlands, 1966–67 (age in years)						
	15–19	20–29	30–39	40–49	50–59	60–69	Total
Systolic
Males, 1966–67	122	128	124	122	124	120	124
Females, 1966–67	128	122	122	126	126	116	124
Diastolic
Males, 1966–67	82	84	84	80	80	76	82
Females, 1966–67	84	80	80	78	78	72	80

Year	Asaro Valley (Gamusi People) (age in years)		
	20–29	30–44	45+
Systolic
Males 1983	114	113	113
Females 1983	110	107	108
Diastolic
Males	68	68	66
Females	65	64	59

Years		Malaita Island, Solomon Islands (Kwaio people) (age in years)				
		15–19	20–29	30–39	40–49	50+
Systolic
Males	1966–72	108	120	117	113	117
	1978–80[d]	112	117	111	111	120
Females	1966–72	115	114	111	110	114
	1978–80	116	115	118	122	123
Diastolic
Males	1966–72	73	78	76	73	74
	1978–80	73	77	76	72	72
Females	1966–72	77	74	71	70	68
	1978–80	77	72	74	72	70

Data are 50th percentiles, for comparison with U.S. data (Table 7.1), except for the Solomon Islands data which are means.
[a]Sinnett and Whyte (1973).
[b]King et al. (1985).
[c]Friedlaender et al. (1987).
[d]The same persons were studied longitudinally in 1966–72 and 1978–80.

or within a country due to internal changes. Blood pressure level and hypertension prevalence among migrants from the Tokelau Islands (Fig. 3.2) to New Zealand, for example, increased (especially among males) even after adjustment for other variables (Joseph et al., 1983). As in Samoans undergoing modernization (McGarvey and Schendel, 1986) or migrating to Westernized areas, such increases are due in part to increases in obesity and salt intake as well as stress (as discussed later).

In Indonesia, age increases in blood pressure were greater in urban than rural groups, and the former also had higher levels of obesity (i.e., body mass index or wt/ht^2) and urinary sodium/potassium ratio (Koyama et al., 1988). In Nigeria, clinical studies suggest that hypertension is becoming prevalent among urbanized and more affluent groups who are acquiring Western habits of diet and smoking (Ogunnowo and Odesanmi, 1986). Rural Zulus, in contrast to urban Zulus, in Natal (South Africa) do not exhibit high prevalence rates for hypertension, probably because of less obesity and more physical activity in the former as well as acculturation effects in the latter (Seedat and Hackland, 1984). These factors are discussed later in this chapter.

Increased rates of congestive heart failure in certain areas of Africa are due in part to the increasing prevalence of hypertension in urban areas. Interpretation is complicated by causes of heart failure other than hypertension (especially rheumatic heart disease, as noted earlier).

In China prevalence rates for hypertension have increased considerably in recent decades, although these rates are still in the lower range (i.e., 3–10 percent of the population) of the worldwide scale (generally, about 5–20 percent). Although prevalence rates are still low in China, the large population at risk results in a large pool of perhaps 25–30 million hypertensives. Surveys suggest that many hypertensives, especially younger male adults, are unaware of their disease (Huang, 1986). In a nationwide survey of blood pressure in China in 1979–80, a north (high) south (low) gradient in hypertension prevalence was observed and may be due in part to differences in salt intake (Liu and Lai, 1986) (see later, under "explanations"). Although populations at high altitude have been presumed to be protected against hypertension, a study in Tibet indicates that this is not uniformly true (Sun, 1986).

In the Soviet Union surveys disclosed prevalences of hypertension (defined as 95+ mm Hg diastolic pressure or use of antihypertensive drugs within two weeks prior to examination) ranging from 17 to 30 percent among more than 80,000 men aged 35 to 54 employed in 22 cities, and 21 to 29 percent among 70,000 men aged 40 to 59 in selected communities (including Tashkent in Uzbek and Moscow) (Oganov et al., 1988). Although the criteria differed from that used in the United States (Table 7.1), these results suggest that hypertension may be at least as prevalent in the Soviet Union as in the United States. These Soviet surveys are part of a national intervention program aimed at reducing hypertension and deaths from related cardiovascular diseases. Mortality rates from stroke in Siberia are discussed later.

In conclusion, many populations undergoing modernization through internal changes or through migration exhibit increases in blood pressure and prevalence of hypertension, due to a variety of life-style changes. Apparent racial/ethnic differences in blood pressure may reflect the intensity and length of time that acculturation and modernization have operated through changes in diet, exercise, and level of stress (as discussed later). Differences within a country or racial/ethnic group may also involve the same mechanisms, as well as internal cultural variation related to diet and possibly genetic heterogeneity among groups.

Cerebrovascular Diseases

Large apparent international variations exist for mortality from cerebrovascular diseases or "stroke." In a comparison of 33 countries, the annual age-adjusted death rate (per 100,000) ranged from 35.8 in the Philippines to 196.7 in Japan

(Fratiglioni et al., 1983), or a 5.5-fold difference. Mortality rates are also high for Finland, Northern Ireland, and Czechoslovakia, while relatively low rates have been reported for Denmark, Sweden, and Poland. The high rates for stroke mortality in Czechoslovakia and certain other Eastern European countries, and lower rates in Denmark and Sweden, are shown in Table 4.5. Rates for England and Wales are intermediate, while Canada and the United States have relatively low rates. Sri Lanka has the lowest death rate. Even disregarding the heterogeneity of "stroke," total stroke or cerebrovascular disease mortality rates for developing countries, including Sri Lanka and the Philippines, are of uncertain accuracy because of inaccuracies in both numerators and denominators (see Chapter 2).

Among the 52 countries listed in Table 4.5, the age-adjusted death rate for cerebrovascular diseases in Japan is only intermediate, though much higher than the rates for the United States and Canada. Relatively higher death rates have been reported for certain Caribbean and Eastern European countries (with Bulgaria having the highest rate). The apparent discrepancy in the ranking for Japan in different studies is due at least in part to a decline in incidence rates for stroke, as discussed later. Within Japan, Koreans who immigrated mostly during the 1940s had higher death rates than other Japanese for cerebrovascular diseases; unfortunately data on mortality in Korea are limited (Ubukata et al., 1986). As we have noted, data on racial/ethnic groups within countries are rare for cardiovascular diseases. Although Koreans and Japanese are closely related genetically (Chapter 3), cultural differences (including diet) may be important with regard to cardiovascular disease mortality.

Japan is not included in the recently established MONICA Project of the World Health Organization (Chapter 4). Table 7.4 shows the five MONICA areas with the lowest and highest mortality rates for cerebrovascular diseases (or "strokes"). For males Eastern European countries again are among the top five, along with Siberia and Beijing. For females there was a fivefold difference from lowest to highest rates in MONICA areas, with highest rates in some of the same areas as for males (i.e., Belgrade and Novosibirsk) (Tuomilehto et al., 1987).

"Stroke" has been divided into several pathological subgroups, including cerebral infarction or intracerebral hemorrhage, but the accuracy of such data depends on the availability of sophisticated diagnostic equipment. The clinical definition of "stroke" encompassing all subtypes, however, appears to be valid (Malmgren et al., 1987), so that international comparisons are justified. In an extensive review of some 72 *incidence* studies worldwide during the past 40 years, Malmgren et al. (1987) judged that only nine were "ideal" (methodologically) for geographical comparisons of stroke incidence. Geographical differences were not great for the studies in Soderhamn (Sweden), Rochester (Minnesota), Shibata (Japan), Tiburg (Netherlands), Espoo-Kauniainen (Finland), Auckland (New Zealand), Oxfordshire (U.K.), and Benghazi (Libya). Although incidence rates tended to be highest in Shibata, Japan, rates for Soderhamn, Sweden, were nearly as high despite the low cerebrovascular disease mortality rates in Sweden as a whole (noted above). Noteworthy is the absence of adequate data from developing countries, with the exception of Libya.

The lack of "race-specific" incidence rates in racially heterogeneous populations was noted by Malmgren et al. (1987). Also noteworthy was the evidence for a decline in a Japanese study (in Hisayama) of about 30 percent in age-adjusted incidence rates for two categories of stroke (i.e., "cerebral hemorrhage" and "cerebral infarction") between 1961–66 and 1972–76. In contrast, Soderhamn, Sweden, showed no evidence for a decline between 1975–78 and 1983–85.

In comparing reported studies similar to those reviewed by Malmgren et al. (1987), Alter et al. (1986) noted that age- and sex-standardized incidence *ratios*, with the United States as the standard population, in 37 regions worldwide showed little variation with the possible exceptions of China and Japan (which had high ratios). Ratios in some areas of Japan were low, however, while the Chinese data were based on house-to-house surveys, which resulted in better case ascertainment than other studies based mainly on hospitalized cases. Thus methodologic differences across studies, along with regional variation of unknown significance, preclude generalizations about variation in stroke incidence. Higher incidence rates may exist in parts of Japan, but reductions in incidence also may be occurring. Further data are needed from China. Since mortality rates for Beijing are also relatively high among the countries in the MONICA Project (Table 7.4), either the incidence rates are in fact higher or the higher mortality is related to lack of treatment of hypertension.

A survey of six cities in the People's Republic of China disclosed cerebrovascular disease *prevalence* rates of about 100 per 100,000 per year (Li et al., 1985), which is higher than the average for the 33 countries compared by Fratiglioni et al. (1983). Although overall prevalence rates in China are lower than that for Japan (i.e., about 200 per 100,000 per year), rates in China varied from 59 to 272. *Intracerebral hemorrhage* appeared to be proportionately common in China, but we have noted problems in comparing rates of subtypes of stroke. Intracerebral hemorrhage, related to underlying raised intracranial pressure, is one of several vascular events that can cause "stroke" or acute onset of focal neurologic deficit such as paralysis.

Another epidemiologic survey, involving a screening examination with high participation rate (i.e., 98.9 percent), characteristic of surveys in China, has been reported in Guangxi province of southern China. After age adjustment to the 1960 U.S. population, the incidence rate for all cerebrovascular diseases was 81.4 per 100,000, and for "completed strokes" 65.4. In apparent contrast to the surveys reported by Li et al. (1985), the majority of strokes in southern China were "nonhemorrhagic" (Yao and Zhuang, 1988). If these differences in type of stroke are real, regional differences in hypertension could be involved. A north–south gradient has been reported in China for prevalence of hypertension (discussed above) and for incidence of stroke (Liu et al., 1985), which may be related to salt intake (as discussed later).

In conclusion, inaccuracies in both mortality and morbidity data on stroke preclude meaningful generalizations. The wide range in *mortality* rates (vs. incidence rates) is due in part to the inclusion of different countries in some mortality comparisons—that is, developing countries such as the Philippines. Variation in mortality rates among the MONICA countries is also considerable. Table 7.4 shows a five-fold difference between the lowest and the highest death rates, excluding the rate for Halifax, which is based on small numbers of deaths and has a large standard error.

Worldwide variation in age-standardized *incidence* rates may not be as great as previously suspected and may reflect inaccuracies and lack of comparability of data. Considerable variation may exist *within* such countries as Japan and China. Surveys from developing countries are needed. More intensive studies are needed on incidence and prevalence within specific populations to examine regional and racial/ethnic variation as well as changes over time. Such intensive regional and racial/ethnic studies should include assessment of diet, as discussed later. Variation may be lower for incidence than for mortality rates (Table 7.4), since the latter are undoubtedly affected not only by stroke incidence but by availability and utilization of health services, especially for hypertension control. It is difficult to explain such variation in stroke mortality among the MONICA (Table 7.4) areas solely on the basis of inaccuracies of certification, and the more detailed analyses promised in that project should be enlightening.

Ischemic (Coronary) Heart Disease

Ostensibly international variation in *ischemic heart disease* (IHD) mortality is considerable, although data from developing or Third World countries are meager even in comparison with cancer data (see Chapter 4). Large international variation in age-standardization mortality (Tables 4.5 and 7.4) include high rates in Siberia, Finland, the United Kingdom (especially Scotland and Northern Ireland), and parts of Eastern Europe. In Caribbean countries mortality rates vary greatly, from among the lowest (e.g., Martinique, St. Vincent/Grenadines, Barbados, Bahamas, and Dominica) to among the highest (Cuba and Trinidad/Tobago); Puerto Rico has intermediate rates and ranks lower than the United States (Table 4.5). Relatively low death rates prevail in parts of Western Europe (i.e., France, Spain, and Portugal) and the Mediterranean (i.e., Greece and Italy, but not Malta), in Beijing, China, and in Japan.

Mortality rates for IHD are much lower in Japan than in most North American and European countries, in contrast to the pattern for cerebrovascular diseases. This emphasizes the diverse patterns for specific major categories of cardiovascular diseases. Studies of Japanese migrants to the United States were discussed earlier. In contrast to the U.S. Japanese migrant findings of changes in IHD death rates, Italian migrants to Australia *maintain* their relatively lower IHD mortality rates versus native-born Australians (Armstrong et al., 1983).

The Greenland Eskimos (Inuit) reportedly have low prevalence rates of IHD but epidemiologic data are limited (Bjerregaard and Dyerberg, 1988); low levels of certain risk factors, especially serum lipids related to diet (see later) may be involved (Milan, 1980). Along with hypertension, IHD has been regarded as rare in traditional, nonurbanized populations in such areas as Africa and the Pacific islands. In the Solomon Islands, for example, there was little ECG evidence for IHD when surveyed in 1966–72 but more recent data are not available (Friedlaender et al., 1987). Increases in IHD prevalence have been observed in South African blacks but not in Nigerians, although we have noted that hypertension (a major IHD risk factor) may be increasing in urban Nigerians. Although hypertension prevalence may have increased in recent years in East Africa, IHD was reportedly still rare in a series of 846 hypertensive patients at Kenyatta National

Hospital (Lule et al., 1985). The process of urbanization may be important, as with hypertension. Other temporal trends are discussed later.

For the more developed countries, data from the Seven Countries Study of males, including regions within some countries, demonstrate large international variations in CHD mortality (and incidence) rates (Table 7.5). Low IHD death rates for Japan, and lower rates for the Mediterranean, as well as high death rates in Finland and the United States (noted earlier) were evident in the Seven Countries Study. Finland includes the minority Lapp population (Chapter 3). In contrast to Finns, Lapps reportedly have a lower prevalence of IHD as well as certain risk factors (i.e., serum triglycerides), according to various medical teams working in the Finnish and Norwegian Lapp populations during the International Biological Program (Milan, 1980).

Within the same region of northern Norway, areas inhabited by Finns had higher mortality rates of IHD than areas populated mainly by Norsemen and Lapps (Thelle and Forde, 1979). Lapps are a distinct "local race" (see Chapter 3 and Table 3.1). Regrettably, routine mortality statistics in Norway do not identify Lapps, but the prospective study of 2,320 men and 2,130 women in Finnmark County, Norway (Thelle and Forde, 1979), which included information on ethnic origin as well as IHD risk factors, should provide interesting data on IHD rates in Lapps as they become slowly integrated with the rest of Norwegian society. In the baseline survey a confirmed family history of myocardial infarction was less frequent, and age-adjusted mean systolic blood pressure was lower, among Lapps; the well-known smaller stature of Lapps was confirmed (Thelle and Forde, 1979).

For men and women aged 45–64 in 26 countries from 1950 to 1978, mortality rates from heart disease varied by a factor of 3, and the north/south gradient of rates in Europe increased, but not all countries experienced a decline in rates. Reasons for these differences are under investigation (Thom et al., 1985). Most of these 26 countries included predominantly white populations, and only U.S. whites were included in comparisons.

In New Zealand, age-adjusted death rates for 1970–77 have been compared for Mormon and non-Mormon Maoris and non-Maoris. IHD death rates were much lower for Mormon than non-Mormon Maoris (especially in males), but also lower in non-Mormon non-Maoris versus non-Mormon Maoris (Smith et al., 1985b). Surprisingly, differences in IHD and other death rates were small between Mormon and non-Mormon non-Maoris. Socioeconomic differences may be involved in Maori versus non-Maori mortality differences, and the low SES of non-Maori Mormons (who include a large number of Pacific Islanders) also may be important.

There is great interest in differences in time trends for cardiovascular disease mortality rates in different populations, as noted earlier for the United States. The trends toward increasing mortality rates from IHD in past decades in Eastern Europe (i.e., Poland and Czechoslovakia) may be expected to appear in developing countries as demands for tobacco and Western diets increase (Shaper, 1986). In Singapore, mortality rates for IHD increased from 1959 to 1983, but there was some decline in younger age groups, suggesting a birth cohort effect (Hughes, 1986). The author has been unable to find data on IHD mortality for the racial/ethnic groups of Singapore.

On the Island of Mauritius off the coast of Madagascar, with its many racial/ ethnic groups (Chapter 3), overall mortality declined 7 percent between 1972 and 1980, but cardiovascular disease mortality rates increased 45 percent and IHD mortality rates more than doubled. The need for health education, regarding dietary and tobacco habits, on Mauritius has been recognized (Brissonnette and Fareed, 1985). According to the latest statistics on mortality from cardiovascular diseases (Table 4.5), Mauritius ranks 50th of the 52 countries in the WHO data base, but data are needed on IHD prevalence in the various racial/ethnic groups.

Declines in IHD mortality in Japan since 1970 *may* be related to concomitant changes observed in national surveys of hypertension (due to treatment) and declines in prevalence of smoking, although smoking rates are still high (Ueshima et al., 1987). This may also be true for the decline in stroke incidence in Japan, discussed earlier. In contrast, mortality trends in Italy from 1968 to 1978 suggested an increase in middle-aged (50- to 59-year-old) men of 1 percent per year, possibly related to smoking. Although IHD death rates remain lower in Italy than in most of Europe (except France), the large declines seen in Japan, Australia, and New Zealand were not evident (LaVecchia and De Carli, 1986).

Incidence (vs. mortality) data on IHD are relatively rare. The Seven Countries Study (Table 7.6) showed a more than 10-fold difference between age-standardized incidence rates for eastern Finland (highest rates) versus Crete (Keys et al., 1980). This pattern follows that found for mortality. Hungary joined the Seven Countries study in 1965 with a separate cohort of 1,088 men 40–59 years of age and "coronary free" at entry. On the basis of the number of "hard events" recorded (Lamm et al., 1985), the rates may be intermediate.

EXPLANATIONS FOR DIFFERENCES

U.S. Blacks and Whites

Errors of Measurement, Age, and Socioeconomic Status

Kuller et al. (1986) have suggested that there is confusion between hypertensive disease and IHD in mortality data on blacks, especially young female blacks. Community-wide studies are needed on the quality of mortality data on IHD in U.S. blacks. The paramount question concerns the contribution of hypertensive disease to the apparent excess of "IHD" in blacks, especially younger women. Accuracy of diagnosis of disease may be related to SES and hence to racial group. IHD was previously believed to be less frequent in U.S. blacks than whites, but even earlier surveys (in 1960–62) showed that "suspect" CHD was slightly more frequent in blacks (Moriyama et al., 1971). Affecting black–white comparisons may be the lower rate of coronary arteriography among blacks than whites in U.S national surveys of hospital discharges (Ford et al., 1988b).

Black/white ratios for IHD death rates, as noted earlier, vary with age and are high for young adults but not in older age groups. Thus studies of the influence of SES differences on black–white mortality ratios for IHD should provide age-specific data.

Table 7.6 Results of the Seven Countries Study of Coronary Heart Disease (CHD): 10-Year Incidence of "Hard" CHD[a] Among Men Free of Cardiovascular Disease at Entry into the Study, Mortality Rates after 15 Years (Age-Standardized Rates per 10,000 Men) and Dietary Characteristics

Cohort	Total No.	"Hard" CHD			CHD death rate		Diet (% calories from fatty acids)	
		No.	Rate	(SE)	Rate	(SE)	Saturated	Monounsaturated
East Finland	728	71	1,074	115	1,202	120	23.7	11.9
U.S. railroad men	2,315	—	—	—	773	56	16.2	16.2
West Finland	806	45	539	80	741	92	19.4	11.3
Zutphen (Netherlands)	845	45	513	76	636	84	20.2	12.5
Crevalcore, Italy	956	43	450	67	424	65	8.9	11.4
Rome, railroad workers	736	25	357	68	515	81	7.6	17.1
Montegiorgio, Italy	708	22	353	69	447	78	9.6	11.6
Corfu, Greece	525	17	337	79	202	61	6.4	18.3
Belgrade, Serbia	516	13	317	77	—[b]	—	—	—
Slavonia, Croatia	680	18	253	60	389	74	13.6	13.3
Zrenjanin, Serbia	476	12	239	70	297	78	9.7	20.1
Ushibuka, Japan	496	11	204	63	127	50	2.9	2.9
Dalmatia, Croatia	662	13	185	52	216	57	9.1	13.4
Tanushimaru, Japan	504	8	148	54	144	53	2.9	2.9
Velika Krsna, Serbia	487	6	132	52	67	37	5.7	14.6
Crete, Greece	655	2	26	20	38	24	7.7	25.8
Total	9,780	351	370[c]	19	—	—	—	—

Data abstracted and modified from Keys et al. (1980, 1986).

[a]"Hard" CHD is definite myocardial infarction or death from CHD.

[b]Belgrade University faculty were excluded because of uncertainties regarding completeness of death records.

[c]The mean of the rates for the 15 groups weighted by the number of men at risk in each cohort. U.S. railroad workers, representing the seventh country, were excluded from incidence data because no 10-year follow-up examination was done.

Ecologic studies indicate that areas with high death rates of cerebrovascular disease are also those with lower SES and/or highest proportions of blacks—as in Philadelphia (Dayal et al., 1986). For IHD, associations with SES are not as clear, and positive associations between income or education have been reported. In Philadelphia, areas with high IHD death rates were predominantly white and represented a spectrum of SES levels (Dayal et al., 1986). In most studies, however, IHD mortality is inversely associated with level of education or occupation (which are used as indices of SES). In male participants in the Multiple Risk Factor Intervention (MRFIT) Trial in Sacramento, California, SES measured by education and occupation was inversely associated with IHD risk factors (or probability of an IHD event), but the association was less apparent in blacks than in other groups (white, Spanish-American, and Asian) (Kraus et al., 1980).

Socioeconomic factors may be involved in explaining the poorer *survival* of U.S. black than white patients with coronary (ischemic) heart disease, since coronary arteriography and surgery are less frequent in blacks and lower-SES groups (Anon., 1985b; Ford et al., 1988b). Mortality from hypertension-related diseases, such as kidney diseases, may be affected by access to kidney transplantation, which is lower in U.S. nonwhites than in whites (Held et al., 1988).

Sociocultural Factors

Higher average blood pressure and higher prevalence of hypertension in blacks versus whites persist when education is controlled, as shown in the U.S. National Health Survey (Drizd et al., 1986) and in the Hypertension Detection and Follow-Up Program (HDFP). In the HDFP, the age-adjusted prevalence of hypertension (diastolic 95+) in the higher education levels was almost twice as high in blacks as in whites (Heymsfield et al., 1977). SES differences do not appear to explain all of the black–white differences in cardiovascular disease morbidity and mortality. In the U.S. HDFP, the higher *mortality* among blacks than whites with mild hypertension was reduced but not eliminated by controlling for education level. This suggests either that education is a poor surrogate for SES and/or that such factors as sociocultural stresses and access to or use of medical care were involved (Tyroler, 1983); differences in obesity with educational group are discussed later.

In a prospective 20-year follow-up of cardiovascular disease in the Evans County (Georgia) population, black women had an estimated 70 percent excess risk of cardiovascular disease mortality compared with white women. Adjustment for SES, by comparing cardiovascular mortality in blacks and low-social status whites, removed some of the excess risk in blacks (Table 7.7). Only after controlling for other risk factors, and especially *hypertension*, was the difference in cardiovascular mortality virtually eliminated. The explanation for higher prevalence of hypertension among U.S. blacks remains a key research issue. Sociocultural factors may operate through attitudes that influence diet (and hence, obesity) or more directly through stress and coping mechanisms.

The joint influence of SES and a psychological–behavioral profile known as "John Henryism" on hypertension in U.S. blacks and whites has been reported (James et al., 1987). The John Henryism scale, named after the legendary black "steel-driving man," attempts to assess active coping with psychosocial stressors. The association between SES and blood pressure was modified by this scale; that is, among persons with high levels of John Henryism, low-SES blacks were almost three times as likely to be hypertensive as higher-SES blacks. Hypotheses for this finding involve occupational, sociocultural, and psychological factors.

Studies on hypertension within low-SES blacks (James et al., 1987) implicate the importance of stresses associated with goal striving and lack of resources

Table 7.7 Evans County, Georgia, Prospective Study of Cardiovascular Disease (CVD) Mortality Among Black and White Women

Groups compared	Excess risk of CVD death in blacks vs. whites
All women (all social status groups)	70%
All black women	
vs. high-social-status whites	100%
vs. low-social-status whites	44%
vs. low-social-status whites and adjusting for risk factors	Little or no excess[a]

Source: Johnson et al. (1986).

[a]Data were presented only as graphs, without actual numbers.

for problem solving, but further research is needed. The effect of low levels of social support on hypertension were specific for low-income blacks in a rural Southern community (Strogatz and James, 1986). There is considerable interest in the role of family linkages and other support systems with regard to hypertension within low-SES blacks. Social support also needs to be studied with respect to coping behavior (i.e., John Henryism) among lower-SES blacks. The underlying mechanism may involve stress and its effects on sodium metabolism, as discussed next.

Diet

In U.S. blacks the importance of dietary habits in the first few years of life is becoming apparent. Higher total fat and cholesterol intakes in black versus white children during the first 4 years of life could influence dietary habits in later childhood and adolescence (Nicklas et al., 1987a) and thus contribute to the emergence of blood pressure differences.

Evidence is increasing for a role of dietary sodium (Na) and potassium (K) in influencing hypertension risk, even within a population. In Southern California, the dietary Na/K ratio was significantly correlated with age-adjusted systolic and diastolic pressure (Khaw et al., 1988). Therefore, population differences in dietary Na/K ratio may influence differences in hypertension prevalence. Although black–white differences in sodium intake have not been reported in the United States (Frisancho et al., 1984), lower potassium intake in blacks may be an important factor (Langford et al., 1985). The interpretation of black–white differences in blood pressure, however, is complicated by racial differences in *excretion* of both sodium and potassium (see next section).

Body Constitution

Morphologic, physiological, and biochemical differences between blacks and whites may be relevant to explanations for differences in cardiovascular diseases. As noted in Chapter 2, the categories of explanations for racial/ethnic differences in disease rates are difficult to separate. Underlying the racial differences in body constitution are complex interactions between environmental factors such as diet and attitudes, as well as possible genetic factors.

Hypertension. An understanding of the explanations for black–white differences in hypertension and cholesterol fractions (mainly HDL) would provide the key for understanding black–white differences in cardiovascular disease incidence and prognosis. In the Evans County study (Table 7.7) (Johnson et al., 1986), the excess mortality in black females was largely due to cerebrovascular disease, and hence it is understandable that adjustment for blood pressure level was responsible for removing the black–white difference in total cardiovascular mortality. The explanation for black–white differences in hypertension, especially among females, remains an important research issue.

The association between centrally deposited or abdominal body fat and blood pressure holds within both U.S. blacks and whites (Blair et al., 1984). The development of this type of fat distribution in adolescence is correlated with total body fat in both blacks and whites (Baumgartner et al., 1986). Thus black–white differences in obesity, especially among young adult females, may be important in explaining black–white differences in hypertension and cardiovascular mortality. Black–white difference in body mass index and obesity in adult females persist within education or income categories, suggesting that sociocultural factors influence these differences.

Overweight U.S. whites had a higher risk of hypertension than overweight blacks (Van Itallie, 1985), and subscapular skinfold, an estimator of upper-body fat, had a stronger association with diastolic blood pressure in whites than in blacks (Blair et al., 1984). Thus *hyperresponsiveness* of blood pressure to overweight in blacks is not involved in explaining hypertension differences (Van Itallie, 1985).

Appropriate stratified or multivariate analyses (see Chapter 1) to test the contribution of overweight or obesity in explaining black–white differences in hypertension, however, have not been done. In view of differences in dietary fat intake between black and white children, diet is an environmental factor that could contribute to black–white differences in total body fat and fat distribution. Sociocultural factors such as attitudes about body weight may be important underlying variables in explaining black–white differences in obesity, and this requires further study.

Factors other than differences overweight and body fat distribution may be involved in the increased risk of hypertension in U.S. blacks. Two factors to be considered are black–white differences in psychosocial stresses (see earlier), and sodium/potassium intake (diet) and/or metabolism (discussed later). These two factors may be interrelated, since stress may act through the autonomic nervous system to reduce sodium excretion and thereby increase the risk of hypertension.

Regarding black–white differences in hypertension, attention has turned to differences in sodium metabolism. In age-matched adult normotensives, blacks excreted significantly less sodium and potassium than whites after ingestion of a salt load (i.e., 2 liters of normal saline solution) (Luft et al., 1977). In Bogalusa, blacks excreted less sodium in the urine (Berenson et al., 1984). Since large dietary differences in sodium in black and white children were not observed, a physiological mechanism may be involved. Sodium concentration within red cells also is higher among U.S. blacks than whites (Trevisan et al., 1984).

Multivariable studies are needed on black and white populations by age group including such variables as dietary Na/K ratios, excretion of Na and K, and obesity and body fat distribution. Ideally, SES and sociocultural factors should be included along with estimates of degree of racial admixture (see below). Among 764 black and 224 white male truck drivers in San Francisco studied cross-sectionally, adjustment for sodium intake and body mass index (along with education and seven other variables) *increased* the black–white differences in hypertension prevalence (Winkleby et al., 1988). Thus, the question of sociocultural and/or genetic factors in black–white differences in hypertension must still be explored.

Ischemic heart disease. We have noted higher mortality rates for IHD among young adult blacks versus whites, especially females. Incidence rates in black females are also higher in some studies of urbanized populations. For males, the excess mortality at younger ages may be related to sudden death rather than to higher incidence of IHD, but this is uncertain. Complicating this picture is the possibility of misclassification of hypertension-related deaths to IHD among blacks (Kuller et al., 1986).

For IHD risk in both U.S. black and white populations depends on multiple risk factors in a "web" of causation, a term used by MacMahon and Pugh (1970). Some CHD risk factors are summarized in Table 7.8. With some exceptions the major risk factors for IHD are similar in black and white populations, as shown by the Evans County studies. Smoking has an independent effect on lipoprotein fractions, increasing the risk of IHD, but less strongly in black than in white young adults (Freedman et al., 1986). As we have noted, hypertension, a risk factor for IHD, appears to be influenced by overweight more strongly in whites than in blacks.

As noted in Chapter 1, racial/ethnic differences in disease may be due to differences in frequency or distribution of risk factors. Black–white differences in hypertension have already been discussed. In recent U.S. national surveys, total serum cholesterol did not differ between black and white adults (20–74 years old), with age-adjusted levels of 209–211 in black and white men and 214–215 in black and white women (Fulwood et al., 1986). The smaller increases in cholesterol with menopause observed in black versus white women, however, could reduce the relative risk of black versus white women at older ages (Baird et al., 1985).

Cholesterol fractions (i.e., LDL and HDL levels), important in interpreting differences in IHD risk, have been measured in these surveys and in several community-based studies. Higher HDL levels in U.S. blacks than in whites, especially in males, have been reported in some but not all studies. In Evans County, Georgia, and in the Cincinnati (Ohio) Princeton School Study of the Lipid Research Clinic, HDL cholesterol levels were higher in black than in white children and adults, especially among men; black–white differences in females were not statistically significant (Khoury et al., 1983; Glueck et al., 1984). In the

Table 7.8 Summary of Selected Risk Factors for Coronary (Ischemic) Heart Disease (CHD)

	CHD risk factors			
Host factor	Hypertension	Total serum cholesterol	HDL fraction	CHD Risk
Sex	F > M	F < M	F > M	F < M
Age	+	+	+	+
Blacks vs. whites (U.S.)	B > W	B = W	B > W[a]	B = W[b]
Body build (fat)	+	+	−	+
Exercise	−	−	+	−
Intake of saturated fats	+	+	−	+
Smoking	+	+	−	+

[a]Mostly in males, while in females differences are smaller.

[b]Incidence lower in black males for total IHD in some studies, while incidence equal in black and white females; mortality rates higher in black than white young adult females (see text). Differences in associations between risk factors and disease for specific manifestations of CHD are discussed in the text.

Key: +: Increase or positive association with risk or risk factor; −: negative association with risk or risk factor.

highly educated population of the Framingham (Massachusetts) study, which includes a Minority Study of 100 randomly selected black adults, however, mean levels of both total serum cholesterol and HDL were *lower* in black than white men and women (Wilson et al., 1983). Noteworthy is the finding that black–white differences in HDL in the Cincinnati study were maintained after adjustment for SES, but in women, black–white differences remained statistically insignificant (Glueck et al., 1984).

The negative association between HDL level and obesity, reported in whites, held for black men but not black women in an urban (Chicago) hospital screening clinic-based population (Ford et al., 1988). The negative association between education and HDL cholesterol in black women in this low-SES population of Chicago and in other studies of black men and women contrasts with the pattern in whites. Thus evidence is emerging that the control of HDL differs between blacks and whites (for unknown reasons).

Two other risk factors should be mentioned in connection with possible mechanisms providing relative protection against IHD in blacks versus whites. In Evans County, apolipoprotein A-I levels were higher, and Apo-CII levels lower in blacks than whites (especially males), even after adjusting for alcohol intake and other variables (Heiss et al., 1984). Additional studies are needed on other black populations, especially in urban and higher-SES areas. Another favorable risk factor in black males in Evans County is higher fibrinolytic activity in blood plasma. Plasma is added to a commercial fibrin plate containing a firbrin clot, and the size of the "reaction zone" or area of lysis (i.e., destruction) of the fibrin clot, due to fibrinolytic enzyme in the plasma, is measured. In black men, social class was negatively associated with plasma fibrinolytic activity, which was comparable only in physically active, low-SES whites and blacks (Dischinger et al., 1980; Szczeklik et al., 1980).

In summary, the higher prevalence of obesity and hypertension in black young adult females may counterbalance any protection from HDL (Curry et al., 1984) and other favorable risk profiles and have led to higher death rates for IHD in certain age groups. It is uncertain whether the apparent IHD differences in blacks and whites represent the effects of higher prevalence of hypertension-related deaths (Kuller et al., 1986), due to high prevalence of obesity and other mechanisms, and/or the independent effects of obesity and hypertension on IHD risk. Incidence studies, described earlier, suggest that for women, differences in IHD risk are involved. For men, the difference in IHD mortality (before age 65 years) may reflect mainly sudden deaths, but the underlying mechanism of black–white differences is unclear.

The interpretation of racial/ethnic differences in IHD risk factors has been complicated by studies of levels of specific fatty acids in the blood and body (i.e., fat) tissues. The fatty acid compositions of fat tissues and serum lipids partly reflect the composition of dietary fats but are affected by risk factors such as smoking and alcohol (Cambien et al., 1988). In a postmortem study of fatty acids in fat tissue in males 25–44 years of age in New Orleans, palmitoleic acid was significantly lower and stearic acid higher in blacks versus whites (Bhattacharyya et al., 1987). Palmitoleic acid is an unsaturated fatty acid; stearic acid is a saturated acid widely distributed in plants and animals. Although diet was not assessed in this study, the authors referred to surveys in New Orleans showing no black–white differences in intake of total fat or percentage of fat derived from animal and plant sources, and were tempted to conclude that racial differences in fatty acid metabolism might be involved. Since other studies suggest that serum level of stearic acid is negatively (and palmitoleic acid positively) associated with alcohol consumption (Cambien et al., 1988), higher alcohol consumption among blacks is not a likely explanation. Further studies are needed to explore the hypothesis of metabolic differences (Bhattacharyya et al., 1987), since the fatty acid pattern of blacks could increase risk of IHD.

Genetics

Hypertension. On the basis of historical evidence, Wilson (1986) suggested that American blacks may be highly sensitive to salt because of their derivation from populations in low-salt areas of West Africa. This hypothesis requires further examination through physiological studies on black populations and studies of racial admixture in the exploration of possible genetic factors in sodium sensitivity and hypertension risk.

Nigerian blacks heterozygous for hemoglobin S (i.e., with sickle cell trait) (Chapter 5) may handle sodium better than blacks with normal hemoglobin (HbAA) (Idahosa and Erhuunwunse, 1984). Idahosa (1986) concluded that genetic and non-sodium-related environmental factors are more important in hypertension than salt intake. Analyses of dietary Na/K ratios and excretion of Na and K in blacks and whites, however, indicate that further studies are needed to assess the independent effects of diet and genetics on physiological mechanisms relevant to blood pressure control changes with age.

Studies of degree of admixture in various black populations in relation to hypertension have been inconsistent. The earlier evidence was reviewed by Tyroler and James (1978), who noted that positive findings in one U.S. study could have been due to confounding of degree of African ancestry with environmental factors (MacLean et al., 1974). Skin color is associated with social status and hence with various stresses and sociocultural factors that might influence risk of hypertension.

Among the black Caribs of St. Vincent Island in the Caribbean, there was no statistically significant association between estimated degree of admixture (in four groups) and frequency of "hypertensive" versus "normotensive" status, although a slight increase in number of hypertensives was observed as African admixture increased (Hutchinson and Crawford, 1981). Mother–offspring correlations in diastolic pressure among black Caribs suggest an environmental effect (Hutchinson and Crawford, 1981) that also requires exploration. Another possibility, though remote, would involve maternal inheritance through mitochondrial DNA.

Future studies in U.S. and Caribbean blacks would have to consider socioeconomic status and sociocultural stresses along with skin color and genetic polymorphisms (for estimation of degree of racial admixture). The ideal studies would consider sociocultural factors including assessment of social stresses and social support, especially in view of apparent urban–rural differences in black–white blood pressure patterns by age. Among the black Caribs of St. Vincent, social variables have been shown to influence male systolic and diastolic, and female diastolic, pressures within blacks (Hutchinson, 1986), and similar studies are needed using blacks and whites in the same region.

Obesity, cholesterol, and HDL. Although the association between HDL and obesity in black females is weak, obesity is an important factor in cardiovascular disease mortality in young black females, and black–white differences in obesity may be important in explaining at least part of the differences in mortality from hypertension and IHD. Studies on the degree of racial admixture in relation to obesity and anatomical fat distribution in black females have been advocated (Kumanyika, 1987) to assess the role of genetic differences in explaining black–white differences in the prevalence of obesity.

Black–white differences in HDL level are most consistent for males, but differences are not consistent across the populations studied. A speculative hypothesis has been advanced regarding genetic factors. The hypothesis involves expression of a former adaptation to the African environment. Genetic factors are involved in the control of HDL and LDL cholesterol fractions. Since HDLs facilitate the immobilization of the spirochete vector for sleeping sickness, which is endemic in equatorial Africa (Chapter 5), natural selection may have favored high HDLs in Africans (Gartside et al., 1984). Such hypotheses are difficult to test directly, although the effect of HDLs on sleeping sickness could be explored in more detail in Africa. A black–white difference in frequency of a gene or genes influencing HDL level would not preclude environmental modulation of HDL and hence changes in black–white differences in HDL according to place and time. Regional variation in black–white differences in HDL level in the United States could reflect such environmental factors, but genetic differences between northern and southern U.S. blacks should be recalled (see Chapter 3).

Studies using RFLPs (see Chapter 3) to examine directly genetic (DNA) differences between racial/ethnic groups and both lipid profiles and IHD risk are a new area of research (Wallace and Anderson, 1987) that offers promise.

Other genetic factors. The Bogalusa Heart Study disclosed ABO associations with systolic pressure among white but not among black adolescents (Fox et al., 1986). These associations, however, have been inconsistent and, at best, weak.

HLA-DR4 has been associated with *giant cell arteritis* or temporal arteritis, an inflammation of arteries. The lower frequency of this disease in U.S. blacks may be related to lower frequency of the HLA-DR4 allele in blacks (Love et al., 1986) (see Chapter 3, Table 3.4). The inflammatory nature of this disease is noteworthy. HLA associations with diseases have involved mainly autoimmune or infectious diseases, along with certain cancers (as discussed later).

Conclusions

Black–white differences in mortality from hypertension-related diseases (including cerebrovascular diseases) and IHD appear to be due largely to differences in hypertension prevalence, especially in young adult females. For males, black–white differences in mortality from IHD in young adults may involve sudden death, and the role of hypertension is probable but uncertain.

The explanation for black–white differences in hypertension prevalence probably involves a complex interaction between environmental factors related to diet, attitudes about obesity, and stress. The existence of a genetic substrate in blacks is not established, but further studies are needed on the degree of admixture that also incorporate individual estimates of SES and indices of social support and coping mechanisms.

Whatever the explanations for black–white differences in hypertension risks, some reduction in black–white differentials in mortality from hypertension and hypertension-related diseases (especially cerebrovascular diseases) has occurred in recent decades. The persistence of black–white disparities in hypertension, cerebrovascular diseases, and IHD (especially in young women), however, argues for intensified primary and secondary prevention programs in black populations. Primary prevention programs should include obesity and smoking control, through educational programs, while secondary prevention should focus on compliance with antihypertensive medication as well as nonpharmacologic methods of hypertension control. These nonpharmacologic methods would involve the same risk factors as those targeted in primary prevention (i.e., diet and exercise).

Time changes in IHD (CHD) mortality among U.S. blacks suggest that beneficial effects of higher HDL levels in blacks (if indeed they existed) have been offset by changes in other risk factors such as obesity. A pattern of higher IHD risks in urban versus rural and/or higher- versus lower-SES blacks is emerging, paralleled by some contrasts in certain risk factors (e.g., total cholesterol, HDL cholesterol, fibrinolytic activity) in these groups. This pattern, however, may not hold for all risk factors, with hypertension showing some associations with stress only in lower-SES blacks. Most important is the conclusion that modification of dietary habits, with regard to fat intake, and exercise habits along with further improvements in drug control of hypertension could reduce CHD incidence and mortality among U.S. blacks (and presumably blacks in urban areas in Africa).

The MRFIT trial has shown that medical care can be effective in diagnosis and treatment, including compliance with drugs, in both blacks and whites, and that similar dietary and smoking changes can be achieved despite the lower educational background of blacks (Connett and Stamler, 1984).

Other U.S. Racial/Ethnic Groups

Japanese Migrants

In Honolulu Japanese, a battery of variables has been assessed as risk factors in multivariate analyses for specific manifestations of CHD in a prospective 10-year follow-up of 7,705 men. Physical inactivity, for example, was associated only with *total CHD* (all manifestations), while smoking was associated with all specific manifestations except uncomplicated angina pectoris (Yano et al., 1984).

Individual studies including two or more racial/ethnic groups living in different areas are rare (Chapter 1). A cohort study comparing the relative importance of specific risk factors in Japanese men in Japan and Hawaii indicated that the age-adjusted 12-year mortality rate was 41 percent higher in Hawaii, that is, the ratio of risk of IHD death, adjusted for age, in Hawaii/Japan was 1.41. More than half of this increase could be attributed to different levels of known risk factors in the two cohorts (Yano et al., 1988). That is, after adjusting for differences in known IHD risk factors, as well as age, the relative risk of fatal IHD (Hawaii/Japan) was 1.17; this ratio was not statistically significantly different from 1.00 (Table 7.9). Small sample sizes of deaths in Japan, which has low IHD mortality rates (as noted above), made analyses of specific risk factors difficult. Comparisons of the strength of association between specific risk factors and CHD mortality in Japan versus Hawaii showed some remarkable similarities (Table 7.9).

These important findings imply that the low rates of IHD death found in Japan could be approached by Japanese in Hawaii, and possibly by other racial/ethnic groups, if risk factor levels could be positively influenced.

Hispanics

Except for hypertensive emergencies, there is little evidence for higher rates of hypertension and IHD among various Hispanic groups in the United States. This holds for Mexican-Americans, despite high prevalences of certain risk factors versus Anglos, including obesity level and salt consumption. In the San Antonio Heart Study, higher triglyceride and lower HDL cholesterol levels in Mexican-Americans versus Anglos were most strongly associated with differences in fat patterning (i.e., central adiposity) (Haffner et al., 1986c). Within high-SES groups, however, obesity and body fat patterns may be more similar in certain Hispanic and white populations (Bogin and Sullivan, 1986; Farrell et al., 1987), again suggesting the importance of environmental factors. The complex interactions between genetic and environmental factors in determining anatomical fat distribution in different racial/ethnic groups require further study.

The number of studies among various Hispanic groups is increasing, including surveys of dietary habits and knowledge, attitudes, and behavior regarding health-related practices (Chapter 4). Also included are various attempts to assess acculturation through scales (Chapter 2). In the San Diego Family Health Pro-

Table 7.9 Strength of Risk Factors for Coronary Heart Disease in a Cohort Study of Japanese Men in Japan and Hawaii, 1965–80

Risk factor	Both groups combined		Separate analysis of each group	
	Relative risk (RR)	Probability RR differs from 1.00	Japan RR	Hawaii RR
Systolic blood pressure	1.96	.0001	2.27	1.88
Serum cholesterol	1.39	.001	1.64	1.20
Serum uric acid	1.20	.09	1.37	1.04
Serum glucose	2.25	.0001	2.53	1.58
Lifetime smoking	1.97	.001	2.20	2.26
Alcohol intake	0.54	.001	0.61	0.57
Hawaii vs. Japan	1.17	>.10		

Modified after Yano et al. (1988).

Multivariate analysis was used to assess the independent effect of each variable adjusting or controlling for age and all other risk factors (including some not listed in this table).

Relative risks are per decade of follow-up and are interquartile risks—i.e., differences in risk between groups based on a distribution subdivided into quartiles.

ject, knowledge of cardiovascular health-related diet (i.e., fat and salt intake) and exercise behaviors was strongly related to acculturation level in Mexican-Americans (Vega et al., 1987). These findings have implications for planning of health behavior interventions.

We have noted that family studies in different racial/ethnic groups may be useful in assessing possible differences in the strength of genetic components and also genetic heterogeneity in disease causation (Chapter 2). In a study in San Diego, familial aggregation of blood pressure was greater in 95 Anglo-American than in 111 Mexican-American families, but the explanation in terms of genetic factors versus shared family environment is unclear (Patterson et al., 1987).

Amerindians

Despite the higher prevalence of obesity and diabetes mellitus among Southwestern Amerindians, lower levels of smoking and serum cholesterol may help to account for lower hospitalization rates for IHD (Coulehan et al., 1986). Studies are needed on trends in hypertension, obesity, smoking, and blood lipid profiles in these populations. Recent apparent increases in hospitalization rates for IHD (i.e., AMI) among the Navajo may be related to increasing prevalence of hypertension and diabetes (Klain et al., 1988). Analytic epidemiologic studies are needed in these groups and in others (e.g., Senecas of New York).

Other Groups

Among U.S. gypsies, both genetic factors (i.e., familial hyperlipidemia), perhaps reflecting inbreeding (see Chapters 2 and 3), and environmental factors may contribute to the pattern of vascular diseases (Thomas et al., 1987), but more systematic studies are needed. Environmental factors may include cultural attitudes toward obesity.

Since obesity, blood pressure, and HDL level were not lower in Californian Seventh Day Adventists, other explanations for low IHD such as social support mechanisms are under study (Fraser et al., 1987). Other dietary factors to be studied include dietary fiber, which has been associated with reduced IHD mortality in a 12-year prospective study in southern California (Khaw et al., 1987).

In Mormons, the relatively low prevalence of cigarette smoking may account for much of the difference in mortality rates for IHD (Lyon et al., 1978). In the Behavioral Risk Factor Surveys of 1981–83 and 1985, involving 28 states and the District of Columbia, Utah had the lowest proportion of current smokers (i.e., 17.9 percent vs. the median of 28.5 percent) among adults (18 years of age and older) (Brooks et al., 1986). Direct studies of cardiovascular disease rates in Mormons and non-Mormons, using data on smoking and other risk factors, appear to be lacking.

International Differences

Errors of Measurement and SES

While some of the differences in relative mortality rates for major categories of cardiovascular diseases may be real, it should be noted that comparability of death rates for such categories as IHD is open to question because of differences in practices and available technology regarding diagnosis of disease, differences in coding of causes of death, different proportions of deaths due to ill-defined causes, and problems with accuracy of denominator data (e.g., age distributions for older age categories). Special projects such as the WHO MONICA Project, and especially the methodologically more carefully controlled Seven Countries Study, however, have confirmed many of the differences discussed earlier.

Errors of measurement hold for comparisons among developed, as well as developing, countries. An example of the complexity of the goal of obtaining comparable data on diagnosis of IHD is a comparison of old and new epidemiologic criteria for "definite" myocardial infarction (MI) used by the World Health Organization, showing that studies using different criteria are difficult to compare (Beaglehole et al., 1987). Combining "definite" and "possible" MI would improve comparability. All studies involved in the MONICA Project (discussed earlier) will use the new criteria, but these criteria involve qualitative evaluations as well as more objective data such as quantitative ECG coding and abnormal serum enzymes. Thus, there is room for inaccuracies and lack of comparability of data across populations.

Socioeconomic status (SES) is an important variable to be considered in comparisons of cardiovascular disease rates across populations and racial/ethnic groups. SES differences may be associated with such risk factors as smoking and diet, and few studies attempt to evaluate the independent effects of these variables.

While most studies in industrialized or Westernized countries worldwide have been consistent in showing negative associations between SES (as measured by education or occupation) and either blood pressure level or "hypertension," results of studies in developing countries have been conflicting. In a community near Kingston, Jamaica, multivariate analysis of data from surveys indicated increasing blood pressure with increasing social class (measured by occupation) in males but an opposite association in females (Dressler et al., 1988).

In industrialized societies IHD incidence and mortality also tend to be higher in lower-SES groups, due in part to associated known risk factors such as hypertension, obesity, and smoking. The British Regional Heart Study, in a region with relatively high IHD mortality, multivariate analyses showed that adjustment for known risk factors (i.e., smoking, blood pressure, serum cholesterol, body mass index, self-assessed physical activity at work) still left a residual effect of SES on IHD risk. IHD was defined as fatal IHD or nonfatal IHD based on defined criteria (Pocock et al., 1987). Although British men in nonmanual labor classes had 24 percent lower IHD mortality than the manual labor classes, the former still had higher rates than most European countries and five times higher rates than Japanese men (Pocock et al., 1987).

Mediterranean countries with low IHD rates are also relatively low in SES, but dietary practices and lower smoking rates may have been protective. Increases in IHD mortality rates in middle-aged men in Italy in 1968–78 may have been related to increased smoking rates as reflected in lung cancer rates (LaVecchia and DeCarli, 1986). A limitation of the Seven Countries prospective study is that risk factors were measured at the beginning of the project, and changes occurred during follow-up. The Italian groups in this project, on the basis of later surveys, underwent an increase in dietary animal fat consumption between 1960 and 1980. In contrast, declines in IHD mortality in New Zealand between 1968 and 1980 were due at least in part to changes in smoking and dietary fat or cholesterol consumption (Jackson and Beaglehole, 1987).

Analyses of the Seven Countries Study data (Keys et al., 1986) have by-passed SES and dealt directly with risk factors largely responsible for the effect of SES on IHD risk. The independent associations between dietary constituents and IHD risk in that study may reflect "different kinds of agriculture imposed by climatic differences" (Keys et al., 1986) and/or sociocultural factors. The apparent retention of dietary habits of migrants from the Mediterranean, including Greeks and Italians in Australia, suggests that whatever the basic explanation for these habits, sociocultural factors influence their continuation.

Sociocultural Factors

Smoking and alcohol. As noted above, both SES and smoking are seldom considered in comparisons of cardiovascular disease rates across countries or racial/ethnic groups. Thus variation in smoking rates across populations may simply reflect underlying SES differences. In Britain cigarette smoking accounted for a large proportion of social class differences in IHD (Pocock et al., 1987).

Excessive, versus moderate, alcohol consumption is related to increased risk of cardiovascular diseases and may in part explain, for example, the higher blood pressures in Australian than U.S. males (MacMahon and Leeder, 1984). In contrast moderate alcohol consumption has been associated with lower risk of CHD, probably through the mechanism of increased levels of HDL cholesterol, which is protective (see earlier). Thus, further studies are needed on moderate alcohol consumption in relation to population differences in CHD risk.

Studies of different ethnic groups within the same country can provide rewarding information on the effects of risk factors on chronic diseases including cardiovascular diseases. In Jerusalem, differences in major cardiovascular disease risk factors including cigarette smoking and alcohol consumption were shown among four country-of-origin groups, while the same inverse relationship between smoking and HDL cholesterol was shown for all groups (Halfon et al., 1984). Lower HDL cholesterol is associated with increased CHD risk, as noted earlier.

Studies of the racial/ethnic groups of similar origin but now located in diverse areas may also be enlightening. Coronary heart disease incidence has been reported as high among Indian populations in various countries, including Trinidad (Beckles et al., 1986) and South Africa (Wyndham, 1982; Sewardsen and Jialal, 1986) as well as in India. In East London a high proportion of smokers was noted among Bangladeshi males (Silman et al., 1985). An increase in blood pressure in Indian migrants to England is not involved, although increased duration of stay may be associated with increases in body weight and blood pressure (Silman et al., 1987). Interest has focused on diet and diabetes mellitus in Indian groups (see later).

Acculturation. Studies in the Solomon Islands (Melanesia) and in Polynesia suggest the importance of degree of acculturation in blood pressure levels and the association between age and blood pressure (Table 7.10) (Page et al., 1974; Harburg et al., 1982). Maupiti is in the Society Islands of French Polynesia (near Tahiti, Fig. 3.2) and has undergone rapid cultural and economic change since the 1970s, but the population is still less Westernized and urbanized than Samoans, Rarotongans or the Maori. In Pukapuka, an isolated island (Fig. 3.2) with a more traditional culture, there was no association between age and blood pressure. In the Solomon Islands (in Melanesia, Fig. 3.2) data from the 1966–72 survey of blood pressure in various groups also showed that the less acculturated groups tended to exhibit little or no increase in blood pressure with age and had a lower proportion of males with higher pressures (Table 7.10). In the 1978–80 resurvey of the same persons, the least acculturated groups, including the Aita and the Kwaio (Table 7.5), showed little increase in average pressures (especially diastolic pressure) with age. The Nagovisi are becoming more acculturated, especially in diet, and increases in blood pressure were noted longitudinally between 1966–72 and 1978–80. The pattern of change in blood pressure over time with acculturation was complex, however, and may be influenced by genetic heterogeneity or clustering of genetic factors influencing blood pressure in certain groups, but direct evidence for this hypothesis is lacking (Friedlaender et al., 1987). An apparent exception to the pattern of higher pressures in more acculturated groups was noted by King et al. (1985) in Papua New Guinea, and the explanation is unknown; genetic heterogeneity among the small groups of this region has been observed, but its role in blood pressure differences is unknown.

The role of acculturation in other populations also may be complex, as witnessed by Samoans residing in Samoa and Hawaii. In Hawaii, Samoans in urban areas had significantly lower blood pressures than those in rural areas,

Table 7.10 Relationship Between Degree of Acculturation and Blood Pressure in Various Studies

| | Solomon Islands Groups | | | | | |
	Nasioi	Nagovisi	Lau	Baegu	Aita	Kwaio
Degree of acculturation	+++	+++	++	+	+	0
Correlation: Age by systolic blood pressure (females)	0.36	0.30	0.36	NS	NS	NS
Percent males with pressure 140/90 or higher	3.4	2.7	7.8	0.8	0	0.8

| | Polynesian Groups (males) | | | | |
	Rarotonga	Samoa	Maori	Maupiti	Puka-Puka
Degree of acculturation (approx.)	Highest	— Intermed. —		Lower	Lowest
Association between age and blood pressure	Strong	— Intermed. —		Lower	None

Redrawn from data in Page et al. (1974) and Harburg et al. (1982). Approximate relative degree of acculturation is rated from 0 (lowest) to +++ (highest) on the basis of eight criteria including diet (Western versus traditional), economy (cash versus other), education, and medical care.

Solomon Islanders are Melanesians (see Chapter 3).

See references in Harburg et al. (1982) and Baker et al. (1986) for details on studies in Polynesians. The Solomon Islands data have been updated by Freidlaender et al. (1987), and the Kwaio remain the least acculturated or most traditional group.

suggesting either selective migration (on the basis of blood pressure) or sociocultural differences (Hanna and Baker, 1979). Other studies suggest that "biocultural adaptation" to modern environments in Hawaii may occur gradually and thus explain the higher blood pressures in migrants from more versus less traditional areas of Samoa (McGarvey and Baker, 1979; Baker et al., 1986) but the evidence is inconclusive. Further studies are needed on the mechanisms of selective migration—for example, the characteristics of migrants by age and year of migration.

In both Samoan and Tokelau migrants, along with other groups, increases in body fat with acculturation may account for part of the change in blood pressure (see later). Among Korean migrants to Japan, a role for the stresses of migration (i.e., social change and acculturation) and occupation has been suggested regarding high cardiovascular disease mortality (Ubukata et al., 1986). Further studies are needed to delineate these factors. High salt intake (see later) and poor medical control of hypertension also may be involved. Thus a model of acculturation processes, involving stresses and salt intake, should be tested among Koreans.

Among Italian migrants to Australia the maintenance of low IHD rates even after long-term residence could reflect the continuation of dietary habits by Italians (e.g., higher intake of vegetable-origin fat and protein, and lower salt intake) (Armstrong et al., 1983). Because there appeared to be some convergence of rates, however, these findings may indicate slow acculturation processes.

The potential importance of both diet (i.e., carbohydrate, salt, and alcohol) and psychosocial factors or stresses in hypertension and hypertension-related diseases is supported by results of studies on Filipinos in California (Stavig et al., 1984) and Pacific Island (Tokelau) migrants to New Zealand (Salmond et al., 1985).

Henry (1988) has marshaled evidence for a primary role of stress with acculturation as the basis for both increased salt intake and increased blood pressure, with psychosocial stress as the most important factor in hypertension. The specific argument that stress leads to increased intake of sodium is debatable. Supportive evidence for the role of stress in affecting physiological factors relevant to hypertension, however, comes from recent data on Samoan men in Western Samoa. Rates of urinary catecholamine excretion were higher in Westernized "cash economy" groups than in traditional groups. Life-style characteristics including life satisfaction and agreement with Samoan customs were also related to variation in catecholamine excretion (James et al., 1987). Catecholamines, or adrenaline (epinephrine) and noradrenaline (norepinephrine), are adrenal medullary humoral factors that act as vasoconstricting agents, and thus are involved in the pathogenesis of hypertension.

There is increasing interest in population differences in patterns of catecholamine excretion in relation to acculturation and urbanization. In the traditional agricultural-based Polynesian population of Tokelau Islanders, mean 24-hour catecholamine excretion was lower than that in urban groups in Westernized countries (Jenner et al., 1987). This humoral hypothesis of stress effects offers promise for a unified theory of hypertension that explains epidemiologic features both within and between populations. Consideration of the role of stress in disease is not new and recalls the early work of Walter B. Cannon on the sympathetic nervous system in the "fight or flight" response which prepares the body for immediate activity but may have long-term adverse health consequences.

It is likely that acculturation operates through several mechanisms to increase current blood pressure, patterns of blood pressure change with age, and risk of related diseases such as IHD. Urbanization may involve acculturation, as when traditional groups migrate to urban areas, or internal changes when residents of areas undergo urbanization with crowding and increased sociocultural contacts. The latter process may be similar in some ways to that described for acculturation, although interactions of distinct cultural groups may not be involved. Increased sodium intake probably has a role independent of its secondary association with stress.

Diet and Cholesterol

In explaining racial/ethnic differences in prevalence or incidence rates for cardiovascular diseases, interest has focused on protein and fat consumption, along with salt intake. Studies of specific racial/ethnic groups continue to provide data relevant to our understanding of the roles of these factors.

International comparisons of dietary risk factors and IHD mortality rates have implicated total dietary fat and type of fat (Keys et al., 1986; Lewis et al., 1986). Table 7.6 shows death rates for IHD and mean (average) levels of dietary constituents from analyses of food consumed by statistically selected subsamples of each cohort in the Seven Countries Study. Multivariate analyses of these data (Keys et al., 1986), using simple regression and multiple linear regression (Chapter 1), have suggested that 96 percent of the variation in death rates from IHD *across* populations may be explained by a combination of risk factors including the ratio of monounsaturated to saturated fats, age, blood pressure, and smoking. The multiple linear regression analyses involved mean values for each risk factor in each of the 15 cohorts or separate groups in the seven countries. Dietary variation alone, in terms of the ratio of monounsaturated to saturated fatty acids, accounted for 44 percent of the variation in IHD death rates across the cohorts.

It should be emphasized that these results refer to *interpopulation* variation in death rates explained by interpopulation variation in average levels of risk factors. They cannot be extrapolated to *within-population* variation. Indeed, the value of such international studies lies in exploiting the wider range of variability in diet to extract conclusions regarding the extent to which other countries might reduce their cardiovascular mortality rates if drastic changes in diet were implemented (Chapter 1).

Keys et al. (1986) observed that dietary changes had taken place in some of the countries since the initiation of the prospective study. Changes such as increased fat consumption and changes in type of fat consumed in Japan could have reduced the differences in cardiovascular mortality. Although the dietary intake of 15-year-old students in Osaka, Japan, was somewhat Westernized in comparison with adults, these students still had a considerably lower intake of fat and a higher polyunsaturated/saturated fatty acid ratio than U.S. students (Ueshima et al., 1982). This also holds for mainland China, where average fat intake (as percent of total calories) is about 38 percent of that in the U.S. (Roberts,

1988). This suggests that worldwide differences in cardiovascular (i.e., IHD) mortality will persist for some time.

Dietary fat as a risk factor for IHD presumably operates mainly through influences on total serum cholesterol and lipoprotein fractions. Experimental studies, including controlled clinical trials, are often done in areas where disease rates are high (Chapter 2). One example is the Oslo (Norway) Study's hypertension trial, in an area with above-average death rates for IHD (Table 4.5). One study in this trial is noteworthy in that it used information on follow-up of *untreated* males, who are often difficult to find in Westernized countries, to draw conclusions about the modification of blood pressure (a major risk factor for IHD, as noted earlier). Among middle-aged men with mild hypertension (mainly 150–179 systolic and 110 or less diastolic pressures) followed for 5 years, rate of change in serum triglycerides, serum cholesterol, and body weight predicted changes in blood pressure (Holme et al., 1988). The main conclusion is that programs to control blood pressure in mild hypertensives should include interventions against serum triglycerides, such as dietary changes. The North Karelia (Finland) studies, also involving an area with high IHD mortality rates (Tables 4.5 and 7.4), have shown that changes in dietary fat composition can decrease serum lipids and blood pressure (Ehnholm et al., 1982; Puska et al., 1983).

More work needs to be done, however, to clarify the role of saturated and total fat intake versus other risk factors such as exercise. Although Keys et al. (1986) found no evidence for an independent effect of habitual physical activity of occupation in explaining population (i.e., cohort) differences in IHD mortality, exercise may operate through these known risk factors as well as independently of them. Prolonged exercise, as among endurance athletes, increases the HDL level, possibly through enhanced fat clearance (Sady et al., 1986). Thus, population differences in exercise and training levels must be considered as underlying factors, in addition to fat intake, in explaining international and racial/ethnic differences in CHD rates.

Very low LDL levels in certain African groups may reflect low intake of saturated fats. In contrast, high intake of saturated fats may contribute to high rates of cardiovascular disease in the Finnish population (Lewis et al., 1986). In various countries migrants from India have high rates of IHD and diabetes mellitus. High intake of total fats, although derived mostly from vegetable oil and hence polyunsaturated, along with cigarette smoking may help to explain the high risk of CHD among Indian migrants (Silman et al., 1985). The total amount of dietary fat, as well as its composition, may be important in IHD risk.

In Jerusalem, Israel, the lower incidence of myocardial infarction in orthodox religious adults may be related to independent effects of cholesterol and LDL level, presumably related to dietary practices, as evident in studies of young adults ranked by degree of religiosity (Friedlander et al., 1987). Offspring of Israeli Jewish fathers of Yemenite origin, who are known to have a low incidence of CHD, have low levels of total plasma cholesterol and show no age-related changes in lipid levels (Zahavi et al., 1987). These studies implicate cholesterol, presumably due in part to dietary habits, in explaining ethnic and religious group differences in CHD risk factors and CHD risk. In a survey of 8,829 men in Israel mean serum cholesterol and mean intake of saturated fatty acid were lowest in those born in Africa and Asia and highest in those born in Africa and Asia and highest in those born in Central and Eastern Europe (Keys, 1988).

The reader should recall the diet "laced with fish oil" of the person least likely to develop IHD, in the thumbnail sketch quoted earlier. Our man in the thumbnail sketch should take heart from the results of recent studies on fish oil. Major attention has been given recently to Eskimo populations, with high protein–fat and low carbohydrate–fiber diets, in relation to ischemic heart disease. The role of fatty fish in lowering plasma triglycerides and raising HDL cholesterol may also hold also for Japanese and West African fish eaters (Robinson and Day, 1986). In the Netherlands a 20-year prospective study of middle-aged men found a more than 50 percent reduction in IHD mortality among those consuming at least 30 g of fish per day (Kromhout et al., 1985), and experimental studies show favorable changes in lipid profiles with fish oils in patients with hypertriglyceridemia (Phillipson et al., 1985). Clinical trials are needed, however, to assess the relative effectiveness of fish oils versus aspirin in prophylaxis of patients with vascular disease, and to verify their role in primary prevention of coronary thrombosis (Anon., 1988c). Those contemplating adoption of the dietary practices listed in the thumbnail sketch will have to decide for themselves.

Sodium. Hypertension, as well as cholesterol, has an independent effect on risk of death from CHD, as shown in the U.S. MRFIT (Multiple Risk Factor Intervention Trial) study (Martin et al., 1986). Interpopulation differences in salt intake appear to be involved in explaining certain racial/ethnic differences in hypertension, as shown in the Solomon Islands (Page et al., 1984) where blood pressures remain low in some ethnic groups which also have low dietary sodium and low urinary excretion of sodium (Friedlaender et al., 1987).

Most studies have failed to show significant associations between salt intake and blood pressure *within* a single population. Daily variation in sodium intake within individuals is an important complicating factor in assessing such associations. Also, within many countries regional variations in diet may not be great. Within Japan, however, regional variations in salt (sodium) intake were significantly associated with regional *mortality* rates for cerebrovascular disease (Ikeda et al., 1986). While the population was "ethnically fairly homogeneous," regional variations in salt intake and in cerebrovascular disease mortality rates were rather wide.

Cerebrovascular mortality rates could be influenced by many factors, including control of hypertension. In the Japanese study (Ikeda et al., 1986), however, examinees with no history of antihypertensive treatment were classified into several "hypertensive" groups. In one group, defined as systolic pressure of 160+ *and* diastolic pressure of 95+, K intake was significantly lower (in men) and the Na/K ratio was significantly higher (in men and women) than in matched controls (Ikeda et al., 1986). It would be interesting to study the factors determining regional variation in dietary Na and K intake, including both availability and local ethnic or sociocultural influences. Regional variation in consumption of miso soup and miso paste, major sources of sodium in traditional Japanese dishes, was mentioned as one contributing factor (Ikeda et al., 1986).

In Japan the average sodium intake in males was 256–272 (depending on age) mmole/day, with regional variations of 215–325 mmole/day or 5–7.5 g. Among southern California men, sodium consumption was 132–171 mmole depending on age (30–79 years), or only 3–4 g. Both studies (Khaw and Barrett-Connor, 1988; Ikeda et al., 1986) considered only sodium from food, with no information on table salt, nor was such information included in NHANES I reports. In Western countries such as Finland, Great Britain, and the United States, however, salt in foods (added during processing) is an important component of total sodium intake (James et al., 1987). Declines in salt intake in Japan in recent decades and possibly in Great Britain have implications for cardiovascular diseases as well as certain cancers (Chapter 8).

Important studies have emerged from China, where random samples of men and women 40–49 years of age from different regions have been studied for urinary excretion of sodium and potassium, as well as blood pressure and height and weight. Significant correlations were found between urinary sodium and mean blood pressure in a substudy of 12 male and 10 females population groups selected as having the "same nationality" and living at similar altitudes (Liu and Lai, 1986). Dietary intake of Na and K was not measured, so the excretion may represent both dietary and physiologic variation. Urinary potassium levels in these regions of China were not correlated with blood pressure, but Na/K ratios were not analyzed statistically.

Salt intake has also been implicated in the differing trends in stroke mortality between Eastern and Western European countries (Tuomilehto et al., 1987), but no data on salt consumption were used; rather, inferences were based on stomach cancer data.

Body Constitution

Populations, including racial/ethnic groups, vary in the amount of body fat and its anatomical distribution as measured by various techniques. These features are subject to change over time, however, especially with acculturation and urbanization. In Papua New Guinean groups undergoing acculturation, apparent changes in body fat over a 15-year period, with evidence for more "central" deposition, may reflect increased acculturation in two groups studied (one on the north coast and the other in the highlands), although acculturation was not directly measured (Norgan, 1987). Thus there is interest in the role of such changes in explaining part of the increases in blood pressure and cardiovascular diseases that accompany acculturation and urbanization in many groups.

The amount and anatomical distribution of body fat have been recognized increasingly as an important risk factor for cardiovascular diseases including IHD, through its association with hypertension and as an independent predictor in most populations. Increases in body fat appear to explain at least part of the increases in blood pressure and hypertension with migration (and acculturation) in such groups as the Tokelau Island migrants to New Zealand (Joseph et al., 1983), Samoans undergoing acculturation (Baker et al., 1986; McGarvey and Schendel, 1986), and Asian migrants in London (Silman et al., 1987).

In describing the independent contribution of "central" obesity (defined by subscapular vs. triceps skinfold) to prediction of IHD in the Honolulu Heart

Program, Donahue et al. (1987) noted that this association might vary across populations. In a 6-year prospective study of American Samoans, a Polynesian population noted for high prevalence of obesity, obesity (defined by body mass index and skinfold measurements) was not associated with total cardiovascular mortality (Crews, 1988). Despite their high levels of obesity, with 46 percent of men and 66 percent of women having a body mass index of 30 kg/m², hypertension prevalence is comparable to that in the United States, and cardiovascular mortality rates are lower than in the United States. One hypothesis requiring exploration concerns the relative amounts of internal versus external deposition of body fat, the latter being measured by skinfolds and the former by computerized tomography, in Samoans versus other groups. Variations in body fat distribution across populations, and changes over time within a population, may reflect dietary patterns as well as interactions with underlying genetic factors.

Genetics

Blood group variation among populations has long been of interest in relation to disease distribution. Among the cardiovascular diseases, ischemic heart disease has been positively associated with group A and negatively associated with group O in some studies (Morton, 1976), and A has also been weakly associated with blood pressure in some studies (Kark and Friedlander, 1984). The effect of these weak associations on population differences in cardiovascular diseases is probably negligible.

The issue of genetic factors in sodium sensitivity appears to be unresolved. Each population may contain a proportion of persons who are genetically salt-sensitive, as in the United States (Jacobson and Liebman, 1980) and Japan (Fujishima et al., 1983). Theoretically, this proportion may vary across populations, owing in part to previous adaptations to the amount of available salt. Sodium *metabolism*, as opposed to sodium intake, is a major issue with regard to certain populations (e.g., blacks and Japanese) in relation to hypertension and cerebrovascular diseases.

Genetic factors are involved in the control of total cholesterol, LDL and HDL fractions, and apolipoproteins. The latter may be most important in predicting IHD, especially in middle-aged men. As discussed above with reference to U.S. blacks and whites, there is considerable interest in racial/ethnic variation in lipoprotein fractions and the role of genetic differences in the explanation of such variation.

After discovery of genetically determined defects in LDL receptors, with no apparent difference in their frequency between U.S. blacks and U.S. whites, interest has turned to the role of genetic factors in determination of LDL and HDL levels. Extensive family studies in the multiethnic Jerusalem Lipid Research Clinic Study have suggested homogeneity in the model of modes of transmission of LDL and HDL levels in serum, which involves a "mixed mode" or combination of both major (recessive) genes and multifactorial inheritance; one exception may have been LDL inheritance in North African groups (Friedlander and Kark, 1987).

Apolipoprotein variation or polymorphism in various populations and racial/ethnic groups represents a new research frontier. Apo-B, the principal component of LDL, has emerged as the strongest risk factor for IHD in some populations, and there is great interest in the role of genetic variation at the apo-B locus as an independent risk factor (Hegele et al., 1986; Durrington et al., 1988). RFLPs have been used in studies of both apo-A and apo-B variants. Some RFLP associations at specific loci have been reported in some but not all populations, and an extensive review of these studies is beyond the scope of this text (see Wallace and Anderson, 1987; Cooper and Clayton, 1988).

One important point concerns direct versus indirect associations between these specific polymorphisms and IHD risk, the latter involving other risk factors such as lipid profiles. RFLPs may simply be markers for alleles genetically linked to varying degrees with gene variants that increase risk of hyperlipidemia or other aspects of unfavorable lipis profiles. In a case-control study of angiographically defined IHD in the population (mostly Mormons) of Utah, genotypes at three apolipoprotein regions (i.e., apo-A, AI, and B) were not directly associated with IHD risk but may have indirect effects through lipid profiles (Ward et al., 1987).

Apolipoproteins are also related to the physiology of clot formation and dissolution, via plasminogen (the precursor of clot-dissolving plasmin); plaminogen is activated by tissue plasminogen activator (TPA). Several prospective studies have shown an independent association between increased plasma fibrinogen concentration and risk of IHD; part of the effect of smoking on IHD risk may be mediated through plasma fibrinogen, which promotes thrombus or blood clot formation through several mechanisms (Meade et al., 1986). Fibrinogen concentration in plasma is under genetic control (Humphries et al., 1987), but genes controlling both fibrinogen formation and fibrinolysis (i.e., dissolution of clots) must be studied in order to understand the genetic control of thrombus formation (and hence risk of IHD). We have discussed fibrinolysis in plasma, due to fibrinolytic activity, among blacks and whites.

RFLPs have also begun to be used in exploring genetic variation in the locus controlling plasma fibrinogen concentration, through polymorphisms in genes that are probably linked to the fibrinogen genes (Humphries et al., 1987). Thus the mechanism for the RFLP associations may be similar to that proposed for apolipoproteins. Further studies of these RFLPs are needed in diverse populations.

CONCLUSIONS

The background of cardiovascular disease epidemiology is that of complex, heterogeneous categories with different risk factors operating in a web of causation. Multiple factors are undoubtedly involved in the causation of hypertension in a given population and in explaining differences across racial/ethnic groups. Studies of hypertension in high-risk groups including Samoan migrants and Bahamians suggest that diet, social stress, physical inactivity, and changes in obesity are important factors. The independent contributions of some of these factors in explaining high risks of hypertension and IHD in certain populations require clarification, in order that effective prevention programs can be developed—for example, aimed at social stress reduction through support groups, as well as education programs involving exercise and weight reduction.

Evidence for independent effects of diet, including intake of fats (especially saturated) in IHD risk and salt/potassium ratios in hypertension (and cerebrovascular diseases), in various populations is considerable. This suggests that modification of dietary habits could have a major influence on risk of IHD and hypertension and stroke. Regional and presumably culturally related variations in dietary habits involving salt consumption have been shown in such areas as Japan and China and may determine regional variation in prevalence of hypertension and cerebrovascular diseases.

The importance of dietary differences in explaining geographic and racial/ethnic differences in IHD morbidity and morality has been established, largely through the work of the Seven Countries Study, which has taken into account the wide variation in diet across countries and cultures. Experimental studies in high-IHD-risk areas such as North Karelia, Finland, have also indicated the importance of diet and dietary modification in IHD risk.

Fraser (1986) observed that international differences in IHD are major evidence for the influence of environmental factors on IHD risk but that such evidence does not preclude an additional component reflecting genetic factors. On the genetic front, increasing evidence from recent studies implicates apoplipoprotein variation, with strong genetic contribution, and fibrinogen–fibrinolysis factors which may also have a genetic component. Undoubtedly there will be an increase in studies comparing population frequencies in these characteristics.

8

Cancers

Although the estimated proportions of all deaths due to diseases of the circulatory system and neoplasms are highest in the developed world, these categories may also account for more than 50 percent of all deaths in developing countries (Hakulinen et al., 1986). Cancers have long been regarded as major diseases of developed countries, where they usually rank second in causes of death, but their importance in developing countries is being increasingly recognized. The World Health Organization has estimated that more than half of the world's approximately 6 million new cancer cases arise in the developing world (Anon., 1984a,b). Recognition of the problem of cancer in the developing world is also witnessed by the appearance of several monographs (e.g., Aoki, 1982; Howe, 1986; Parkin, 1986).

Because of the existence of many population-based cancer registries throughout the world, data on geographic and racial/ethnic differences are more numerous for cancers than for other chronic diseases. Information on disease rates in racial/ethnic groups within a single country and on various migrant groups is also more abundant for cancers. Finally, there is an increasing number of analytical epidemiologic studies (especially case-control studies) in various racial/ethnic groups, thus allowing comparison of risk factors among these groups.

DESCRIPTION OF RACIAL/ETHNIC DIFFERENCES

United States

Blacks and Whites

Systematic comparisons of cancer incidence and survival among major ethnic groups in the United States are a rather recent phenomenon. Burbank and Fraumeni (1972) documented a trend toward higher age-adjusted mortality rates for all cancers combined among U.S. nonwhites (who were mostly blacks) than for whites. In 1976 Mason et al. published an atlas of cancer mortality among "nonwhites," about 92 percent of whom were blacks, but the inclusion of other groups such as Amerindians resulted in high rates for "nonwhites" in some regions (e.g., thyroid cancers in the Southwest). An updated atlas on cancer mortality in nonwhites is in preparation, to accompany the recently published atlas for whites (Pickle et al., 1987).

Total cancer *death* rates in 1985 were higher in blacks than in whites in all age groups except the oldest (i.e., 85+ years), and this same pattern holds for the heterogeneous category of cancers of the digestive system (Table 4.1). Lung cancer mortality rates are also higher in blacks, up to age 75 years. Black–white differences in mortality rates for female breast cancer vary by age group (Table 4.1), reflecting differences in incidence rates by age (discussed later). Cervical cancer death rates (not shown) are about three times higher in black than in white females. Mortality rates are influenced by *survival* rates as well as by *incidence* rates, and survival rates are poorer for certain cancer sites among blacks (see later). Examination of incidence rates is more informative with regard to the formulation of hypotheses for explanations of racial/ethnic differences in cancer development.

Increases in both incidence and mortality rates have occurred in recent decades for certain cancer sites among blacks—for example, prostate, esophagus, and colon–rectum. The sharp increase in incidence rates for colorectal cancers from about 1937–39 to 1969–71 in blacks, at many times the rate of increase for whites, especially at ages under 60 years, suggests a cohort effect possibly related to dietary changes (Ziegler et al., 1986). This change is particularly noteworthy in view of the time changes in heart disease among U.S. blacks (Chapter 7) because of the possibility of a common underlying dietary explanation.

Using data from the U.S. Third National Cancer (Incidence) Survey of 1969–71, Goldson et al. (1981) tabulated cancer sites that show higher, lower, or similar age-adjusted incidence rates in blacks versus whites. Cancers of the esophagus, cervix uteri, prostate, and stomach; multiple myeloma; and a few other cancers were at least 50 percent more frequent in blacks. Similar findings (Tables 8.1 and 8.2) have been reported on incidence rates for more recent years from the population-based cancer registries in the U.S. Surveillance Epidemiology and End Results (SEER) Program, which covers about 13 percent of the population but is more weighted by nonwhite groups (see Chapter 4). Higher incidence rates for cancers of the lung and bronchus among blacks versus whites and other groups are noteworthy. American blacks, including those in Newark, New Jersey, have higher age-adjusted incidence rates than African blacks (see below) for most cancers, except the uterine cervix and a few other sites (Thind et al., 1982).

The contrast incidence rates for certain cancer sites are lower for U.S. blacks than whites. Examples are malignant melanoma of the skin; cancers of the testis, breast (see later), corpus uteri, bladder, and brain; Ewing's sarcoma; neuroblastoma; and acute lymphocytic leukemia (ALL). Average age-adjusted incidence rates of testicular cancer in 1973–81 were lower in blacks than in all other racial/ethnic groups, and four to five times lower than in whites except during childhood (Brown et al., 1986). Lower incidence rates for ALL in U.S. blacks also have been reported in a childhood cancer registry in the Philadelphia area (Kramer et al., 1983), although rates are even lower in Africa. Using U.S. mortality data and incidence rates from both the Third National Cancer Survey (1969–71) and SEER (1973–76), Pratt et al. (1988) noted that incidence rates for ALL were lower in black than in white children while mortality rates had declined in whites but not in blacks; thus ALL mortality rates were similar in the two races (Pratt et al., 1988).

Table 8.1 Average Annual Age-Adjusted Incidence Rates per 100,000 Population for Cancers at Selected Sites in the U.S. SEER (Surveillance, Epidemiology, and End Results) Program Areas by Race, for 1973–77 (Sexes Combined)

Site(s)	White (all areas)	Black (all areas)	Chinese (Calif.)	Chinese (Hawaii)	Japanese (Calif.)	Japanese (Hawaii)	Amerindian (NM)[a]	Utah
All	325.7	359.4	306.0	259.3	218.2	260.0	185.4	200.4
Buccal cavity, pharynx	10.7	12.5	17.6	7.3	3.1	5.3	0.5	12.1
Digestive system	75.9	92.9	97.4	88.0	91.3	102.7	71.9	57.2
Esophagus	3.0	10.0	5.9	4.2	5.5	3.1	1.0	1.7
Stomach	8.6	15.4	15.0	12.0	31.7	31.4	21.6	7.2
Pancreas	9.5	14.4	8.4	9.3	5.9	8.5	10.8	7.4
Liver	1.8	3.5	12.9	7.0	2.2	4.8	3.3	1.1
Gallbladder	1.4	1.2	1.2	2.6	0.9	1.8	13.8	1.3
Biliary	1.3	0.9	2.3	2.7	1.0	3.9	4.7	1.0
Colon	31.0	33.0	32.3	33.5	31.9	29.1	8.6	24.5
Rectum	11.5	11.7	18.0	15.7	11.0	18.4	6.2	10.7
Lung	45.4	62.5	53.5	35.9	20.3	30.4	7.3	23.5
Breast	46.9	40.2	30.7	31.8	35.2	27.1	10.8	40.1
Cervix uteri	5.8	14.1	7.2	4.5	3.0	4.1	10.0	4.3
Corpus uteri	16.1	8.1	10.0	15.8	9.7	11.7	1.9	13.6
Ovary	7.7	5.2	5.4	4.1	7.7	4.3	5.8	7.2
Testis	1.8	0.4	1.0	0.3	1.1	0.4	0.7	2.2
Prostate	26.7	46.1	15.5	20.1	7.0	22.1	25.4	34.6
Bladder	15.5	9.0	8.8	5.8	5.4	8.6	1.6	12.9
Brain	5.3	3.2	2.6	3.6	2.1	1.7	2.4	5.0
Thyroid	4.0	2.8	6.9	11.3	5.5	6.3	0.6	4.3
Melanoma (skin)	6.3	0.7	0.6	—	0.7	0.1	0.6	8.1
Lymphoma	12.3	7.9	8.5	6.4	5.8	6.9	4.0	8.1
Multiple myeloma	3.5	7.9	2.5	1.7	—	1.5	2.9	3.3
Leukemia	9.9	8.6	7.2	4.5	3.4	6.9	5.4	8.9

Data abstracted from Young et al. (1981). Rates were age adjusted to the total 1970 U.S. standard population. See Chapter 4 for description of SEER Program.

[a] Amerindian population of New Mexico.

Table 8.2 Average Annual Age-Adjusted Cancer Incidence Rates per 100,000 from 1978–81, SEER Program

Site(s)	Whites	Blacks	Hispanics (N.M. only)	Filipinos	Native Hawaiians
All sites	335.0	372.5	246.2	222.4	357.9
Breast, female	86.5	71.9	54.1	43.4	111.1
<40 years	8.2	10.7	7.9	7.1	7.1
40+ years	221.1	179.3	134.9	117.0	300.0
Cervix uteri	8.8	20.2	17.7	8.8	14.1
Corpus uteri	25.1	13.4	11.1	11.7	27.1
Lung					
Male	81.0	119.0	34.3	38.1	100.9
Female	28.2	30.5	13.0	18.4	38.6
Stomach	8.0	13.8	15.7	7.0	32.4
Pancreas	8.9	13.6	10.8	6.7	10.0

Data selected from Baquet and Ringen (1986).
N.M.: New Mexico

Incidence rates for colon cancer are now about equal in blacks and whites, but rectal cancer rates are still lower in blacks (Ziegler et al., 1986); this black–white pattern is in contrast with that in parts of Africa (see below). A study at St. Jude's Children's Research Hospital in Memphis, Tennessee, however, suggests that colon cancer may be more frequent in black than in white children (Koh and Johnson, 1986). Further studies are needed on this issue using data from population-based cancer registries.

Age-specific rates should be examined in comparisons of cancer incidence in blacks and whites. Several studies have shown similar or higher incidence rates for female breast cancer among U.S. "nonwhites" or blacks in comparison with whites (Gray et al., 1980) for ages under 40 years, with lower rates for blacks after age 40. Clinical stage of disease as well as age at diagnosis should be considered in black–white comparisons of incidence rates because of implications for survival (and hence mortality) rates. In New York State, incidence rates for breast cancers diagnosed at a *later clinical stage* (i.e., metastatic or widespread) were higher in black than in white females in some age groups (<40, 40–49, and 50–59 years) (Polednak, 1986a) (Table 8.3). Even at older ages, black–white differences in incidence rates were smaller for later clinical stages (regional or metastatic) than for early-stage (localized) cancers which have a better prognosis. In Detroit, incidence rates for late-stage breast cancer were high in black versus white women at all ages (Satariano et al., 1986). These findings are relevant to prognosis or survival in black and white patients (discussed later). Death rates for breast cancer in 1985 were higher in U.S. black than white women at younger ages (less than 55 years) (Table 4.1).

Black–white differences also depend on histologic types of cancer. Ewing's sarcoma, one histologic type of primary bone cancer, was mentioned above as being less common in U.S. blacks (and African blacks, as discussed below) than in whites. In contrast, higher incidence rates for osteosarcoma in black versus white adolescents but not in adults have been confirmed (Huvos et al., 1983; Polednak, 1985).

Table 8.3 Incidence Rates (per 100,000 per year) for Breast Cancer in Black and White Females by Age and Clinical Stage at Diagnosis in New York State (1976–81)

Age (years)	Total (all stages)			Clinical stage 3 (metastatic)		
	White	Black	White/black	White	Black	White/black
20–39	19.88	19.36	1.03	3.09	3.78	0.82
40–49	138.03	101.37	1.36	21.29	21.59	0.99
50–59	203.03	154.46	1.31	37.59	39.50	0.95
60–69	256.02	182.49	1.40	51.57	44.63	1.16
70–84	317.71	231.37	1.37	61.12	52.50	1.16
85+	367.05	284.10	1.29	61.12	58.22	1.06

Data from Polednak (1986a).

The relative incidence of some cancers in blacks and whites has been investigated less extensively. Differences in incidence rates for various cancers of soft tissues in U.S. blacks and whites have recently been suggested. These cancers include neurofibrosarcoma and malignant neurilemmoma, both cancers of nervous tissue, and leiomyosarcoma (Polednak, 1986b). Leiomyosarcomas are malignant tumors of smooth muscle that occur most often in the uterus and stomach. Higher age-specific incidence rates for leiomyosarcoma have been shown for blacks than whites in New York State (Table 8.4). The Mantel–Haenszel summary chi-square test (Chapter 1) for combining data from age strata yielded a statistically significant association between race and incidence of leiomyosarcoma (chi-square = 53.11, $p < .001$).

In summary, comparisons of mortality and incidence rates for specific cancer sites or groups of sites in U.S. blacks and whites should consider age, sex, histologic type, and stage at diagnosis.

Japanese, Chinese, Other Asians, and Pacific Islanders

U.S. Japanese have lower rates for buccal cavity and pharynx, lung and bronchus, female breast, cervix uteri, brain, malignant melanoma, and lymphoma. Rates are higher for stomach and (in Hawaii) liver cancer (Table 8.1).

Studies of Japanese migrants to the United States have a special place in the development of migrant studies of disease. Results are complex and vary with cancer site, undoubtedly reflecting the different risk factors involved in these sites and the rapidity of change in these factors. Major findings include the retention of high risk of stomach cancer in the first-generation migrants ("Issei") but not in the second-generation ("Nisei") born in the United States. In contrast, Issei rates for colon cancer increased in the *first* generation relative to the low rates in Japan (Haenszel and Kurihara, 1968; Haenszel et al., 1972; Haenszel, 1982).

Other cancer sites showed different patterns among Japanese migrants. Breast cancer rates, for example, remained low in Issei and Nisei, while cervical cancer rates declined and ovarian cancer rates increased relative to rates in Japan. Retention of rates of gastric and breast cancer similar to those in Japan suggest the possible importance of either genetic factors or environmental factors operating *early* in life in cancer causation.

Table 8.4 Incidence Rates per 100,000 per Year for Leiomyosarcomas in Black and White Females in New York State by Age Group (1978–81)

Age (years)	Whites		Blacks		
	No.	Rate	No.	Rate	Ratio (W/B)
0–29	24	0.129	4	0.098	1.3
30–39	40	0.680	16	1.346	0.5
40–49	104	2.309	40	4.475	0.5
50–59	148	2.810	31	4.068	0.7
60–69	158	3.485	40	7.596	0.5
70–79	127	3.926	29	10.383	0.4
80+	55	3.193	4	3.969	0.8

Data from Polednak (1986b). For results of statistical tests, see text.

More recent incidence data have been compiled for gastrointestinal cancers in Japanese and various racial/ethnic groups in Los Angeles County. Annual age-adjusted incidence rates for stomach cancer in 1972–82 in Japanese males (Table 8.5) and females, although lower than for Japan, were about twice as high as in blacks and Spanish-surnamed whites, and four times as high as in non-Spanish-surnamed whites (Shimizu et al., 1987). An important finding was the even higher rates of sigmoid colon and rectum in California Japanese versus non-Spanish-surnamed whites (Table 8.4) and versus the well-known lower rates in Japan.

Chinese populations in California versus Hawaii show some interesting differences in incidence rates for certain sites, as well as differences in comparison with whites (Table 8.1). In comparison with whites, incidence rates for stomach, liver, biliary tract, and rectum cancer are higher in Chinese, while rates for breast and uterine corpus, ovary, bladder, and a few other sites tend to be lower. Noteworthy are the higher incidence rates in Californian versus Hawaiian Chinese for buccal cavity and pharnyx and for lung. Largely due to these sites, total age-adjusted incidence rates are higher in Californian than Hawaiian Chinese.

Cancer mortality rates for specific sites were compared in U.S. Chinese (in California, Hawaii, and New York City), Hong Kong, and Guangdong (in the People's Republic of China) (King et al., 1985). Guangdong province (formerly written as "Kwantung" in English) is located in southeastern China (Fig. 3.2) and represents the "homeland" of the majority of Chinese in the United States and Hong Kong. The Guangdong mortality data for 1973–75 were obtained from a survey of national mortality statistics in China (China Map Press, 1979). U.S. Chinese, like Japanese migrants, have been separated into foreign-born ("idai") and U.S. born ("erdai").

Displacement of death rates occurred in U.S. Chinese (especially the erdai), who had a reduction in rates for sites showing high rates in Guangdong (e.g., esophagus, nasopharynx, liver) and an increase for sites with low rates in Guangdong (e.g., colon, lung, breast, and leukemia). Lung cancer death rates were especially higher for idai and Hong Kong males at all ages versus Guangdong, and both idai and erdai Chinese females had higher rates than U.S. white women. Although stomach cancer mortality in Guangdong (the homeland area) was lower

Table 8.5 Age-Adjusted Incidence Rates for Cancers of the Gastrointestinal Tract by Race in Los Angeles County, California (1972–82)

Racial group	Stomach	Sigmoid colon	Rectum
Males			
Spanish-surnamed whites	24.9	10.3	15.3
Blacks	22.6	10.9	15.3
Non-Spanish-surnamed whites	11.9	14.0	17.1
Japanese	50.8	25.0	30.3
Females			
Spanish-surnamed whites	11.0	7.2	8.0
Blacks	10.4	9.1	10.0
Non-Spanish-surnamed whites	5.7	9.7	10.3
Japanese	22.3	16.5	19.0

Data selected from Shimizu et al. (1987).

than in other parts of China, rates did not differ between Guangdong and U.S. Chinese. Thus, U.S. Chinese resemble Japanese migrants in showing retention of stomach cancer risks, presumably reflecting the influence of cultural (especially dietary) habits. Displacement of cancer mortality rates among migrants toward the rates in the U.S. population, as evident for increases in lung cancer among Chinese migrants (King et al., 1985), indicates the effect of changes in such environmental factors as smoking habits (as discussed later).

Although death rates for nasopharnygeal cancer (not shown) have decreased in recent decades among Chinese-Americans (especially males), rates remain 7–10 times higher in Chinese than other groups (including Japanese and Amerindians) (Levine et al., 1987). Incidence rates for nasopharyngeal cancers in Chinese worldwide are discussed later.

Filipinos, persons whose ancestry is from the Philippines, are another Asian group, aligned with Southeast Asian populations with respect to their physical anthropological characteristics (Chapter 3). They have remarkably low incidence rates for total cancers and for most major specific sites except for cervix (Table 8.2) and thyroid (Table 8.8). Data on cancer rates in Filipinos are mainly from Hawaii and California. Migrants from the Philippines have increased in California in recent decades. The issue of selective migration, with regard to health, must be recalled in interpreting health statistics. The addition of data on cancer incidence in the Philippines to *Cancer Incidence in Five Continents* (Muir et al., 1987) is noteworthy. Total mortality from all causes is also remarkably low in Filipinos versus other racial/ethnic groups in California (i.e., Los Angeles County) (Frerichs et al., 1984).

Cancer incidence data on *Pacific Islander* populations in the U.S. are relatively limited. Polynesians, represented by native Hawaiians (Table 8.2), have relatively high cancer incidence rates for all sites combined—female breast (after age 39 years), uterine cervix, lung, and stomach.

Hispanics

U.S. Hispanic populations have only recently received attention with regard to cancer incidence and mortality. Surprisingly, there are still no national mortality statistics on causes of death for all Hispanics (Chapter 4). However, a national program on cancer control among Hispanics has been initiated by the National Cancer Institute, and an annotated bibliography of studies on cancer has been prepared (Montes, 1986). Cancer survival patterns among Mexican-Americans and Anglos have been compared as part of the SEER Program reports (see later).

Incidence data on Hispanics have been available for Mexican-Americans in New Mexico, as part of the SEER Program (Young et al., 1981; Baquet and Ringen, 1986) (see Chapter 4). In this population the total age-adjusted cancer incidence rate (1978–81) was almost as low as that for Filipinos (Table 8.2). Noteworthy are low incidence rates for lung cancer and female breast cancer (age 40+ years), but high rates for cervix uteri and stomach.

In the SEER Program, New Mexico and Puerto Rico are the only areas for which population data for Hispanics are available. In a study of bone cancer incidence rates using SEER data from Puerto Rico for 1973–81, New Mexico was excluded because fewer than 30 incident cases were available; for Puerto Rican Hispanics, incidence rates for both osteosarcoma and Ewing's sarcoma were lower than those for "whites" (Spitz et al., 1987). Interestingly, higher osteosarcoma incidence rates were found among black versus white adolescents (<20 years of age at diagnosis), as previously reported (Polednak, 1985), but not among Hispanics.

In Los Angeles County, the cancer pattern in Mexican Americans was generally similar to that in American Indians. Incidence rates were high for gallbladder, liver, cervix uteri, and stomach, and low for lung, buccal cavity, and female breast (Menck et al., 1975). The probable importance of environmental factors is indicated by differences between immigrant and indigenous Mexican-Americans.

Using Spanish surnames to identify Mexican-Americans in Texas, cancer mortality in 1969–80 was 25 percent lower in males but only 4 percent lower in females in comparison to other whites. While lower mortality in Hispanics was found for lung, colon, breast, and prostate, higher mortality prevailed for stomach, liver, and gallbladder (Martin and Suarez, 1987). Mortality and incidence rates for liver cancer are more than twice as high in Mexican-Americans than in other whites, and dietary factors, hepatitis B infection, and environmental exposures (see below) need to be investigated (Suarez and Martin, 1987).

As with Japanese migrants, Puerto Rican migrants in New York City retained excessive mortality rates for stomach cancer (1969–71), along with high cervical and esophageal cancer mortality rates (Rosenwaike, 1984). Warshauer et al. (1986) found that stomach cancer death rates were somewhat lower, however, for migrants than for Puerto Rico in 1958–79, while colon cancer death rates increased greatly in migrants. For 1979–81 Puerto Rican-born New York City residents also showed colon cancer mortality rates that were higher than previous periods though still lower than those for other New York City residents (Rosenwaike and Shai, 1986). Not all Puerto Rican groups, however, may have higher mortality rates for cancers of stomach and cervix, as suggested from preliminary data in a high-income area of New York State (i.e., Long Island) (Polednak, 1988c).

Mortality rates for total cancers and a few selected sites have been compared for the entire Puerto Rican-born, Cuban-born, and Mexican-born populations in the United States for 1979–81 (Rosenwaike, 1987). Age-adjusted death rates for total cancers, ages 5 years and older, were slightly lower in all three Hispanic migrant groups (i.e., about 150 per 100,000 per year) versus whites (193 per 100,000) and blacks (244 per 100,000). Death rates were lower in Hispanics, especially the Puerto Rican-born, for lung cancer in both males and females and for female breast cancer. Mortality data on other cancer sites were not reported.

Rapid changes in cancer risk across a single generation may have occurred in the largely U.S.-born, Spanish-surnamed population of Colorado (Savitz, 1986). Between 1969–71 and 1979–81, incidence rates increased among the Spanish-surnamed population for cancers of various sites (e.g., colon and rectum, lung, female breast) and converged toward rates in other whites. The higher rates for other sites among Spanish-surnamed females (e.g., stomach, cervix, pancreas) did not converge, however, possibly because of small sample sizes or to maintenance of risk factors such as diet and sexual habits.

Noteworthy is the general finding among migrant studies that colon cancer rates increase rapidly, while stomach cancer rates tend to increase much more slowly after migration. This suggests that dietary habits early in life may be important in stomach cancer while risk of colon cancer is more readily modified by habits adopted in later life.

American Indians

American Indians in New Mexico (Table 8.1) are noteworthy for their low overall incidence rates for cancers and low rates for many specific sites—for example, buccal cavity and pharynx, lung and bronchus, female breast, urinary bladder, and melanoma of the skin. A few sites show higher rates than in U.S. whites—liver, gallbladder, other biliary tract, and cervix uteri (Black and Key, 1980; Black and Wiggins, 1985). The limitations of using broad racial groupings such as "American Indians" were discussed earlier (Chapter 3). Thus, considerable diversity in cancer rates can be shown for specific subgroups of American Indians. Although esophageal cancer rates are not high in New Mexican Indians (Table 3.1), very high rates have been noted in Inuit (Eskimos) of Alaska (as well as Greenland), Canadian Eskimos, and Aleuts (Lanier et al., 1985). Alaskan natives are composed of three racially and geographically distinct groups—Eskimos, Indians, and Aleuts. The genetic separation of Eskimos and Aleuts from Amerindian groups was discussed in Chapter 3.

Cancer surveillance in a remote Indian population in northwestern Ontario (Young and Frank, 1983; Sievers and Fisher, 1983) showed high rates of kidney cancer and gallbladder cancers. Gallbladder cancer is common in other Amerindian groups. Low-risk sites such as lung, breast, and skin also followed the general pattern as for most American Indian groups. Gallbladder cancers are particularly interesting, because the strength of the relationship between antecedent gallstones and risk of gallbladder cancer is much stronger for southwestern American Indians (Lowenfels et al., 1985).

U.S. Jewish Groups

Published studies of cancer incidence and mortality among U.S. Jewish groups are surprisingly few in number. Estimated cancer death rates for 1953–58 for New

York City residents aged 45 years and older showed lower rates for cervical cancer in females and various smoking- and/or alcohol-related sites in males (i.e., lung, tongue, larynx, pharynx, esophagus) in the Jewish versus Catholic and Protestant groups (Newill, 1961). In contrast, death rates were higher among Jews for stomach, pancreas, large intestine, lymphosarcoma, and leukemia. Also in New York City, Seidman (1970, 1971) reported similar patterns of mortality in Jews for 1949–51. Greenwald et al. (1975) examined cancer mortality in 1969–71 among Russian immigrants, as an indirect estimate of the Jewish population, in New York State exclusive of New York City; the mortality experience of the entire population was used to calculate expected numbers of cancer deaths among the Russian-born. Statistically significant findings were low mortality for buccal cavity and pharynx among males, higher mortality for stomach cancer in both sexes and pancreatic cancer in females, and lower mortality for cervical cancer. Proportional mortality ratios for specific cancer sites showed a significantly lower proportion of lung cancers in male (but not female) Russian-born Jews versus non-Jews, and lower proportions of breast and cervical cancer in Jewish females. These findings were consistent with those of other studies.

Lower death rates for lung cancer have been reported in Jewish males in various U.S. cities—for example, New York City, Baltimore and Pittsburgh. In Canada, where religious enumeration is part of the official census, average annual age-adjusted death rates for lung cancer in Montreal for 1959–63 were lower for Jewish than British or French males but not females (Segall, 1963). Horowitz and Enterline (1970) confirmed these findings for Jewish males in Montreal.

There is a need for further studies, using data from more recent years, comparing cancer incidence and mortality rates by site in U.S. Jews versus non-Jews and relating any differences in patterns of smoking and alcohol, sexual and reproductive patterns, and dietary habits.

Various Migrant Groups

Similarities between rates among certain migrants and rates in their countries of origin—for example, Finnish migrants for esophageal cancer and Russian migrants for stomach cancer—suggest that risk factors such as dietary habits were maintained by the migrants (Haenszel, 1962).

Among migrants of Czech descent to rural Nebraska, colon cancer rates have declined (relative to the high rates in Czechoslovakia) with gradual acculturation (Pickle et al., 1984). These changes implicate environmental factors, especially changes in diet (as discussed later). Diet may also be involved in the transition to higher colorectal cancer rates among migrants to Melbourne, Australia (Kune et al., 1986). In contrast with Japanese migrants to the United States, Polish migrants have shown more rapid increases in breast cancer rates (Staszewski and Haenszel, 1965; Haenszel, 1982).

Certain immigrant populations in the United States may retain their low socioeconomic status, which in turn affects their risk or stage at diagnosis of cancer. Caribbean immigrant women from Haiti, for example, have an unfavorable distribution of stage at diagnosis of cervical cancer compared to other women in New York City. This is probably attributable to infrequent cancer screening among lower-SES groups (Fruchter et al., 1986).

Rates of cervical cancer in Haitian immigrants are difficult to estimate because the total population at risk (e.g., in New York City) is uncertain. This also holds for estimation of rates of other diseases such as AIDS and AIDS-related cancers among Haitian immigrants in Miami (Hardy et al., 1985). Late stage at diagnosis of cervical and other cancers, and high relative frequency of cervical cancer, is also characteristic of Haiti, an extremely poor Caribbean country (Laguerre, 1981; Mitacek et al., 1986).

Other U.S. Religious and Cultural Groups

Cancer patterns in other U.S. ethnic groups will be discussed briefly. Included among "low-risk populations" for cancers, in a symposium published in the U.S. *Journal of the National Cancer Institute* in 1980, were Mormons (Utah and California), Hutterites, and Seventh Day Adventists.

Significantly lower overall cancer death rates in U.S. Hutterites from South Dakota (Martin et al., 1980) have also been confirmed for Hutterite brethren of Canada (Morgan et al., 1983). Stomach cancer rates were higher, however, perhaps reflecting the original Ukrainian migrant groups who also have high rates for this cancer (see below).

Utah Mormons, especially the most devout groups, have much lower rates than other groups for lung cancer and for all other smoking- and alcohol-related cancers (Gardner and Lyon, 1982a,b). Cancer incidence rates for Utah (Table 8.1) reflect, at least in part, the large proportion of the population comprised of Mormons. In Utah the age-adjusted rate for all sites is much lower than that for all whites (in SEER areas) and almost as low as that for Amerindians in New Mexico, due to lower rates versus all whites for most sites (especially lung and colon); exceptions are prostatic cancer and melanoma of skin. Seventh Day Adventists (Phillips et al., 1980) also have lower total cancer death rates, and this group is of special interest with regard to digestive (e.g., colorectal) cancers because of their ovolacto vegetarian diet (Schiffman, 1986).

Racial/Ethnic Differences in Cancer Survival Rates in the United States

Comparative data on prognosis of cancers appear to be rare worldwide. The most reliable statistics are from the United States. Data from the Surveillance, Epidemiology, and End Results (SEER) Program of the National Cancer Institute have been used to evaluate cancer patient survival for eight racial/ethnic groups in the U.S. population: Anglos, blacks, Hispanics, American Indians, Chinese, Japanese, Filipinos, and Hawaiians (Young et al., 1984). Among 402,752 patients with first primary cancer diagnosed in 1973–79, survival rates for Hispanics were almost identical to those for Anglos. In 1973–81 Japanese had the highest survival rates and American Indians the lowest for many cancer sites (Baquet and Ringen, 1986) (Table 8.6).

In comparison with whites, blacks showed distinctly lower 5-year relative survival rates for bladder, corpus uteri, and breast cancer. Studies on breast cancer survival in U.S. blacks and whites are most numerous. Lower survival rates for black than white women with breast cancer are well established. Later stage at diagnosis in blacks is a definite factor, but other factors are involved, because

Table 8.6 Five-Year Relative Survival Rates (%) for All Cancers and Specific Cancer Sites in U.S. Racial/Ethnic Groups, 1973–81

Group	Relative survival in percent by site				
	All sites	Colon-rectum	Female breast	Cervix	Corpus uteri
Japanese	51	59	85	72	86
Anglo	50	51	75	68	88
Hispanic	47	46	72	69	86
Filipino	45	41	72	72	78
Chinese	44	50	78	72	87
Hawaiian	38	51	76	73	80
Black	38	44	63	63	57
Native American	34	37	53	67	66

Data from U.S. SEER (Surveillance, Epidemiology, and End Results) Program (see Chapter 4), reported by Baquet and Ringen (1986).

Relative survival is the observed survival corrected for expected mortality from all causes, based on general population death rates.

black–white differences exist within stage at diagnosis groups (Young et al., 1983; Baquet and Ringen, 1986) (Table 8.7).

Also noteworthy are black–white differences in survival of patients with certain childhood cancers (Haddy, 1982). Poorer prognosis of black children with acute lymphocytic leukemia (ALL), in contrast with the lower risk of ALL in black children (see earlier), had been described in 1972 (Walters et al., 1972) and confirmed by later studies. Although survival differences may be narrowing in some regions (Szklo et al., 1978), they apparently still persist in the SEER Program populations (Pratt et al., 1988).

International Comparisons

Variation in *mortality* rates for total cancers and selected cancer sites is indicated by the limited data on 52 countries published by the World Health Organization

Table 8.7 Breast Cancer Survival by Clinical–Pathologic Stage at Diagnosis in U.S. White and Black Females, 1975–81

Stage at diagnosis	Five-year relative survival (%)	
	White	Black
All stages	75	63
< 2 cm, negative nodes	96	93
2–4.9 cm, negative nodes	89	84
< 2 cm, positive nodes	85	78
5+ cm, negative nodes	79	71
2–4.9 cm, positive nodes	72	66
5+ cm, positive nodes	56	44
Stage IIIB	46	37
Distant	17	13
Unknown	80	71

Source: Baquet and Ringen (1986).

(WHO, 1987; see Chapter 4). Table 4.5 shows age-adjusted death rates for stomach cancer, lung cancer in males and females, and female breast cancer. Stomach cancer death rates are highest in Japan, with high rates for Singapore, parts of Central and South America (especially Chile), Iceland, and Eastern Europe. Lowest rates are for the United States, Canada, and Sri Lanka. In contrast, lung cancer death rates are high in the United States (especially for females) and Canada, Scotland and the rest of Great Britain, and Hungary; rates are also high for females in Iceland, Denmark, and Singapore and for males in Belgium, Luxembourg, and the Netherlands. Rates are low in most of Central and South America and the Caribbean (except Cuba and Dominica). Breast cancer death rates are lowest in Guatemala and other countries in South America, along with Japan, and highest in Dominica, Iceland, and Great Britain.

With the advent of atlases of cancer mortality from various countries including China (see Chapter 4), exploration of regional differences in cancer death rates has recently become possible. Although analyses of such data rarely include consideration of racial/ethnic groups, regional comparisons correspond to some extent to such groups—as shown in Iran (Nadim and Nasseri, 1986). A major question requiring collaboration between anthropologists and epidemiologists is the extent to which regional differences in cancer rates are related to sociocultural factors (e.g., dietary and sexual habits) and whether the distributions of environmental factors relate to definable ethnic groups or more directly to degree of urbanization and socioeconomic and geochemical differences. Even when data are available on ethnic groups, broad categories such as Chinese or Malay and Indian in Singapore and Southeast Asia obscure within-group differences in culture and environment (Armstrong, 1986) and, to a lesser degree, in genetic background.

Much of the interest in worldwide cancer *incidence* rates is due to awareness of the periodically updated *Cancer Incidence in Five Continents* (Waterhouse et al., 1982; Muir et al., 1987), which includes data from all population-based cancer registries in the world. The range of variation in cancer incidence rates is wide, as shown for some major sites (Table 8.8). Large variation is evident, for example, for cancers of the lung and the colon, with less variation for rectal cancer. The interpretation of such wide variability in rates has proved to be a major challenge and impetus for further work. In addition, there is interest in the "blank" spaces on the cancer map, for many countries do not have population-based or even hospital-based cancer registries. Kuwait has replaced Dakar, Senegal, as the area with lowest rates for some cancers.

Along with data on U.S. ethnic groups discussed above, *Cancer Incidence in Five Continents* includes specific ethnic groups within other countries—for example, in Singapore (Malaysia), Israel, and New Zealand. Thus, within a given multiracial population or geographic area, considerable variation in cancer incidence may be apparent. Unfortunately, no data are available from African populations (Muir et al., 1987).

Relative to Chinese in Singapore, for example, age-adjusted incidence rates are lower in Malays and Indians for a number of cancer sites—for example, nasopharynx, stomach, bladder, colon and lung. Indians and Malays also differ, with very high rates for cancer in the *mouth* (i.e., oral cavity) (Table 8.9) (Shan-

Table 8.8 Ranges from Highest to Lowest Age-Standardized[a] Annual Incidence Rates for Selected Cancer Sites from Population-Based Cancer Registries

Site	Males			Females		
	Lowest	Highest	Ratio[b]	Lowest	Highest	Ratio
Stomach	3.7 (Kuwait)	82.0 (Nagasaki)	22	1.6 (Kuwait)	36.1 (Nagasaki)	23
Colon	0.2 (Kuwait)	34.1 (Conn., U.S.)	171	0.7 (Kuwait)	29.0 (Detroit, blacks)	41
Rectum	1.5 (Martinique)	21.9 (FRG, Saarland, urban)	15	1.3 (India, Madras)	13.9 (FRG, Saarland, urban)	11
Liver	0.1 (Ireland, Southern)	34.4 (Shanghai)	344	0.2 (Kuwait)	11.6 (Shanghai)	58
Pancreas	0.7 (India, Bangalore)	16.4 (Los Angeles, Koreans)	23	0.4 (India, Madras)	9.4 (U.S., Alameda, Calif. blacks)	24
Prostate	1.3 (China, Tianjin)	91.2 (U.S., Atlanta, blacks)	70	—	—	—
Lung, bronchus	5.8 (India, Madras)	110.0 (Blacks, New Orleans)	19	0.5 (India, Nagpur)	68.1 (Maori, New Zealand)	136
Breast	—	—	—	14.0 (Israel, non-Jews)	93.9 (Hawaiians, U.S.)	7
Cervix	—	—	—	3.0 (Israel, non-Jews)	83.2 (Brazil, Recife)	28

[a]Rates are standardized to a world age distribution; data derived from Muir et al. (1987). Rates based on fewer than 10 cases are excluded from this table.
[b]Ratio of highest to lowest.

Table 8.9 Cancer in Singapore: Relative Risks[a] by Ethnic Group after Adjustment for Age, Using Chinese as the Reference Group (1973–77)

Site	Chinese world adjusted rate per 100,000	Relative risks for		
		Malays	Indians	Others
Mouth				
Males	1.9	0.89	4.13	0.58
Females	0.7	1.93	13.79	1.32
Males				
Nasopharynx	19.2	0.24	0.04	0.22
Esophagus	19.9	0.08	0.34	0.11
Stomach	44.8	0.23	0.41	0.19
Colon	13.4	0.35	0.45	1.16
Rectum	12.6	0.47	0.51	0.67
Liver	33.2	0.52	0.43	0.42
Lung	64.4	0.37	0.22	0.39
Females				
Breast	20.9	0.77	1.14	1.62
Cervix uteri	18.4	0.60	1.25	0.63
All sites				
Males	278.1	0.41	0.45	0.56
Females	163.5	0.65	0.96	0.96

Sources: Modified after Shanmugaratnam et al. (1983); data for 1968–82 may be found in Lee et al. (1988b).

Relative risk is the rate in each ethnic group (Malay, Indian, and others) divided by the rate in the Chinese (reference group), after age adjustment (see Chapter 1). For example, rates for all sites in males for Malays, Indians, and others are only about half the rates for Chinese.

mugaratnam et al., 1983). The low relative risks for stomach cancer in Malays and Indians versus Chinese persist in more recent data (Lee et al., 1988b). Some explanations for these differences, including use of tobacco and other chewing products, are discussed later. The Singapore Chinese are not homogeneous ethnically and recent data show lower cancer incidence rates for Hainanese and Hakka versus Hokkiens (the predominant group) while Cantonese have higher rates for nasopharynx and female lung cancers (Lee et al., 1988a).

Table 8.10 indicates the populations with the highest age-standardized incidence rates for specific cancer sites, among groups for which data are available (Muir et al., 1987). The populations and ethnic groups covered in Volume V of *Cancer Incidence in Five Continents* are indicated in Table 8.11, which ranks these groups on the incidence rate for stomach cancer age-adjusted to the estimated total world population. Noteworthy additions to Volume V are Kuwaitis in Kuwait, Pacific Islanders in New Zealand, Tianjin in northern China, a Philippines registry, new registries in Brazil, and Korean and Filipino groups in California. Senegal in Africa has been deleted (Muir et al., 1987).

Starting with stomach cancer, some highlights of worldwide variation in cancer incidence rates will be discussed including racial/ethnic comparisons where available. The interested reader is referred to other compendia cited in this chapter and an earlier review by Muir and Nectoux (1982). Our discussion will concentrate on the most common cancer sites worldwide.

Table 8.10 Countries or Groups with Highest Incidence Rates for Specific Cancer Sites Among Countries with Population-Based Cancer Registries

Cancer site	Sex	Population	Rate per 100,000
Lip	M	Canada, Newfoundland	15.1
Tongue	M	India, Bombay	9.4
Mouth	F	India, Bangalore	13.5
Oropharynx	M	France, Calvados, rural	14.5
Nasopharynx	M	Hong Kong	30.0
Hypopharynx	M	France, Calvados, rural	17.7
Esophagus	M	Israel, Asian-African born	35.8
Stomach	M	Japan, Nagasaki	82.0
Colon	M	U.S., Connecticut	34.1
Rectum	M	FRG, Saarland, urban	21.9
Liver	M	China, Shanghai	34.4
Gallbladder, etc.	F	Israel, Asian-African born	23.6
Pancreas	M	U.S., Los Angeles, Korean	16.4
Nose, sinuses	M	Kuwait, non-Kuwaitis	3.4
Larnyx	M	Brazil, Sao Paulo	17.8
Lung	M	U.S., New Orleans, blacks	110.0
Bone	F	Brazil, Porto Alegro	3.3
Connective tissue	M	U.S., Hawaii, Hawaiians	4.3
Melanoma of skin	M	Australia, Queensland	30.9
Breast	F	U.S., Hawaii, Hawaiians	93.9
Cervic uteri	F	Brazil, Recife	83.2
Corpus uteri	F	U.S., San Francisco Bay, whites	25.7
Ovary, etc.	F	New Zealand, Polynesians from Pacific Islands	25.8
Other female genital	F	Brazil, Recife	5.7
Prostate	M	U.S., Atlanta, blacks	91.2
Testis	M	Switzerland, Vaud, urban	9.9
Penis	M	Brazil, Recife	8.3
Bladder	M	Switzerland, Basel	27.8
Other urinary organs	M	Canada, NW Terr. and Yukon	15.0
Brain	F	Israel, African-Asian born	15.7
Thyroid	F	U.S., Hawaii, Filipinos	18.2
Lymphosarcoma	M	U.S., San Francisco Bay, Japanese	9.5
Hodgkin's disease	M	Canada, Quebec	4.8
Myeloma	M	U.S., Alameda, Calif. black	8.8
Lymphatic leukemia	F	Israel, African-Asian born	30.6
Myeloid leukemia	F	New Zeland, Polynesian Islanders	7.7

Source: Data abstracted from Muir et al., 1987.
Excludes data based on 10 or fewer cases and a few sites for which rates are very low.

Stomach

At least until the 1980s, stomach cancer was the most common site worldwide, although lung cancer incidence rates are increasing while rates for stomach cancer are declining in many (but not all) countries. High incidence rates for stomach cancer are found in parts of Europe (including Eastern Europe), parts of the Soviet Union, Iran, East Asia (especially Japan, China, and Mongolia), and South America (see also Parkin et al., 1984; Howe, 1986).

Table 8.11 Stomach Cancer Annual Incidence Rates for Males in the Countries and Racial/Ethnic Groups Included In *Cancer Incidence in Five Continents,* from Highest to Lowest

Japan, Nagasaki City	82.0
Japan, Miyagi Prefecture, rural	80.1
Japan, Hiroshima	79.9
Japan, Miyagi Prefecture, urban	79.2
Japan, Osaka Prefecture	76.9
Costa Rica	58.8
China, Shanghai	58.3
Brazil, Sao Paulo	53.6
Colombia, Cali	49.6
Brazil, Fortaleza	46.6
U.S., Los Angeles, Koreans	44.8
Italy, Parma	44.0
Poland, Nowy Sacz	43.7
Italy, Varese	39.0
Singapore, Chinese	37.3
China, Tianjin	36.4
Romania, County Cluj, rural	35.7
Yugoslavia, Slovenia	34.9
New Zealand, Pacific Islanders	33.0
Poland, Cracow City	32.9
Romania, County Cluj, urban	32.6
Hungary, Szabolcs, urban	32.6
Czechoslovakia, Slovakia, rural	32.0
Spain, Navarra	31.6
Iceland	31.4
Hungary, County Vas	31.4
U.S., Hawaii, Hawaiians	31.2
Czechoslovakia, Slovakia, urban	29.9
New Zealand, Maori	29.8
U.S., Hawaii, Japanese	28.4
U.S., California, Los Angeles, Japanese	25.5
Martinique	25.3
Canada, Newfoundland	25.3
German Democratic Republic	25.2
Finland	24.6
Federal Republic of Germany, Saarland, urban	24.5
U.S., California, San Francisco Bay, Japanese	24.3
Federal Republic of Germany, Hamburg	23.7
Poland, Warsaw	23.2
United Kingdom, northwestern region	22.0
United Kingdom, Scotland east	22.0
United Kingdom, England and Wales, Mersey region	21.8
United Kingdom, Scotland west	21.7
Federal Republic of Germany, Saarland, rural	21.4
Spain, Zaragoza	20.8
Netherlands, Eindhoven	20.7
Scotland	20.4
United Kingdom, Trent	20.4
United Kingdom, Birmingham	20.3
United Kingdom, England, Oxford	20.2
Italy, Ragusa	19.8
United Kingdom, Scotland southeast	19.6

Table 8.11 *(continued)*

Switzerland, Basel	19.6
U.S., Connecticut, blacks	19.4
Hong Kong	19.2
U.S., California, San Francisco Bay, blacks	19.1
Netherlands Antilles	19.1
United Kingdom, England and Wales, urban	18.9
Norway, urban	18.5
Israel, Jews born in Europe or America	18.3
Israel, Jews born in Europe or America	18.3
U.S., New Mexico, American Indian	17.9
Switzerland, Neuchatel	17.9
Norway, rural	17.8
Puerto Rico	17.6
United Kingdom, Scotland northeast	17.5
U.S., Louisiana, New Orleans, blacks	17.5
Spain, Tarragona	16.9
France, Calvados, rural	16.9
U.S., Michigan, Detroit, blacks	16.9
Canada, New Brunswick	16.7
U.S., California, Alameda County, blacks	16.7
France, Doubs, urban	16.4
Israel, all Jews	16.2
Switzerland, Vaud, rural	15.8
U.S., Georgia, Atlanta, blacks	15.8
United Kingdom, S. Thames	15.7
U.S., New Mexico, Hispanics	15.7
U.S., California, Los Angeles County, blacks	15.6
Singapore, Indians	15.5
France, Bas Rhin	15.5
Canada, Quebec	15.3
France, Calvados, urban	15.2
Australia, West	15.1
Sweden	15.0
Australia, Cap. Terr.	15.0
United Kingdom, England and Wales, rural	15.0
Switzerland, Zurich	14.8
Australia, Victoria	14.8
U.S., California, Los Angeles County, Latino	14.7
United Kingdom, N. Scotland	14.7
Switzerland, Vaud, urban	14.3
Denmark	14.3
Canada, Manitoba	14.0
U.S., California, Los Angeles, Chinese	14.0
New Zealand, non-Maori	13.7
Australia, New South Wales, urban	13.6
Switzerland, Geneva	13.5
Canada, Maritime Provinces	13.5
France, Doubs, rural	13.1
Australia, South	13.1

Table 8.11   (*continued*)

Australia, Queensland	13.0
Canada, Prince Edward Island	12.7
India, Bangalore	12.6
Australia, Tasmania	12.6
New York City	12.4
Israel, Jews born in Israel	12.4
Ireland, Southern	12.4
Israel, Jews born in Africa or Asia	12.3
Canada, British Columbia	11.9
U.S., Hawaii, whites	11,8
Canada, Alberta	11.8
Canada, Saskatchewan	11.7
Canada, Ontario	11.5
France, Isere	11.5
U.S., Hawaii, Chinese	11.2
Australia, New South Wales, rural	10.9
U.S., Connecticut	10.8
U.S., California, Alameda County, whites	10.7
India, Poona	10.5
U.S., California, San Francisco Bay area, whites	10.4
U.S., Michigan, Detroit, whites	10.2
U.S., California, Los Angeles County, whites	9.6
U.S., New York State (excluding New York City)	9.4
Singapore, Malays	9.4
Philippines, Rizal	9.4
U.S., California, San Francisco Bay area, Chinese	9.1
India, Bombay	8.9
Kuwait, non-Kuwaitis	8.7
U.S., Washington, Seattle	8.0
Israel, non-Jews	7.9
India, Nagpur	7.8
U.S., Louisiana, New Orleans, white	7.3
U.S., Georgia, Atlanta, white	7.3
U.S., Iowa	6.8
U.S., Hawaii, Filipino	6.8
U.S., New Mexico, other white	6.3
U.S., Utah	6.3
Canada, Northwest Territories and Yukon	5.3
U.S., San Francisco Bay, Filipinos	4.7
U.S., Los Angeles, Filipinos	4.1
Kuwait, Kuwaitis	3.7

Data abstracted from Muir et al. (1987), and arranged from highest to lowest age-standardized incidence rates. Rates are per 100,000 per year and have been age-standardized by using
the age distribution of the world population.

Variation in stomach cancer incidence rates in populations and ethnic groups is great (Tables 8.8 and 8.11), with the highest rates in Japan. In fact, the risk of gastric cancer in Japan is so great that screening by endoscopic examination has been provided by statutory regulations. More than 5 million persons in Japan are screened for stomach cancer annually (Hirayama, 1988; Hisamichi et al., 1988).

Incidence rates for stomach cancer are lower in Japanese in Hawaii than in Japan (i.e., 30.0 vs. about 75.0–82 per 100,000 per year, respectively), although rates in Japanese in Hawaii are higher than those for other Hawaiian groups (Tables 8.1 and 8.2) except for Hawaiians (Table 8.11). Retention of high rates of stomach cancer, as described in U.S. Japanese, also occurs in Australia among migrants from Greece, Poland, southern Europe, and other areas versus the Australian-born population (McMichael and Giles, 1988).

Thus in the same geographic area stomach cancer incidence rates vary considerably by ethnic group. Stomach cancer incidence rates, for example, are about 2.5 times higher in Jews than in non-Jews in Israel. In New Zealand, incidence rates for stomach cancer are higher in Maori than in non-Maori groups (i.e., 41.7 vs. 16.3 per 100,000). Incidence rates are about four times higher in Chinese than in Malays in Singapore (Tables 8.9, 8.11). For other parts of Southeast Asia, where data are limited to hospital registries, relative frequencies (or the proportion of total cancers) among males are high in Rangoon, Burma, and Vietnam (Armstrong, 1986). The lowest known rates worldwide were previously shown for Senegal (Waterhouse et al., 1982) and more recently for Kuwaitis in Kuwait (Table 8.11).

Gastric cancers have been classified into two histologic groups with the "diffuse" type, more common in younger persons and associated with blood group O, showing less variation in frequency across populations than the "intestinal" type, which is more common in areas with high rates. The frequency of the intestinal type has also declined among Japanese migrants to the United States and over time among various populations worldwide (Howson et al., 1986).

Another region of high rates is Central and South America, including Chile, Brazil and Colombia, (Table 8.11) where large-scale studies have focused on dietary factors and precursor lesions (Correa, 1982; Correa et al., 1983). Gastroscopic studies of hospital patients in Chiapas, Mexico, suggest that the same histologic type (i.e., "intestinal") may be common among the indigenous (Mayan) population (Halperin et al., 1988), but epidemiologic studies are needed.

As with cardiovascular diseases, time trends in incidence and mortality rates for specific cancers are of great interest with regard to the crude assessments of the role of environmental factors. By analyzing time trends in population data on suspected causal agents such as dietary components and smoking or alcohol consumption, clues can be provided for more detailed (i.e., analytic) studies in various populations. Remarkable declines in stomach cancer mortality have been documented from the early 1950s to the late 1970s for various European countries, the United States and Canada, Australia, England and Wales, Scotland, and Japan (which still had the highest rates) (Howson et al., 1986). In another high-risk area, Chile, death rates have declined since the late 1950s (Haynes, 1986). In Scotland, however, there was no evidence for a continued decline in incidence rates from 1976–78 to 1983–85 (Prabhu et al., 1988). It will be important to continue to monitor time changes in specific countries and regions within countries including Japan where major efforts are being made at primary and secondary prevention.

As evidenced by the Sixth Annual Symposium of the European Organization for Cooperation in Cancer Prevention Studies (in 1988), which dealt with gastric carcinogenesis, interest in explaining regional differences in stomach cancer incidence and mortality continues, and ongoing studies emphasize dietary factors and the role of precursor lesions.

Lung and Larynx

Lung cancer has reportedly overtaken stomach cancer as the most prevalent cancer site worldwide. Available data on worldwide mortality rates were noted above. Variability in lung cancer incidence rates is also great (Table 8.8). For males, highest incidence rates are for U.S. blacks while lowest rates were for African blacks (in Senegal) and in India (Table 8.11). Greater variation is evident among females, with highest rates among the Maori of New Zealand. High incidence rates are also well known for Chinese females in Shanghai (i.e., about 20 per 100,000 per year) and in other areas including Cantonese in Singapore (Lee et al., 1988) and in the United States. The higher incidence rates in U.S. Chinese versus certain other groups (for both sexes combined; Table 8.1) reflect this female excess. The histologic type predominating among Chinese females is unusual (i.e., adenocarcinoma). Although cigarette smoking is also a causal factor among Chinese women, other studies have implicated "passive" exposure to smoke from cigarettes and from cooking, as well as previous tuberculosis (see later). Intriguing findings on Chinese residing in Japan, who originated mostly from southeast China and Taiwan, include high mortality rates from female lung cancer (and liver cancer) as in other Chinese populations. Because length of residence in Japan could not be established from routinely collected statistics (Kono et al., 1987), this pattern deserves further study.

Cancer of the *larnyx* is noteworthy for the male predominance, but there are increasing rates in females related to changing smoking rates. The highest recorded incidence rates are in Brazil (Sao Paulo) and in Doubs, France, with high rates also in Italy, Spain and Bombay, India (including females). In Thailand, larnygeal cancer ranks eighth among cancers in males, higher than nasopharynx but lower than stomach and esophagus (Somboomcharoen, 1986). In northern Thailand, the relative frequency of cancers of the larnyx and hypopharynx is higher in males, but the proportion of cancers in females in this category is also high (Menakanit et al., 1971).

Liver and Bile Ducts

Although primary *liver* cancer may account for less than half as many cancers worldwide as lung cancer, it is very common in Africa and eastern Asia. China accounts for over 40 percent of the global total (Parkin et al., 1984). There are perhaps 250,000 new or incident cases of primary hepatic cancer per year worldwide (WHO, 1983; Anon., 1987g).

The highest incidence rates worldwide are for Shanghai (Table 8.8) and Hong Kong, although Taiwan and Mozambique also have very high rates. In Singapore, incidence rates are higher in Chinese than in Malays or Indians (Table 8.9). Racial/ethnic differences in age-standardized rates per 100,000 per year were larger among males than females in 1978–82—40 in Chinese, 20 in Malays, and 15 in Indians (Jin, 1987). We have noted the higher incidence rates among Chinese in California (Table 8.1). Guangxi Province of China (Fig. 3.2) has the highest crude *mortality* rate from primary hepatic cancer. Hepatocellular carcinoma is reportedly common in both the Chinese and aboriginal Senoi groups (see Chapter 3) in West Malaysia (Sumithran and Looi, 1985). Recently, high incidence rates have been shown for Polynesian Islanders living in New Zealand (Muir et al., 1987).

Relative frequencies, or proportions of total cancers accounted for by liver cancers, are high in Thailand (Armstrong, 1986). Liver cancer, which includes hepatocellular carcinoma, adenocarcinoma, and cholangiocarcinoma (or intrahepatic bile duct carcinoma), may be the most common cancer site in males in Thailand (Ayuthya, 1982). In Thailand, liver cancer appears to be more frequent in northern or northeastern areas, as noted in a study of relative frequency of cancers in Chiang Mai Province (Menakanit et al., 1971) and in cancer statistics for 1981 reported by the National Cancer Institute (Sombooncharoen, 1986). There may be difficulty in distinguishing the diagnosis of hepatocellular carcinoma versus intrahepatic bile duct cancers (i.e., cholangiocarcinomas) in Thailand. Reliable cancer incidence rates cannot be calculated for Thailand because of the absence of population-based cancer registries.

As with stomach cancers, histologic type should be considered in population comparisons, but such data are not routinely available (Waterhouse et al., 1982). In areas with low incidence of hepatocellular cancer, a histologic variant, called fibrolamellar cancer, is more common in some studies, especially in younger persons, but is rare in high-risk groups such as Africans and Orientals (Anon., 1987g).

Cancer of the bile ducts are relatively rare, and incidence data are limited but suggest considerable worldwide variation. Thailand may have the highest worldwide frequency of cholangiocarcinomas, which are mainly intrahepatic (i.e., hilar or at the entry of the bile ducts into the liver) as opposed to extrahepatic (as in Japan and Western countries) (Juttijudata et al., 1983, 1984). Cancers of the gallbladder and extrahepatic bile duct are often grouped together in descriptive statistics, although their etiology differs. For this combined category the highest known incidence rates are among Israeli females (born in Africa and Asia) Amerindians females (Tables 7.10, 8.8 and 8.11), with high rates also in females in Poland. Gallbladder cancer is common in Chile and in other Amerindian populations, and rare in New Zealand Maori and Nigerians. Post mortems suggest that these cancers in Chileans, Swedes and Czechoslovakians may reflect (in part) the effects of gallstone disease (Nervi et al., 1988).

Colorectal Cancers

Another digestive system site showing considerable variation in incidence worldwide is colorectal cancers, which rank high (i.e., third or fourth) in estimated order of frequency among cancers worldwide (Parkin et al., 1983). Colorectal cancers are comprised of at least two major subcategories (colon and rectum), with some differences in epidemiologic characteristics. Worldwide variation tends to be greater for colon than for rectal cancer, as noted above (Table 8.8). Large-bowel cancers are rare in most areas of Asia (including India), Africa, and South America, in comparison with North America and Eastern Europe (Waterhouse et al., 1982). The highest known rates for colon cancer in males are in Connecticut (Tables 8.8 and 8.10), with lowest rates in Kuwait and (at least in previous years) in Senegal.

Colorectal cancer mortality rates have been decreasing in the Maori and are now less than half the non-Maori rates (Smith et al., 1985; Muir et al., 1987). Although colon cancer incidence rates are relatively low in Chinese in Singapore, rates for Malays and Indians are even lower (Table 8.9). Incidence rates for colon and rectum cancers have increased between 1968 and 1982 among Singapore Chinese (Lee et al., 1988). These are important observations, indicating the probable role of environmental influences that need to be identified.

As with stomach cancer, the importance of investigating precursor lesions in colorectal cancers (i.e., adenomatous polyps) and their variation in frequency among populations has become increasingly evident. Endoscopic examinations of a selected series of patients suggest low prevalence rates of adenomas in India, Africa, and South America (Bhargava and Chopra, 1988).

Esophagus

Esophageal cancers probably rank sixth or seventh in frequency among cancers worldwide (Parkin et al., 1983), and high incidence rates are found in diverse populations. We have noted higher rates and increases in rates in recent decades in blacks than in other racial/ethnic groups in the United States. The highest incidence rates are in Israel and Shanghai (Table 8.10). Incidence rates are higher in China (especially in northern China) and in Chinese versus other groups (especially Malays) in Singapore (Table 8.9) as well as in Hong Kong. Relative frequencies or proportions of total cancers are also high for males in Burma and Vietnam (Armstrong, 1986).

A distinctive feature of the distribution of this cancer is the large regional variation within countries, as shown by high rates in Brittany and Normandy in France (Picheral, 1986); in northern parts of Iran (Nadim and Nasseri, 1986); in parts of Africa (i.e., Kenya in East Africa and in Transkei vs. Transvaal in South Africa); in Turkemia, Kazakhstan, and Uzbekistan in the Soviet Union (Howe, 1986) and in northern China (China Map Press, 1981). Differences in several dietary and nutritional factors have been suggested as explanations for these variations, as discussed later.

Breast and Cervix

Breast and cervical cancers are the most frequent types of cancer among women worldwide, and therefore among the top five worldwide for both sexes combined (Parkin et al., 1983). Mortality rates among 52 countries were discussed earlier (Table 4.5). For breast cancer the highest incidence rate is among Hawaiians in Hawaii, and the lowest rates are in Israel (Table 8.8), Japan, and Shanghai. Variation is also evident in a single country or multiethnic city—for example, in Singapore (Table 8.9) where incidence rates have increased among Chinese (Lee et al., 1988). In Bombay the order of incidence rates from highest to lowest is

Parsi, Christian, Moslem, and Hindu (Jussawalla et al., 1985). Worldwide variation, however, is less than for cervical cancer.

Cervical cancer incidence is highest in Brazil and Colombia and lowest in Israeli non-Jews and Israeli Jews born in Europe or America. Low mortality rates among U.S. Jews were discussed above. In Singapore incidence rates for cervix are higher among Chinese than among Malays but not Indians (Table 8.9). In Bombay, the order of incidence rates is the reverse of that for breast cancer (i.e., highest in Hindus) (Jussawalla et al., 1985). Relatively high rates also occur in Central and East Africa. Relevant differences in marriage patterns and sexual and smoking habits across countries and cultures are discussed later.

Oral Cavity, Oropharynx, and Nasopharynx

Also showing wide variation within a single country or city, as well as worldwide, are cancers of the mouth (including lip, tongue, and mouth) and oropharynx. Incidence rates for mouth and oropharynx are highest in Indian females and France (i.e., the Department of Bas-Rhin). Oral cancer incidence rates are much higher in Indian males and (especially) females than in Chinese in Singapore (Table 8.9). The relative frequency or proportion of total cancers is high in the Philippines (Manila), Vietnam, Malaysia, and especially Indonesia (i.e., Surabaya, east of Jakarta), but not Rangoon, Burma (Armstrong, 1986).

Nasopharyngeal cancer is generally rare except among Chinese and Southeast Asian populations, with highest incidence rates recorded for Hong Kong (Table 8.10). In Singapore, incidence rates are high for Chinese, intermediate for Malays, and lowest in Indians (Table 8.9); within Singapore Chinese the Cantonese dialect group has the highest incidence rates (Lee et al., 1988). Chinese groups originating from southern China, including Cantonese from Kwantung (i.e., Guangdong) Province (Fig. 3.2), have the highest rates. Nasopharyngeal cancer rates are said to be intermediate in other Asiatic groups, including such countries as Thailand, Malaysia, and the Philippines, although data are limited to relative frequency comparisons rather than actual rates. Within Thailand, the relative frequency is highest in the northeast (Somboonjaroen, 1986) and among "Chinese" versus "Thai" in Chiang Mai Province in the northwest (Menakanit et al., 1971).

Incidence data from Kuwait, despite probable incompleteness, suggest high rates for nasopharynx in males, not attributable to smoking (Bissada and Al-Ghussain, 1986), and for nose and sinuses (Table 8.10). Other high-risk groups include Icelanders, Eskimos (Inuit) in various areas, and Tunisians. Greenland Inuit migrants in Denmark also have a high proportional mortality ratio for this cancer (Prener et al., 1987).

Pancreas

Pancreatic cancer does not rank high among cancers worldwide, although it is common along North American and European males. Comparisons of incidence and mortality rates for pancreatic cancer across countries, and even within developed countries, is complicated by problems of accuracy of diagnosis due to confusion with other digestive cancers in determination of primary site. The range of variation in incidence rates worldwide (Table 8.8) is apparently less than that for many other cancer sites. The highest incidence rates are in U.S. blacks (California) (Table 8.10), and rates are also high among Hawaiian males and in the Maori of New Zealand. We have noted increases in rates among U.S. blacks in recent decades and higher mortality rates in some studies of U.S. Jews.

Burkitt's Lymphoma (BL)

BL deserves separate attention for its place in the history of epidemiology and the important roles of infectious agents. Dr. Denis Burkitt's famous "long safari" across Africa, involving a 10,000-km automobile journey, and the simple data collection method of mailing leaflets with illustrations of children with jaw tumors, led to the definition of a "lymphoma belt" across equatorial Africa and down the East Coast. As with infectious diseases, temperature and humidity were recognized as the determining factors. Burkitt does not know who first suggested the analogy with insect-vectored diseases such as yellow fever and trypanosomiasis (see Chapter 6), but the importance of Epstein-Barr virus (EBV) in endemic areas has been demonstrated. These endemic areas include parts of Papua New Guinea as well as Africa—that is, malarial areas. Malaria has been regarded as a precipitating factor in BL, probably by increasing the division rate of cells (i.e., B lymphocytes) infected with EBV (Morrow, 1985), but this remains controversial. BL cases in nonendemic areas, such as the United States, Europe, and Japan, rarely involve EBV (Lenoir et al., 1985).

Other Lymphomas, Kaposi's Sarcoma, Multiple Myeloma, and Leukemias

Population differences in *Hodgkin's disease* (HD) and *non-Hodgkin's lymphoma* include the higher proportion of children with HD, especially males as in most series, in parts of East and tropical Africa and in Egypt. The predominant histologic subtype, however, differs (Gad-El-Mawla, 1983). The role of infectious agents requires greater exploration. Orientals (including Japanese), Amerindians, and some U.S. black populations blacks appear to be at lower risk for HD, although blacks have poorer survival in the United States. Jews and Italians may be at higher risk (Grufferman and Delzell, 1984). Complicating interpretations of these apparent racial/ethnic differences are north–south gradients in distribution of HD that resemble the pattern for multiple sclerosis.

   Kaposi's sarcoma (KS) is endemic in equatorial Africa, with eastern Zaire having the highest recorded relative frequency—9 percent of all cancers. KS is classified as a cancer of connective or soft tissue, but its histologic origin is a matter of great debate; there is evidence that it may originate from the lymphatic endothelium (Beckstead et al., 1985). The clinical course was generally indolent or chronic in classical endemic KS, while cases diagnosed since 1983 have increased in frequency and severity. The more aggressive course probably reflects the influence of acquired immune deficiency syndrome (AIDS) (Bayley, 1984). The virus associated with AIDS-related diseases is human immune deficiency virus (HIV) (Chapter 6). While earlier cases of KS were responsive to therapy with certain drugs (e.g., actinomycin D and vincristine), more recent cases with weight loss, lymphadenopathy, and absence of nodules or plaques on the limbs have failed to maintain an initial response to chemotherapy (Bayley, 1984). In San

Francisco, vinblastine has proved to be somewhat effective in treating KS related to AIDS, although only 30 percent of patients showed more than temporary arrest (Volberding et al., 1985).

A somewhat similar transition for KS, in numbers and severity as well as in age distribution and clinical presentation, is historically well documented in the United States from about 1979, when KS emerged as a sequela of AIDS (Friedman-Kien et al., 1983; Dowdle, 1983). Previously, the disease has been known among older males of Ashkenazic-Jewish and Mediterranean origin (Oettle, 1962). The probable importance of environmental factors in Kaposi's sarcoma and in Burkitt's lymphoma is evidenced by the rarity of these cancers in U.S. versus African blacks. The absence of black–white differences in incidence rates for other cancers of lymphatic origin (i.e., *lymphangiosarcoma*) in New York State (Polednak, 1986b) and in the SEER areas (Young et al., 1981) is also noteworthy.

Leukemias show racial/ethnic differences in distribution by subcategory. The low incidence of acute lymphoblastic (or lymphocytic) leukemia among U.S. blacks, and even lower incidence in African blacks, was mentioned earlier; the possible role of genetic factors will be discussed later. The incidence of *chronic* lymphatic leukemia is low in Japan and China, while "lymphatic leukemia" incidence rates are highest in Israelis born in Africa and Asia (Table 8.10). The highest incidence rates worldwide for myeloid leukemia have been recorded in New Zealand Polynesian females (Table 8.10), Hawaiian males and the Maori of New Zealand. The emergence of certain leukemias (i.e., T cell) and lymphomas, associated with HIV viruses, in the Caribbean, Japan, and other areas is also noteworthy (Chapter 6). *Lymphosarcomas* are most common in Japanese in California, and in Israelis born in Africa or Asia, while somewhat less frequent in U.S. blacks than whites.

Multiple myeloma was mentioned earlier with reference to U.S. blacks (Table 8.1), but incidence rates are also high in parts of Africa, in Quebec (Table 8.10) and among the Maori of New Zealand, while low in Indians and Japanese. Owing at least in part to improvements in diagnosis, incidence rates are increasing in many countries.

Polycythemia vera (PV) involves excess production of red blood cells and was formerly classified as a disease of blood (see Chapter 9). The higher prevalence among Jewish populations has been confirmed, but this excess does not occur in patients under age 40 years, who comprise only 5 percent of all PV cases but whose disease is clinically more severe than that among older patients (Najean et al., 1987). The etiology of PV, as opposed to secondary polycythemias, which are related to high altitude (hypoxia) and other factors, is obscure.

Various Other Sites

Prostatic cancer shows wide variation in incidence rates worldwide (i.e., 125-fold; Table 8.8). High rates in U.S. blacks including those in Atlanta (Table 8.10) and Detroit have already been noted (Table 8.1), but higher rates in U.S. Chinese groups than in Shanghai are noteworthy. Because of its high ranking among cancers in males, prostatic cancer also ranks among the top 10 worldwide (Parkin et al., 1983). Large increases in incidence over time among U.S. blacks, and changes in rates with migration among Chinese and Japanese, indicate the importance of environmental factors.

Bladder cancer ranks among top 8–12 cancers, with higher incidence rates in males, and highest recorded incidence rates in males in Switzerland (Basel) and in Doubs, France (Table 8.10). Rates are also high in Belgium, along with lung cancer, suggesting the importance of smoking (see below). In contrast to whites in Hawaii, rates are lower in Orientals and especially Filipinos, while also lower in U.S. blacks versus whites in all cities with registries (Muir et al., 1987). Noteworthy are the associations with schistosomiasis (Chapter 5) in certain developing countries and with previous multiple urinary tract infections.

Ovarian cancers are most common in Europe (especially Norway, Sweden and Denmark) and North America, and least common in Asia (especially Japan) and in various Chinese populations. Polynesian Islanders in New Zealand and Israeli Jews born in Europe and America have the highest incidence rates. Also common in the latter group is cancer of the *corpus uteri*, although the highest incidence rates recorded are for whites in California (Table 8.10), while U.S. blacks have lower rates (see earlier). Incidence rates among Maoris are twice those of non-Maoris in New Zealand, and incidence rates are low in Africa and Japan. Japanese living in Hawaii (Table 8.1), however, experience rates comparable to those of U.S. whites.

Testicular cancer incidence rates are low in Africa, and, though somewhat higher than African rates, U.S. blacks (Table 8.1) have lower rates than whites. Highest incidence rates are in Europe, especially Vaud, France (Table 8.10). Noteworthy epidemiologic features of testicular cancer are the peak in early life (i.e., in children and young adults) and an association with a specific condition (i.e., cryptorchidism, or lack of descent of the testis).

Cancer of the *penis* exhibits high incidence rates in parts of the Caribbean, with highest recorded incidence in Jamaica (Waterhouse et al., 1982) and Brazil (Table 8.8). Relative frequency appears to be high in Haiti, especially in coastal versus mountain areas (Mitacek et al., 1986). The relative frequency varies across Africa, with large numbers of cases in Uganda and western Tanzania but a lower frequency in Kenya and eastern Tanzania (Cook-Mozaffari, 1986). Noteworthy are the associations with lack of circumcision in some populations and with poor hygienic practices, which is also relevant to differences in cervical cancer rates in women (as discussed below).

While *thyroid* cancer incidence rates are generally low in North America and Europe, female Filipinos and Hawaiians in Hawaii have the highest known incidence rates (Table 8.9; Muir and Nectoux, 1982). Rates were also high among Chinese in Hawaii, relative to U.S. whites (Table 8.1) (Young et al., 1982), but not in more recent data (Muir et al., 1987). In Filipinos in California, in Polynesian Islanders in New Zealand, and in Iceland, females also have high rates.

The rarity of *melanoma* of the skin in various nonwhite versus white groups in the United States (Table 8.1), including American Indian groups (Black and Wiggins, 1985) and Hispanics, and in other countries such as Africa, is well documented. Rates are low in the Maori. In contrast, Australians have the highest incidence rates (Table 8.10). Also established is the tendency for these tumors to occur on the soles of the feet in Africans as well as U.S. blacks

(Crombie, 1979; Reintgen et al., 1982), in Japanese (Takematsu et al., 1984), and possibly in other groups. Explanations involving pigmentation are discussed later. Melanomas of the uveal tract of the eye are less frequent in blacks and other heavily pigmented races, such as the Japanese and the Maori of New Zealand, than in various Caucasian populations for which incidence rates are generally similar (Hyman et al., 1987).

Rate of cancers of the *brain* and *central nervous system* are difficult to compare across populations because of problems of accuracy of diagnosis and coding. The highest recorded incidence rates are among Israeli Jews born in Europe and America (Table 8.10), or Africa and Asia, while relatively low rates have been reported in China and Asia and among U.S. Japanese, Chinese, Filipinos, Koreans and blacks (Table 8.1). Relatively high incidence rates also occur in Iceland and Sweden. In a comparison of age-specific rates of cancers of the central and peripheral nervous system, the *age pattern* was similar across populations covered by *Cancer Incidence in Five Continents*, but the *magnitude* of incidence rates varied—it was highest in Israel and lowest in Asia (Velema and Walker, 1987).

Among the rare cancers, *choriocarcinoma* should be mentioned. Choriocarcinoma and its precursor or major risk factor, hydatidiform mole, are diseases of the trophoblast or layer of ectodermal tissue that binds the embryo to the uterus. The rarity of choriocarcinoma and diagnostic difficulties have made definitive studies difficult. Geographical variation may be smaller than once believed, ranging from four per 100,000 per year in the U.S. to 10–20 in the Far East (i.e., Singapore, Japan, and the Philippines) and in Jamaica (Buckley et al., 1988). As for other diseases, such as Hodgkin's disease, it has been difficult to separate regional variations or gradations in incidence from racial/ethnic differences. Although an excess risk of choriocarcinoma among Orientals has been widely accepted, only data from Japan show a consistent excess, along with certain African and Central American countries (Bracken et al., 1984). Hydatidiform mole, the precursor lesion, was not found to be greatly increased among pregnancies in a large survey in China, but rates were higher in minority groups (i.e., Zhuang and Mongolians) than in Han Chinese (Song and Wu, 1986).

EXPLANATIONS

Errors of Measurement

We have already noted the problems of imprecision in both numerator and denominator data for rates of chronic diseases such as cancers. Incidence and mortality rates cannot be calculated for many areas of the world, because of the absence of comprehensive cancer registration and incompleteness of death registration. Comparability of death certificate data is affected by differences in clinical interpretation by physicians, availability of diagnostic tests, recording practices in certification regarding selection of an "underlying" cause of death, and differences in coding of causes of death by country or smaller geographic area.

Comparability of certification and coding practices in European countries were studied together by sending sets of case histories of cancer patients to samples of certifying physicians and completed certificates to national or regional coding offices and to a WHO coding center (Mackenbrach et al., 1987). The average proportion of cases correctly classified as to cause of death (I.e., one of five cancer sites) across the eight countries was 83 percent, with Ireland having the lowest rate. In a similar study, involving case histories of five cancer deaths, accuracy for three-digit ICD codes was high for bladder cancer, stomach cancer, and melanoma of the skin, but cervical cancer was often misclassified as uterine cancer; the latter error was shown to affect official statistics on cervical versus uterine cancer in European countries (Kelson and Farebrother, 1987). Also important to note is that response rates from physicians selected in both studies were 70 percent, despite the offering of a payment as an incentive; thus, accuracy of cancer diagnoses and death certification practices may have been overestimated.

Data on relative frequency, or proportion of total ascertained cancers attributed to a given site, are available for some areas as derived from hospital registries or other sources, as an interim basis for comparisons. Registries covered by *Cancer Incidence in Five Continents* provide the most comprehensive data source, including some specific racial/ethnic groups within countries. Even the latter, however, have limitations in terms of comparability of cancer diagnoses and coding, related to such factors as diagnostic facilities and practices. The limited data on histologic type of cancer within each site have been noted by Waterhouse et al. (1982).

Although age-standardized rates are widely used, including those based on estimated world populations (Waterhouse et al., 1982), there is considerable imprecision in estimates of population size and age structure, especially in developing countries. Since cancer rates tend to be highest at older age, at least for total cancers and for many sites, inaccuracies in estimation of populations at older ages, and the large proportions of these deaths attributed to ill-defined causes, are problematic.

Socioeconomic Status

The most extensive on the influence of socioeconomic factors, including education and income levels, in explaining racial/ethnic differences in cancer rates has been done in the United States. In other areas it is extremely difficult to separate the effects of underlying differences in SES among countries or groups from sociocultural factors, because few studies have considered these variables simultaneously. Some examples of such studies are discussed below.

Despite the lack of data on SES for comparison of cancer rates across populations, much of the apparent variation in cervical cancer rates, for example, is undoubtedly related to SES. Case-control studies *within* various populations, including such diverse areas as Thailand (Wangsuphachart et al., 1987) and Los Angeles County (Peters et al., 1986), indicate that level of education is a significant risk factor for *invasive* cervical cancer. Another risk factor for invasive (vs. in situ) cervical cancer is lack of regular cytologic ("Pap") screening, as shown by numerous case-control studies in various countries, and SES-related access to or use of medical care is a major underlying factor. Thus, much variation in cervical cancer rates worldwide and across racial/ethnic groups may be largely explained by SES differences. These SES-related factors may operate secondarily through sociocultural variables involving sexual and hygienic habits along with adequacy of medical care. The only detailed studies of SES and other risk factors in multiethnic settings appear to be in the United States (see later).

In a case-control study of invasive cervical cancer women in Los Angeles County, number of years of *education* was the greatest contributor to the difference in risk between Spanish-speaking and English-speaking groups, while age at first sexual experience and number of sex partners were not involved (Peters et al., 1986). Education may be related to more specific risk factors such as personal hygiene, and hence exposure to a virus such as papillomavirus, or dietary habits (as discussed below).

Risk of stomach cancer within populations also tends to be associated with lower SES. In some populations level of education is associated with risk of stomach cancer which in Poland was related to rural versus urban residence (Jedrychowski et al., 1986). In this Polish case-control study, SES-related variables may have been related to diet, food storage (i.e., refrigerators), and hygienic standards; dietary factors persisted as risk factors after adjusting for SES variables. It is probable that some part of the worldwide variation in stomach cancer incidence rates, as well as the decline in incidence and mortality in many countries (Howson et al., 1986), is related directly to SES, through such intermediary variables as refrigeration. Another component of variation, however, is diet, as emphasized by high incidence rates among Japanese migrants in Los Angeles County (discussed later). The importance of SES, along with climatic and other ecologic factors, is evident with regard to cancers in which infectious diseases play a major causal role, as discussed later.

The direction and strength of the association with SES-related factors vary by cancer site and for incidence versus mortality rates, within countries such as the United States and Great Britain. SES-related variables are positively or inconsistently associated with pancreatic cancer incidence rates. While cervical cancer incidence rates are higher in lower social classes, the reverse holds for breast cancer. We have noted that breast cancer incidence rates in U.S. black versus white women tend to be lower (after age 40), while cervical cancer incidence rates are higher. Analyses of cancer *incidence* rates from the Third National Cancer Survey of 1969–71 indicated that crude adjustment for SES differences, using income and education level of the census tract of residence of black and white cancer cases, removed large fractions of the racial differences in rates of breast and cervical cancers (Devesa and Diamond, 1980) (Table 8.12). For cervical cancer, adjustment for income had a stronger effect than adjustment for education. For the United States as a whole, cervical cancer *death* rates remain about three times higher in black (vs. white) women, despite a higher frequency of Pap smear within the past 2 years in national surveys, within educational level and adjusting for age (Bloom, 1986). Still, only about 55 percent of black women with a high school education have had a Pap smear during the past 2 years; thus, to

Table 8.12 Breast and Cervical Cancer Incidence Rates in U.S. Black and White Women (1969–71), Adjusting for Age and Variables Related to Socioeconomic Status

Type of rate	White	Black	Relative risk	
Breast cancer				
Crude rate	77.5	46.7	1.66	(white/black)
Adjusted for age	73.8	61.6	1.20	
Adjusted for age, income, and geographic area	73.4	63.2	1.16	
Adjusted for age, area, and education	72.6	66.5	1.09	
Adjusted for age and area				
Specific for income: < $6,000 per year	102.0	61.4	1.66	
Specific for education: < 9.0 years	67.6	58.9	1.15	
Cervical cancer				
Crude	18.4	28.9	1.57	(black/white)
Adjusted for age	17.6	32.1	1.82	
Adjusted for age, area, and income	19.5	24.7	1.27	
Adjusted for age, area, and education	18.6	28.4	1.53	

Data from Devesa and Diamond (1980).

decrease the death rate from cervical cancer among blacks, the proportion of black women screened must be increased.

Although some black–white differences remained in incidence rates after SES adjustment (Table 8.12), the adjustment was based on group (vs. individual) data, which probably do not adequately measure SES. Interpretation of these findings is affected little by intercorrelations of SES-related variables with smoking and alcohol (see later), although a role for smoking has been suggested in cervical cancer, and alcohol has been associated with breast cancer risk in some (but not all) studies. Also in other studies some correlations with SES and cancer incidence hold even after adjustment for smoking habits (Williams and Horm, 1977).

Using the same data base, Devesa and Diamond (1983) showed that the higher lung cancer incidence rates in U.S. blacks versus whites could be removed by adjusting for geographic area, income, and education. In fact, adjusted rates were significantly lower in black than white females (Table 8.13). Education and income are surrogates for cigarette smoking (discussed later), although an "urban factor" related to environmental and occupational exposures to lung carcinogens has been shown in some epidemiologic studies.

Mortality rates for breast cancer are similar in U.S. black and white women (Table 4.1) despite lower incidence rates in blacks after age 40 years (see above). This reflects in large part differences in clinical stage at diagnosis, related in part to differences in exposure to cancer screening tests, as well as to differences in survival within stage at diagnosis (see later). Regarding breast cancer screening, in a 1987 national survey, knowledge of mammography was poorer in black than white women 40 years of age and older, and the percentage of women who had ever had a screening mammogram was lower in blacks than whites (i.e., 25 percent versus 32 percent) (Anon., 1988d). Detailed analyses of the effects of socioeconomic differences on these black–white differences in knowledge and practices have not yet been reported, but a role for SES differences is probable.

Table 8.13 Lung Cancer Incidence Rates in U.S. Blacks and Whites (1969–71) Adjusting for Age and Socioeconomic Factors

Type of adjustment	Males			Females		
	White	Black	Black/white	White	Black	Black/white
Age and geographical area	73.5	80.6	1.10*	16.7	15.8	0.95
Age, area, income, education	75.7	71.8	0.95	17.0	14.6	0.86*

Modified after Devesa and Diamond (1983).

*Statistically significant relative risks (see Chapter 1) for these large sample sizes from the Third National Cancer Survey.

SES and Cancer Survival Differences by Racial/Ethnic Group

Black–white differences in survival from cancer of the breast, prostate, and corpus uteri have been investigated in detail, although major issues remain unresolved. The U.S. National Cancer Institute is sponsoring studies on the roles of various factors including histologic type and clinical stage at diagnosis of the cancer, nutrition, and socioeconomic status.

For breast cancer socioeconomic differences appear to explain at least part of the black–white differences in clinical stage at diagnosis (Table 8.14) and in survival even within stage at diagnosis. In the generally high-SES population of upstate New York, black–white differences in survival of breast cancer cases were small, especially within stage-at-diagnosis groups, with the apparent exception of younger women diagnosed at the metastatic stage (Polednak, 1988a). Within a group of uniformly lower-SES breast cancer cases with regional-stage disease, no differences in absolute survival were observed between blacks and whites (Sutherland and Mather, 1985). In western Washington State, adjustment for black–white SES differences by using 1980 census block-group data virtually eliminated racial differences in breast cancer survival, and low SES was an important factor in poor survival within each race (Bassett and Krieger, 1986).

In the metropolitan Atlanta Cancer Surveillance Center, an affiliate of the SEER Program, the survival advantage of white versus black breast cancer cases (diagnosed in 1978–82) was greatest among advanced-stage cases, and a higher proportion of black women did not receive surgery. In multivariate analysis race was a significant prognostic factor even controlling for stage, type of surgery, and county of residence (Bain et al., 1986). Although Bain et al., (1986) concluded that SES did not explain black–white differences in survival, it should be emphasized that county of residence is a poor surrogate for SES, and SES data on individual cases were not available. These investigators are conducting a biracial population-based prospective study of breast cancer survival, including consideration of such factors as nutritional status, social support, prescribed therapy, and compliance with therapeutic regimens. Such studies should include detailed data on income and education in order to determine the influence of SES on these variables and any factors that might operate independent of SES (e.g., patient delay in seeking care or noncompliance with therapies) in explaining racial differences in breast cancer survival. Less aggressive breast cancer therapy in blacks was also shown in a study of SEER cases diagnosed in 1978–82, with

Table 8.14   Clinical Stage at Diagnosis of Breast Cancer in Black and White Women in New York State by County and SES Rank

Region	Mean family income			Breast Cancer: black–white difference in percent stage 3[a]
	White	Black	Black–white/white (%)	
Total state	$25,504	15,898	−37.7%	+24.6%
Upstate	25,877	18,184	−29.8%	+19.7%
New York City	24,660	15,161	−38.5%	+27.6%
Manhattan	37,479	13,514	−63.9%	+47.4%

Data from Polednak (1986a).
[a]Stage 3 is metastatic cancer.

blacks being treated less aggressively (including less surgery) (McWhorter and Mayer, 1987). These differences in therapy may be related to SES, but this requires more intensive study (as noted above). Finally, certain biological features of the cancers may also be involved, as discussed later.

In summary, U.S. black–white differences in survival of breast cancer cases in other series, even within the same clinical stage at diagnosis, may be due to a variety of factors. Socioeconomic factors appear to be important. After "controlling" for SES differences in various ways, and considering stage at diagnosis, some studies still find poorer survival in black women. Imprecise individual data on SES, differences in death rates from other causes (related to SES), failure to control for important prognostic factors, differences in treatment (in turn due to SES and possibly sociocultural factors), and biological differences in tumors may be involved.

Studies on the improved survival of Japanese breast cancer patients in Hawaii suggest that better survival is related to earlier stage at diagnosis (Anon., 1985d; LeMarchand et al., 1985) and not to differences in intrinsic tumor growth rates, as suggested in previous studies. Multivariate analyses indicated that controlling for stage at diagnosis removed most of the differences in survival, although Filipinos and Hawaiians still had significantly poorer survival than Japanese or Caucasians, while SES had little effect on survival.

Turning to other cancer sites, SES indicators and not race were found to be a significant prognostic factor in multiple myeloma (Savage et al., 1985). In contrast to the findings on breast cancer, black–white differences in survival with multiple myeloma appear to involve not patient delay but rather response to chemotherapy. Low SES may affect biological behavior of this cancer, as well as colon cancer and Hodgkin's disease (Savage et al., 1985), possibly through nutritional and/or immunologic mechanisms. Five-year relative survival rates for cervical cancer are only slightly lower in U.S. black than white women (Table 8.6). Thus, the higher incidence rates for cervical cancer in blacks, due largely to SES-related factors (see above), combined with nearly equal cervical cancer screening frequencies in blacks and whites, are responsible for the three-fold excess in cervical cancer mortality in blacks.

On the basis of data from the SEER Program, poorer survival of U.S. black versus white women with adenocarcinomas, but not sarcomas, of the uterus was evident even after adjustment for stage at diagnosis and SES indicators of census tract of residence (Steinhorn et al., 1986). Again, nutritional or immunological factors and previous disease history were suggested as factors requiring exploration in future studies. In general, the importance of economic factors in survival from cancer is becoming increasingly recognized. Berg et al.'s (1977) suggestion that poverty may be associated with host factors prior to treatment that affect survival within each race may also apply to racial differences. For uterine cancers, racial differences in survival should also be considered with reference to factors that affect risk, such as excess body weight (Steinhorn et al., 1986).

The demonstration of independent effects of economic factors on survival with digestive cancers among U.S. white males has led to the suggestion that other sex–race groups also be studied (Chirikos and Horner, 1985). Studies of other cancers, such as multiple myeloma, suggest that SES may influence racial differences in survival through factors other than stage at diagnosis. As with female breast cancer, these factors may involve nutritional and immune status, as well as access to treatment and compliance. Again the independent effects of SES and sociocultural factors, including attitudes regarding cancer and its curability, need to be explored.

Sociocultural Factors

Smoking and Alcohol

The lower frequency of various smoking-related cancers in Jewish populations was noted above. Horowitz and Enterline (1970) conducted a 2 percent random sample survey of smoking behavior among Jews and non-Jews in the Montreal area (i.e., for 28 census tracts) for which death rates were calculated. Jewish males and females were not only found less frequently to be cigarette smokers, but also to smoke less heavily if they did smoke. The high lung cancer death rate among Jewish women, however, could not be explained by cigarette smoking, because they smoked infrequently. Bulka (1986) has observed that Jewish law regarding self-destruction and the harming of others (as in exposing others to passive smoking) is consistent with an antismoking policy.

Other religious groups such as Mormons, whose members follow church doctrines regarding use of tobacco and alcohol, show lower rates of certain cancers, such as lung, pancreas, and cervix (Gardner and Lyon, 1982a,b). Utah, with its large Mormon population, has the lowest proportion of smokers among all states (Anon., 1987e). The contribution of black–white differences in smoking habits to differences in lung cancer rates is currently under investigation; the possible contribution of factors other than smoking (such as diet, occupational exposures, and prior tuberculosis) also should be considered.

Recent changes in lung cancer mortality in the United States are largely due to changes in smoking haits (Burbank, 1972; Cummings, 1984). Dramatic worldwide changes in cigarette smoking prevalence are of major public health importance, and some examples will be cited. The case of Japan (Kristein, 1986), where smoking among males had increased markedly along with lung cancer mortality rates, may be informative with regard to the rising epidemic of lung cancer and other smoking-related cancers in developing countries. The marketing of tobacco has been called the "new slave trade" (Anon., 1984c). In India and China, which include a large fraction of the world's population, about one-fourth to one-third of young adult males are addicted to smoking, and the WHO is launching programs to prevent the approaching epidemic of smoking-related diseases (Stanley, 1986). The largest smoking survey in the world, comprising a sample of 500,000 persons, was recently conducted in China, showing that 69 percent of males and 8.3 percent of females over age 20 years were smokers. Another survey showed a higher smoking rate among females. Yet another survey in Beijing in 1981 found that the highest proportions of smokers were among factory (i.e., textile mill) workers (86.4 percent) and doctors (38.7 percent) (Wan-Sheng et al., 1986). Among students at industrial colleges in Shanghai (average age about 30 years), however, only 0.33 percent of 2,440 women (and 50.5 percent of 4,899 men) were smokers (Li et al., 1988). Smoking was reportedly influenced by social factors related to hospitality and friendship.

We have noted that Chinese women in various countries have high rates of lung cancer (mainly adenocarcinomas) that are not attributable mainly to smoking. Both active smoking and exposure to passive smoke have been shown to be factors in case-control studies in Hong Kong Chinese (Koo et al., 1987; Lam et al., 1987). Other studies have implicated prior tuberculosis in Shanghai Chinese women (Zheng et al., 1987) and cooking oil vapors or smoke (Gao et al., 1987) (as discussed later).

Turning to other tobacco-related cancers, recent increases an oral cancer in the United States suggest a role of tobacco chewing and use of smokeless tobacco. One group at high risk of oral cancer may be Native Americans in Washington state, since prevalence of smokeless tobacco use was high among male (and especially female) students in grades 6–8 (Hall and Dexter, 1988). There is a well-known association between chewing betel nut and slaked lime in western India and Southeast Asia (Malaysia) in relation to oral cancers and precancers. *Primary prevention* programs involving personal and public education aimed at reducing tobacco use offer promise in reducing precursor lesions (i.e., leukoplakia) and oral cancer in India (Gupta et al., 1986). *Early detection* or secondary prevention programs for oral cancer in India involve basic health workers trained by dentists to screen high-risk persons (Mehta et al., 1986), and there is interest in the United States in programs involving dentists. In India, where chewing and use of local cigarettes ("bidi") has been traditional, practices have shifted toward the use of cigarettes, although the latter do contain health warnings (Stanley, 1986).

In Thailand the practice of smoking a local cigar (called "keeyo") in the northeast, but not in Bangkok, has been associated with regional differences in the relative frequency of hypopharyngeal–laryngeal cancers (Menakit et al., 1971). High rates of esophageal cancer in China are also related to smoking.

Among ethnic groups within South Africa (McGlashan and Harrington, 1985), the Xhosa have long been known to smoke commercial and home-grown tobacco, in contrast to the Zulus, and rates of esophageal and lung cancers are higher among the Xhosa. In Bombay, India, rates of various cancers (e.g., oral and pharyngeal, bladder) are related to tobacco-chewing and smoking habits of the ethnic groups—that is, Moslems and Hindus (high) versus Parsis and Christians (low) (Jussawalla et al., 1985). In Belgium, where bladder cancer rates are high and increasing, smoking and occupational exposures may explain most of the risk (Schifflers et al., 1987).

Alcohol plays a role in the high rates of various cancers in parts of Africa (e.g., South Africa), either directly or indirectly (through nitrosamines), and in high rates of oral cancers in parts of France (Picheral, 1986). In a population-based case-control study of a large number of oral and pharyngeal cancer cases in the U.S. SEER areas, the higher risk association with the combination of high levels of smoking and alcohol reportedly held within blacks and whites (although the detailed data were not presented) (Blot et al., 1988). The higher prevalence of heavy smokers and/or drinkers, mainly due to the latter, among black versus white male controls suggests that some of the black–white difference in oropharyngeal cancer rates among males can be attributed to differences in alcohol consumption.

A major research issue is the magnitude of the causal role of alcoholic cirrhosis, and its carcinogenic mechanism, in various populations at intermediate or lower risk of hepatocellular carcinoma (HCC) (Anon., 1987g). Heavy alcohol consumption may also be involved in postcirrhotic liver cancers in Japan (Nonomura et al., 1986). In areas where hepatitis B virus infection is not prevalent, alcohol may account for a significant proportion of liver cancers. In a low-risk area (i.e., London), 41 consecutive Caucasian HCC patients (Dunk et al., 1988) showed a diversity of possible risk factors including presence (i.e., in 80 percent) of cirrhosis, and serologic evidence of past hepatitic B exposure (21 percent) (see later). This was not a case-control study, so estimates of associated risks (i.e., odds ratios; Chapter 1) could not be calculated. In Kingston, Jamaica, histological data suggest that the majority of HCC cases identified involve alcoholic cirrhosis (Hamilton and Persaud, 1981). Thus, the contribution of specific causal agents to HCC incidence varies across populations.

Lower rates of both alcohol- and smoking-related cancers occur among religious/ethnic groups that proscribe these habits, including Mormons and Seventh Day Adventists. Racial/ethnic differences in a variety of cancers may involve differential alcohol consumption, in view of increasing evidence for the role of alcohol in such cancer sites as rectum, colon, and lung (Pollack et al., 1984; Potter and McMichael, 1986). Further studies are needed on the role of alcohol in various cancers in multiethnic settings. The independent effects of SES and sociocultural factors on alcohol use should be explored. Racial/ethnic differences in susceptibility to alcohol-related cancers, perhaps involving alcohol metabolism, also need to be explored (Chapter 9).

Environmental Factors Relevant to Infectious Agents

Exposure to infectious and parasitic agents involved in cancer etiology may vary by racial/ethnic group, largely due to socioeconomic and ecologic factors but also to sociocultural patterns (Chapter 6). The worldwide patterns of cancer rates reflect to a considerable extent the burden of infectious diseases in such major worldwide cancers as liver, cervix, and nasopharynx. The role of infectious agents in various cancers is becoming increasingly recognized.

In Guangxi Province, China (Fig. 3.2), it is estimated that hepatitis B accounts for at least 80 percent of liver cancer cases (Yeh et al., 1985). In general, liver cancer rates tend to be higher among males than females worldwide, and hepatitis B is more common among males in most studies (Chapter 6). In West Malaysia (Malay Peninsula) the sex ratio and the association with hepatitis B may be greater in the "aboriginal" Senoi than in Malays (Sumithran and Looi, 1985). The proportion of cancers related to HBV may vary with time. In Chapter 6 we cited some evidence that hepatitis B seroprevalence may be declining in Japan. In a necropsy analysis of 271 HCC cases in Nagasaki University Hospital in 1964–84, there was a decreasing linear trend with time in the proportion of HBsAg-positive cases (Senba et al., 1988).

The association between intrahepatic bile duct cancer occurrence and levels of infestation with the liver fluke, *Opisthorchis*, has long been noted (Menakanit et al., 1971). Typhoid fever (*Salmonella typhi*) carriers may be at higher risk of cancers of the liver and bile ducts, according to a small prospective study in Denmark (Mellemgaard and Gaarslev, 1988). Bladder cancer has been associated with schistosomiasis, as in coastal Mozambique, where eggs of the parasite have been found in tumors of squamous cell origin (Cook-Mozaffari, 1986). Malaria, another parasitic disease, may have a role in susceptibility to Burkitt's lymphoma (discussed later). Thus certain cancers may be more frequent in populations living in areas where these infections are common (see Chapter 6).

There is considerable interest in the risk of cancer among leprosy patients, as evidenced by a study in Japan (Tokudome et al., 1981). This interest is due in part to the poor cell-mediated immune response among patients with lepromatous leprosy. Prior tuberculosis infection has been associated with lung cancer in a case-control study in Shanghai (Zheng et al., 1987). The odds ratios for tuberculosis diagnosed less than 20 years prior to interview were adjusted for age, education, and sex and were high within each category of smoking (Table 8.15); summary odds ratios were calculated by using the Mantel-Haenszel procedure and logistic regression analyses (see Chapter 1). Although not noted by Zheng et al. (1987), there appeared to be a synergistic relation between level of smoking and prior tuberculosis (Table 8.15) with increasing odds ratios for tuberculosis as smoking level increased. The authors observed that only a small part of the excess rates of adenocarcinoma of the lung among nonsmoking Chinese women could be attributed to tuberculosis. This is related in part to the small proportion of nonsmokers who had a history of tuberculosis (Table 8.15). Results of studies of the association between prior tuberculosis and lung cancer in Western countries have been conflicting, although an association has long been suspected with regard to "scar cancers" of the lung. Recency of active tuberculosis infection may be an important factor in influencing the risk of lung cancer.

Another mechanism for associations between infectious diseases and cancer risk involves effects of antibiotics. Chloramphenicol, a broad-spectrum antibiotic, has been associated with risk of acute lymphocytic leukemia in a case-control study in Shanghai, China, but the causality of the association is uncertain—that is, it may reflect recall bias in cases or an association with the underlying infections (Shu et al., 1987).

The emergence of cancers related to the human immune deficiency viruses (HIV) (Chapter 6) is also evident in the distribution of Kaposi's sarcoma and Burkitt's and other lymphomas. Certain leukemia/lymphoma cancers in the Caribbean, Japan, and other areas have been associated with HTLV-I virus.

Table 8.15 Lung Cancer in Relation to Prior Tuberculosis Infection and Smoking: A Case Control Study in Shanghai China

Prior tuberculosis (TB) diagnosis	Cases	Controls	Odds ratio (adjusted)
Nonsmokers			
No TB	415	714	1.0[a]
TB <20 years ago	18	9	3.5 (1.5–8.0)[b]
Light smoker			
No TB	257	331	1.0
TB <20 years ago	14	15	1.5 (0.7–3.1)
Moderate smoker			
No TB	310	197	1.0
TB <20 years ago	31	6	4.2 (1.7–20.3)
Heavy smoker			
No TB	113	37	1.0
TB <20 years ago	9	0	—
Total			
No TB	1,105	1,279	1.0
TB <20 years ago	72	30	2.7 (1.7–4.3)

Modified from Zheng et al. (1987).
[a]Reference category for calculation of odds ratio.
[b]Adjusted for age, education, and sex.

Burkitt's lymphoma (BL) is frequent not only in Africa but in other tropical areas, such as West Malaysia and Papua New Guinea, where climatic factors and altitude influence the endemicity of many infectious agents including Epstein-Barr virus (EBV) and malarial parasites (Chapter 6). In these areas EBV is commonly associated with BL, while in areas of low prevalence of BL this association is weaker. Prospective studies indicate the importance of EBV in BL, and other studies suggest an interaction with dietary carcinogens (see later), while the causality of the association between BL and malaria has been questioned (Henderson, 1988). EBV has also been implicated in the causation of nasopharyngeal cancer, and interactions with dietary carcinogens have been suggested in Tunisia (Arrand et al., 1988; Henderson, 1988). High rates of EBV occur in children in Greenland, where nasopharyngeal cancer is also frequent, especially among Inuit residents. Inuit migrants to Denmark also have high rates of this cancer (Prener et al., 1987).

With regard to cervical cancer, high rates among certain groups such as South American populations, with Colombia showing the highest incidence rates, the Puerto Rican and black populations, have been known for some time. Socioeconomic and possibly sociocultural factors influence age and frequency of exposure to the putative viral agents, especially human papillomavirus (see later).

Sexual Habits and Reproductive Factors

It was once believed that male circumcision was causally associated with low rates of cervical cancer in Jewish females, but this is no longer accepted. Rather, hygienic practices of male partners may be important in cervical cancer, as in male penile cancer (see later), presumably operating through an infectious agent.

There is evidence for a role for sexual practices of male partners in influencing risk of cervical cancer. High rates of cervical cancer in parts of Latin America may be related to high rates of prostitution and penile cancer, as well as male "promiscuity" (Reeves et al., 1984). In parts of Latin America female virginity is valued, and young men tend to visit prostitutes (Zunzunegui et al., 1986). This background may be similar to that discussed with reference to AIDS (Chapter 6).

Findings on the association between multiple sex partners in women and risk of cervical cancer have been inconsistent across populations studied, and the explanation for this apparent inconsistency is unclear. Having multiple sex partners appears to be a key variable in risk of cervical cancer in Panama (Reeves et al., 1986) but not in a case-control study of Hispanic women in San Francisco (Zunzunegui et al., 1986). As noted for Hispanic women in Los Angeles, level of education, presumably as a surrogate for some exposure variable, may be crucial in explaining ethnic differences in risk of invasive cervical cancer. Puerto Rican-born migrants to New York City in 1969–71 still had an excess mortality 3.3 times that of other whites (Rosenwaike, 1984), suggesting maintenance of some environmental exposures which require examination through analytic studies.

We have noted the lack of cross-cultural data on sexual habits including premarital sexual activity (Chapters 2 and 6). The Eskimo (Inuit) women of Greenland reportedly have an early age of first coitus and a large number of sexual partners, which might explain the high rates of cervical cancer in Greenland and in Inuit migrants to Denmark (Prener et al., 1987). In some African societies, customs of polygynous marriages and freedom of sexual activity may influence rates of both sexually transmitted diseases and cervical cancer (Cook-Mozaffari, 1986). As noted in Chapter 6, however, there is considerable variation in sexual patterns across African groups, and further studies are needed of the direct and indirect effects of female prostitution. In Bangkok, Thailand, where cervical cancer is the major cause of cancer death among women and where female prostitution is common, risk factors included previous venereal and other infectious diseases as well as early age at first coitus, multiple sexual partners, high parity, and husband's history of venereal diseases (Wangsupchachart et al., 1987).

These observations on cervical cancer epidemiology have implicated multiple viral exposures. Early work involved herpes simplex virus (type 2), but more recent evidence (including prospective studies) supports the role of human papillomavirus (HPV) (Campion et al., 1986; Grubb, 1986). Rates of HPV infection differ among populations, probably reflecting differences in sexual habits. Guangxi province in South China (Fig. 3.2), for example, reportedly has limited sexual "promiscuity" and low HPV rates (Boon et al., 1986). HPV transmission, however, may occur "vertically" (i.e., from mother to child) rather than sexually in areas of China were venereal disease is rare but HPV has been found in cervical cancer tissue samples (Xiao et al., 1988).

Marriage and reproductive habits, including age at first pregnancy, are related to risk of various cancers of the female reproductive tract. Early marriage is a risk factor for cervical cancer, but pregnancy at an early age is protective against breast cancer. The order of cervical cancer risk by religion from lowest to highest in Bombay, India, is Parsi, Christian, Moslem, and Hindu; the absolute incidence rate in Parsis (i.e., 5.6 per 100,000 per year) is low relative to rates worldwide (Table 8.8) and to the highest rate in Bombay (i.e., 25.7 in Hindus). The ethnic pattern in Bombay is expected on the basis of differences in certain risk factors (i.e., age at marriage and parity) (Jussawalla et al., 1985), with average age at marriage being later in Parsis versus all groups and in Christians versus Hindus and Moslems (Jayant, 1987). The lower rate of cervical cancer in Moslems than Hindus, despite earlier age at marriage and "multiple partners" in Moslems, may be related to "universal" male circumcision; the latter is associated with better penile hygiene as assessed by amount of smegma (i.e., sebaceous gland secretion found mainly beneath the prepuce). In Parsis, who are more Westernized and in whom circumcision is rare, penile hygiene is also relatively better than in Hindus and Christians (Jayant, 1987).

Multivariate analyses, however, are needed to examine the independent contribution of these factors in Bombay, including socioeconomic status, as assessed for individuals in a case-control study approach to cervical cancer. This also holds for Iran versus Kuwait, where circumcision is common, but the relative frequency of cervical cancer is lower in the latter (Bissada and Al-Ghussain, 1986). The independent effects of age at first intercourse and number of sexual partners also require further study in different populations worldwide (Brinton and Fraumeni, 1986).

National surveys of U.S. women 15–44 years old have indicated higher prevalence of married women living with husbands and greater use of barrier contraceptive methods among Jewish versus other religious groups (Hendershot, 1983). Although these characteristics might be associated with lower risk of cervical cancer, the effect of religion independent of socioeconomic status was not considered.

In Bombay the pattern of age-specific incidence rates for *breast* cancer among the racial/ethnic groups is the reverse of that for cervical cancer, again as expected on the basis of differences in risk factors among these groups (Jussawalla et al., 1985). The decrease in incidence of cervical cancer and slight increase in breast cancer rates in Bombay from 1964 to 1983 may be due in part to a trend toward increasing age at marriage (and hence at first pregnancy) (Jayant, 1986). In Singapore recent increases in breast cancer incidence rates may be due in part to declining fertility rates among Chinese (Lee et al., 1988). Similar increases in breast cancer might be expected in China due to changing fertility.

In the United States fertility in nonwhites (i.e., blacks and Hispanics) continues to be greater than that in whites, but some convergence may be occurring; higher fertility at younger ages in nonwhite women (Westoff, 1986) has implications for cervical and breast cancers, but SES must be considered. Later maternal age at the time of the preceding pregnancy and multiple marriages have been associated with the rare cancer choriocarcinoma, but for this disease the association may reflect the opportunity for the expression of ABO blood group incompatibility on reproductive outcome (see Chapter 9) rather than sexually related factors (Buckley et al., 1988).

Two reproductive variables showing inconsistency in associations with cancer across studies are use of oral contraceptives, with regard to both breast and cervical cancers, and lactation with regard to breast cancer. The negative association between duration of lactation and breast cancer risk in a case-control study in Shanghai, China (Yuan et al., 1988), may reflect in part the longer duration of lactation in this population than in many others studied previously. The reader should recall a recurrent point made in this text (see Chapter 1) regarding population differences in the range of variation in relation to the ability to detect an association. In U.S. surveys, reported intentions to breastfeed expected infants are highest in Anglo women, considerably lower in Hispanics (in Texas), and lowest in blacks (Young and Kaufman, 1988). SES and educational differences must be considered in population comparisons of associations with breast cancer.

In a southern Italian case-control study, a statistically insignificant association between breast feeding for 6 months or longer and breast cancer was reported, but the odds ratio was 0.74—that is, in the direction expected if a protective effect of longer duration of breast feeding existed. In Shanghai the amount of variation in duration of breast feeding (and hence in lactation) is greater, and thus an association (possibly real) can be detected. Byers et al. (1985) have noted some consistency in the findings of studies on lactation and breast cancer risk, especially for premenopausal cancers. The possibility of a threshold effect with longer durations of lactation needs to be explored.

The underlying hypothesis for a protective effect of longer durations of lactation, which postpone ovulatory cycles, involves the increased risk of breast cancer associated with factors that increase the cumulative number of ovulatory cycles. Thus earlier age at menarche and late menopause are associated with increased risk of breast cancer in most studies (see later), although age at diagnosis of breast cancer tends to influence these associations; the underlying mechanism may involve levels of total estrogen or specific estrogen subtypes. Further studies are needed in other populations with long durations of lactation.

U.S. black–white differences in cancers of female reproductive organs are also due in part to differences in reproductive pattern (e.g., age at first pregnancy), but other factors are involved such as age at menarche and body weight (see later). Known risk factors for breast cancer, including late age at first childbirth, do not fully account for the difference in breast cancer rates between Caucasian and Japanese women in Hawaii (Nomura et al., 1984). Within a population, these risk factors also account for only a small proportion of breast cancers.

In contrast to breast cancer, one hypothesis for causation of *chorio-carcinoma*, based on several risk factors, involves low estrogen levels. Lower estrogen levels in Japanese and Chinese versus Caucasian women could be involved in population differences in incidence of choriocarcinoma (Buckley et al., 1988). The significant negative correlations between provincial urbanization level and mortality rates for choriocarcinoma in China (Haynes, 1986) require further examination, in terms of regional differences in reproductive patterns.

Penile cancer, mentioned earlier relative to cervical cancer and characteristics of male partners, has been associated with degree of penile hygiene which may or may not be associated with circumcision status in specific populations. Within Africa penile cancer frequency varies considerably among groups without circumcision, possibly because of differences in penile hygiene or in sexual behavior including exposure to prostitutes, but systematic studies apparently have not been carried out. In Haiti circumcision is reportedly rare and penile hygience poor, but further studies are needed including consideration of apparent regional differences in relative frequency of penile cancer (Mitacek et al., 1986). Circumcision was offered as an explanation for the apparent rarity of penile cancer in Kuwait (Bissada and Al-Ghussain, 1986), but penile hygiene should be studied. Thus further studies are needed within and between populations regarding the effects of penile hygiene and sexual activity patterns on penile cancer risk.

Dietary Factors

The design and analysis of ecologic studies were discussed in Chapter 1. Many international studies have used broad correlations involving only estimates of average or total intake of a single dietary constitutent (such as "fat" or "fiber") in relation to cancer rates, and the limitations of this approach are well known. Thind (1986), for example, has presented correlation coefficients between age-adjusted death rates for specific cancers and levels of consumption of protein, fat, and total calories among a variety of developed and "underdeveloped" countries. Each separate coefficient may be influenced by confounding, or the associations between protein and fat consumption (after adjusting for calories), and multivariate analyses are needed as for cardiovascular diseases (Hartz et al., 1988). The problems with ecologic studies (Chapter 1) include intercorrelations between intakes of dietary constituents (and total calories), as well as the existence of other known (as well as unknown) differences between countries with high and low cancer incidence or mortality rates.

Analyses comparable to those employed regarding cardiovascular disease incidence and mortality rates in the Seven Countries Study (Chapter 7), using multiple linear regression involving several dietary and nondietary risk factors, are needed for specific cancer sites. Such studies would again take advantage of the wide international variation in diet, as opposed to the more restricted ranges among regions or groups within countries such as the United States.

The intensive study of diet in groups with relatively *low* risks for certain cancers, such as Hispanic-Americans with regard to breast and colon cancers (Newell and Boutwell, 1981), as well as pregnancy-related factors (Markides and Coreil, 1986), may prove rewarding. Further studies on vegetarian groups, such as Seventh Day Adventists, with regard to colorectal and other cancers are also warranted.

Major leads have been provided by migrant studies with regard to the role of diet in cancer causation as well as explanations for racial/ethnic differences. The conclusions from these migrant studies, especially in terms of the age at which significant environmental causal factors must operate, depend on the specific cancer site. Interest has focused on dietary fat and fiber intake with regard to colon and breast cancer, and on salted or pickled foods with regard to stomach and nasopharyngeal cancers in various ethnic groups. Specific dietary constituents have been investigated in connection with other cancers, such as iron in esophageal cancer (Isaacson et al., 1985) and arsenic in bladder and kidney cancers in the Far East (C. J. Chen et al., 1985) and in other cancers in Chile (Haynes, 1986b). Some highlights of recent research will be discussed.

Esophagus. Regional differences in frequency and in sex ratio of esophageal cancer, along with various descriptive and analytic epidemiological studies, suggest that not only tobacco and alcohol but dietary components (e.g., teas) and nutritional deficiencies, perhaps related to soil characteristics, are involved in explaining these differences. In mainland China, a high-risk area, alcohol and tobacco have not been major risk factors (although the prevalence of smoking has been increasing, as noted earlier).

An experimental epidemiologic study (defined in Chapter 1) involving an intervention trial has been initiated in China to determine whether a combined treatment with riboflavin (vitamin B), retinol (vitamin A), and zinc could lower the prevalence of precancerous esophageal lesions within 1 year (Wahrendorf et al., 1988). Multivariate analyses showed that individuals with higher blood levels of these nutrients at the end of the trial were more likely to have a histologically normal esophagus, although there was no difference in the frequency of actual precursor lesions. Also noteworthy were the relatively low baseline levels of dietary retinol intake but lack of evidence for gross vitamin A deficiency on the basis of plasma retinol levels in the Chinese population. Longer follow-up studies with higher doses of retinol and zinc are needed to examine the effects on regression of precancerous lesions of the esophagus. Zinc deficiency in animals results in low plasma vitamin A levels despite adequate dietary vitamin A, but the situation in humans is unclear (Smith, 1980). Also in animals riboflavin deficiency produces squamous metaplasia of the esophageal epithelium, so that further studies in high-risk areas such as Iran should consider interactions between dietary deficiencies and local exposures including hot tea consumption (Ghadirian et al., 1988).

Although differences in prevalence of heavy alcohol consumption and smoking may help to explain U.S. black–white differences in esophageal cancer incidence and mortality rates, the role of dietary differences is unclear. Median dietary vitamin A intakes, and median intakes expressed as percent of the dietary standard, were somewhat lower in black than white adults in some age groups in the NHANES (see Chapter 4) (Abraham et al., 1977).

Thus esophageal cancer risk may be associated with nutritional deficiencies that commonly occur in different areas such as China and parts of Africa (Cook-Mozaffari, 1986), and hence are associated with racial/ethnic groups living in these areas, as well as local factors related to cultural practices such as hot teas (as well as alcohol and tobacco habits).

Stomach. Studies of dietary factors in gastric cancers have implicated specific dietary constituents in the progression from precursor lesions to overt cancer. Intestinal metaplasia, the precursor to gastric cancer, has been linked to consumption of dried salted fish and low vitamin A intake (Nomura et al., 1982). Migrant studies in the United States and Australia suggest that dietary habits in early life may be important in the retention of higher stomach cancer rates in certain racial/ethnic groups. Retention of the habit of high salt intake may be involved in the maintenance of high rates of stomach cancer among Japanese immigrants and their descendants in Los Angeles (Shimizu et al., 1987). In Australia, migrants from higher-risk areas such as Greece retain their higher stomach cancer rates (McMichael and Giles, 1988). Again the independent influence of SES and sociocultural factors in influencing dietary habits is unclear.

An important observation is the continued higher mortality rates for stomach cancer in U.S. Chinese versus whites, although the stomach cancer mortality rate in the homeland area (i.e., Guangdong Province) was lower than that for other provinces in China (King et al., 1985b). Also noteworthy is the finding, in a regional survey of salt excretion and blood pressure in China, that both males and females from the Guangdong region had the lowest average urinary sodium levels of all areas studied (Liu and Lai, 1986). This emphasizes the importance of data on the homeland population in the interpretation of findings from migrant studies. Within China an ecologic study showed significant statistical correlations between regional patterns of quantity of salt sold and age-adjusted mortality rates for gastric and esophageal cancer by subarea within Henan province (Lu and Qin, 1987). Although we have discussed the problems involved in interpretation of ecologic studies, these findings provide impetus for analytic studies including assessment of intake of multiple dietary constituents.

Colorectal. Worldwide variation in colorectal cancer incidence rates is considerable. Ecologic studies, usually involving one or a few dietary components, overlook the complexity of dietary factors. As with esophageal and stomach cancers, studies of histologically defined lesions that are precursors to cancer are important in colorectal cancers. High fat and low fiber intake may be associated with higher fecal bile acid concentrations, which in turn may explain racial/ethnic differences in both precursor lesions (i.e., adenomatous polyps) (Thompson, 1982) and cancers. In a case-control study in Australia, the increased risk of colorectal cancer associated with high protein intake was limited to those also consuming low fiber, and vegetable versus cereal fiber was protective (Potter and McMichael, 1986). These findings require confirmation in other populations. Comparisons across populations should be made in terms of colorectal cancer rates and proportional components of the diet. Another promising lead concerns the independent protective effect of dietary calcium intake, shown in a case-control study in Utah (Slattery et al., 1988a), which suggests the need for studies in other populations.

In contrast to stomach cancer migrant studies of colorectal cancers in the United States and other areas have indicated the importance of diet and other environmental agents operating later in life versus during childhood. An interesting apparent parallel between cardiovascular disease (Chapter 6) and colorectal cancers is seen in southern European migrants in Australia. Retention of lower rates of these chronic diseases and analysis of diets (high in fiber) in homeland countries (Greece and Italy) suggests that these migrants have brought with them a distinct dietary culture (McMichael and Giles, 1988). There were some dietary changes in these migrants and some convergence in cancer rates in longer duration-of-residence groups, but rates were still lower.

Among Japanese migrants in Los Angeles County (Table 8.5), the most striking findings were increased incidence rates for sigmoid colon and rectum in Japanese in Los Angeles County versus rates in the homeland and in U.S. whites, implicating environmental factors such as diet. In Japan colon cancer rates have been low despite relatively low fiber intake, possibly reflecting previously low (but increasing) fat consumption (Kuratsune et al., 1986).

Within American blacks the same associations between colorectal cancer and less fiber and more saturated fat intake, as also shown in some studies in whites, have been reported in a small case-control study (Dales et al., 1979). Larger-scale case-control studies are needed in blacks, as incidence rates for these cancers are increasing. In adults some dietary differences between blacks and whites are relevant to colorectal cancer risk, including lower consumption of red meat but lower intake of high-fiber foods (perhaps reflecting SES differences) (Patterson and Black, 1988). A prospective study in a low-risk group (i.e., Seventh Day Adventists in California) showed the usual associations with animal fat intake and a negative association with consumption of beans and lentils (Morgan et al., 1988).

The high-fiber diets, despite high protein intake, of the Finns may explain their lower colon cancer rates versus other Europeans (Weisburger et al., 1983). Known dietary factors, however, do not appear to explain differences in colorectal cancer mortality between Maoris and non-Maoris in New Zealand, where rates are highest in the world but have been decreasing among the Maori (Smith et al., 1985).

The results of studies on colorectal cancer have emphasized the complexity of analyses needed to examine multiple dietary constituents, and their possible interactions, in the etiology of colorectal cancers at various subsites in the large bowel. The U.S. National Cancer Institute is supporting several trials of beta-carotene, and vitamins C and E, in the development of colon and other cancers (Hennekens, 1986).

Finally, the independent association between level of physical activity, not confounded by dietary intake of total calories (or fats and proteins), and risk of colon cancer in Utah (Slattery et al., 1988b) provides impetus for additional descriptive and analytical studies.

Liver. The role of dietary factors in liver cancer is less clear. Aflatoxin, a fungal toxin that contaminates staple food such as peanuts in developing areas including Africa, may be carcinogenic, and a putative mechanism involves immunosuppressive effects (Enwonwu, 1984). The evidence for aflatoxin as a human carcinogen, however, is inconclusive. Preliminary studies from Africa suggested no differences in aflatoxin-B levels between hepatic cancer cases versus controls or in family contacts versus controls (Martin et al., 1985).

An *ecologic* study of aflatoxin levels and hepatic cell carcinoma (HCC) in Swaziland, an independent kingdom located between South Africa and Mozambique, merits some discussion. In Swaziland aflatoxin levels in food were measured by sampling diets in randomly selected villages in each area of the country, and prevalence of HBsAg positivity (see Chapter 6) was assessed through data on blood donors in the Blood Bank of Swaziland. HCC incidence rates were based on a cooperative arrangement with medical practitioners and on regular visits to hospitals and clinics. For 10 subregions in which data were available for all three items (i.e., aflatoxin levels in food, HBV seroprevalence, and HCC incidence), the effect of aflatoxin levels remained after controlling for HBsAg-positive prevalence

(Peers et al., 1987). The authors noted some limitations of the study, including the small number of cases (i.e., 52) distributed among the 10 subareas, lack of data on confounders such as alcohol consumption, and lack of individual data on HBV and individual exposures to aflatoxin. These problems are common in ecologic studies, which are still useful in providing a basis for more definitive studies (i.e., analytical epidemiologic studied with data on individual exposures).

Breast. Dietary and reproductive factors may explain low breast cancer risk in Finnish women (Rose et al., 1986), but these factors need to be delineated. Ecologic studies of correlations between nutritional intake and cancer death rates in various countries have suggested interesting leads. An example is the correlation between total protein and fat intake and certain cancers (including breast) in various countries (Thind, 1986). Case-control studies of recent dietary fat consumption in relation to breast cancer risk *within* a population have not been supportive. Negative findings regarding *recent* dietary fat intake and breast cancer risk (Willett et al., 1987) underscore the possibility that dietary habits early in life may be involved in associations between breast cancer and stature, as well as early age at menarche (see below), both within and between populations.

Dietary habits in early life including fat consumption may differ across populations, including U.S. blacks versus whites (Nicklas et al.,), and these differences may be important in the development of breast cancer. As with cardiovascular diseases, the amount of dietary variation across countries is great, whereas within countries, variation is smaller and intraindividual variation in diet is a problem.

Other sites. With regard to *nasopharyngeal* carcinoma (NPC), Hong Kong Chinese have the highest known rates (see Table 8.10), and 90 percent of cancers may be attributable to childhood consumption of salted fish (Yu et al., 1986). In Guangxi Province of southern mainland China, a case-control study also showed significant associations between NPC and early-childhood intake of salted food items (e.g., fish, duck eggs, and mustard greens) (Yu et al., 1988). Thus population differences in consumption of certain salted food, especially during early life, may help to explain differences in NPC incidence, although the separate roles of SES and cultural factors in explaining dietary differences have not been explored. Interactions between Epstein-Barr virus (EBV) exposure (discussed earlier) and nitrosamines may be important in certain high-risk areas such as Tunisia, Greenland, and South China, and again SES factors may underlie some of these differences in EBV prevalence. In an unpublished anthropological study in Tunisia, South China and Greenland, comparable groups of preserved foodstuffs were consumed, and subsequent chemical analyses revealed detectable amounts of nitrosamines in food items frequently consumed in these areas (Poirier et al., 1987). Genetic (HLA-associated) factors may also modulate susceptibility in these high-risk populations (see later).

Prostatic cancer in males may involve both dietary and reproductive factors, differences which in turn may explain high rates of this cancer in such groups as U.S. blacks (see earlier) in San Francisco and New Jersey (Thind et al., 1982). A small case-control study of prostatic cancer in U.S. blacks implicated dietary factors including higher vitamin A consumption (Heshmat, 1985), but larger-scale studies are needed. As noted earlier, dietary intake of vitamin A in the United States is not higher in blacks than whites, so this factor may operate to increase risk *within* populations, but differences in rates between blacks and whites are not explained (see Chapter 1 for methodologic considerations in comparing studies). The National Cancer Institute is supporting research in this area of frequent cancer sites in U.S. blacks. Obesity has been associated with prostatic cancer risk, and population of racial/ethnic differences in obesity must be considered (see later).

In a case-control study of Japanese in Kyoto (Ohno et al., 1988), estimated dietary intake of both vitamin A and beta-carotene (its precursor) were *protective* against prostatic cancer (Ohno et al., 1988). A hypothesis offered involves both dose-response considerations and interaction with fat intake. That is, very high dietary intake of vitamin A, estimated at three to four times higher in certain urban U.S. populations versus Japanese groups, and the high average intake of fat in the United States (i.e., about a twofold difference) may explain the higher rates of prostatic cancer in the United States (Ohno et al., 1988). As noted earlier (Chapter 1), comparisons of studies of populations may be affected both by population differences in the distribution of risk factors and by the dose response pattern. Further studies are needed to determine if very high levels of vitamin A intake, modulated by higher fat intake, increase susceptibility to prostatic cancer, and if moderate levels are protective. Thus, prostatic cancer is another example of the need to considerable multiple dietary constituents in examination of cancer risk and in explaining population differences in rates.

Cooking practices have not been mentioned, but may contribute to exposure to various carcinogenic agents such as nitrosamines. As discussed earlier, the explanation for higher rates of lung cancer (especially adenocarcinomas) in Chinese females in various areas may involve exposure to passive smoking and previous tuberculosis. Another contributing factor may be exposure to cooking oil vapors, as suggested by a case-control study using the Shanghai Cancer Registry (Gao et al., 1987).

Work Environment

The percentage of worldwide variation in cancer incidence rates related to occupational exposures is probably small, but some of these exposures may be modifiable, and hence excess cancer risks can be reduced. Lung cancer in non-smoking Navajo males working in uranium mines in the U.S. Southwest is largely attributable to their hazardous occupation. Although radiation exposure has been reduced, workers exposed in the 1950s will continue to develop lung cancer (Samet et al., 1984).

In a population-based study of adenocarcinoma of the stomach in Los Angeles County, California, the highest risks from dust exposure were observed in blacks versus whites and Asians (Wright et al., 1988). Various types of dusts have been implicated in the causation of stomach cancers. Mortality rates from cancer of the stomach are high among South African "coloureds," and rates are more than doubled in areas where exposure to the crocidolite variety of asbestos occurs due to occupational and/or environmental contamination (Botha et al., 1986). The role of occupational exposures in disease in South Africa has been discussed elsewhere (WHO, 1983; Parry, 1984). The effects of occupation on cancer risks should be separated from life style or urbanization influences, as suggested by a study of other chronic diseases in Nigerian civil servants and policemen (Idahosa, 1987).

The relation between occupation and bladder cancer was compared in epidemiologic studies in Boston (Massachusetts), Manchester (U.K.), and Nagoya (Japan), and the lack of associations in Japan may reflect differences in exposures to hazardous agents involved in jobs with the same titles as those in other countries (Morrison et al., 1985). In Hong Kong, previously reported associations between nasal cavity cancers and several occupations (e.g., textile working, fishing) were confirmed (Ng, 1986), indicating the general role of environmental exposures in this cancer. Logan (1982) compared data on cancer mortality for 25 sites in England and Wales (1851–1971) by occupational group with studies from other countries, but the confounding effect of socioeconomic status was not considered. Additional international and interethnic comparisons of occupation–disease associations should be made.

Body Constitution

As we have noted, studies within a population can assess the influence of certain risk factors occurring within the range of variation exhibited by that population. In a prospective follow-up study of the U.S. NHANES I population sample, originally studied (including stature and sitting height) in 1971–75 and then followed to 1982–84, stature was positively associated with breast cancer in women, after adjustment for cigarette use and body mass index (Albanes et al., 1988). Dose-response relationships were unclear, and a threshold effect predominated for most cancer sites, with persons in the lowest quartile for stature having the lowest cancer risk. One hypothesis involves nutritional factors influencing growth and development in early life (Albanes et al., 1988).

Population differences in height of women have been associated with differences in breast cancer risk, as shown in the early studies of F. DeWaard and in comparisons across various populations and racial/ethnic groups (reviewed by Micozzi, 1985). The populations with shortest stature such as Japan, India, and other Far Eastern groups have lowest incidence rates for breast cancer. The factors underlying these population differences in height, such as maturational/hormonal factors influenced by dietary habits early in life, require further study. Studies of sociocultural and socioeconomic factors and their interactions in determining specific dietary habits, such as intake of fats, proteins, and total calories, *early in life* in different ethnic groups should prove rewarding.

Adult body weight is influenced by genetic and environmental factors, the latter including diet and physical activity throughout the lifespan. Genetic factors and dietary changes have probably interacted in producing high rates of various cancers such as gallbladder cancer in Amerindians.

Characteristics of menarche and menopause. Within most populations studied, earlier age at menarche is associated with increased risk of breast cancer, especially (or only) in premenopausal women. A large case-control study of U.S. blacks, for example, found an association between early age at menarche and breast cancer *within* this race (Schatzkin et al., 1987). The underlying biological mechanism for the association between earlier age at menarche and increased risk of breast cancer has been much debated. Briefly, higher urinary estrogens in adolescents are associated with earlier menarche (MacMahon et al., 1982), and lower plasma concentration of sex-binding hormone (which binds estrogen) in premenopausal women who have had an early menarche also may be involved in increasing the amount of estrogen available to breast tissue and hence increasing the risk of breast cancer (Moore et al., 1987).

We have noted the considerable worldwide variation in age at menarche including a north–south cline (from later to earlier ages) in Europe and later ages in certain circumpolar groups. Factors underlying racial/ethnic differences in age at menarche are uncertain but may involve past adaptation to unknown environmental influences and/or interactions between SES and environmental factors related to dietary habits early in life. Among South African Bantu girls, for example, later average age at menarche (vs. whites) could reflect inadequate nutrition, which could in turn help to explain their relatively low incidence rates for breast cancer (Hill et al., 1980).

Differences in breast cancer risk between populations by age at diagnosis of cancer have been examined in relation to age at menarche in various populations including black populations, Maoris in New Zealand, and various Japanese and Caucasian groups (Micozzi, 1985). In New Zealand, for example, Maori women have earlier age at menarche and higher breast cancer incidence rates than Europeans, irrespective of SES. With regard to U.S. black–white differences in premenopausal breast cancer, the slightly earlier mean age at menarche among blacks could be a factor (Gray et al., 1980). Specifically, the earlier average age at menarche in U.S. blacks could play a role in black–white differences in the incidence of premenopausal breast cancer. The importance of this factor is uncertain because of temporal changes in relative incidence of breast cancer among younger black and white women (Austin et al., 1979).

Within Europe, comparative studies are needed on breast cancer incidence rates, especially among premenopausal women, in northern and southern countries, including population data, on age at menarche. Methodologically, we have noted that the ability to detect an association between a variable such as age at menarche is related to the range of variation within the population and the underlying dose-response relationship between the variable and risk of the disease under study, as well as the sample sizes available for study. In a case control study of breast cancer in southern Europe (i.e., Palermo, Sicily), the tendency toward early menarche in the population, with 40 percent having menarche before or at age 12 years, was noted as a possible explanation for the lack of a *statistically significant* association between age at menarche (i.e., 11–15 and 15+ years vs. <11 years) (Brignone et al., 1987). There was a clear trend toward an association, however, with lower odds ratios in the later age at menarche groups than the <11-year group (used as a reference for calculation of odds ratios). In a northern Italy case-control study, menarche before age 15 was more common among cases, but there was no trend in risk with decreasing age at menarche, thus suggesting a possible threshold effect (i.e., at or around age 15 years) (La Vecchia et al., 1987).

The relationship between body weight or obesity and age at menarche is complex and incompletely understood. In most populations, risk of premenopausal breast cancer is associated with earlier age at menarche, while postmenopausal breast cancer has been associated with greater body weight (or body mass index). A possible exception has been reported in a case-control study from northern Italy in which higher body weight was related to risk of premenopausal cancer (La Vecchia et al., 1987), but further studies are needed. The common underlying model involving all of these risk factors in breast cancer is estrogen level, since in postmenopausal women most available estrogen is derived from conversion of precursors in peripheral body fat.

In contrast to breast cancer, risk of the rare cancer choriocarcinoma has been positively associated with later age at menarche in a case-control study comprised of cases from several U.S. areas, which is one observation providing a basis for the low estrogen hypothesis (Buckley et al., 1988). Thus, higher rates for this cancer in some areas, such as Japan, could be related to differences in average age at menarche (which tends to be later in some parts of Japan) (MacMahon et al., 1982), along with other reproductive variables.

Skeletal growth rates. U.S. black–white differences in skeletal growth rates, especially in stature and length of long bones, during childhood and adolescence have been suggested as one factor explaining higher age-specific incidence rates for osteosarcoma in black versus white adolescents (Huvos et al., 1981; Polednak, 1985). In one study in New York State, osteosarcoma incidence rates in persons under age 20 years were twice as high in blacks as in whites for the leg (i.e., 0.46 vs. 0.23 per 100,000 per year) but not for the arm (Polednak, 1985). Black–white differences in body proportions, including longer length relative to trunk length (or sitting height), are well known to physical anthropologists, although U.S. and African blacks also differ in these ratios (Hamill et al., 1973; Eveleth, 1978). These racial differences may in turn reflect, in part, differential growth rates that may involve hormonal factors related to environmental (i.e., dietary) factors or genetic differences.

In Mexican-Americans, trunk length is similar to that in Anglos (Malina et al., 1987), but data on osteosarcoma incidence rates in Mexican-American adolescents have not been reported. The only data on bone cancer incidence are for Puerto Rico, where osteosarcoma incidence rates during childhood (i.e., <20 years) were similar to those for whites in the United States, while rates were higher in black children (Spitz et al., 1987), as reported in other studies.

Other anthropometric and morphologic variation. Anthropometric variation in the nasal passages, including frequency of septal deformities, among ethnic groups has been proposed as a factor influencing the attachment of carcinogens to the nasopharyngeal mucosa and the risk of nasopharyngeal cancer (e.g., among Chinese groups) (Clifford, 1967; Preston-Martin et al., 1982). Apparently, there have been no anthropometric studies to explore this hypothesis (Shanmugaratnam, 1982). American-born Chinese have been shown to differ from Chinese-born immigrants in anthropometric features of the nose and face (Lasker, 1946). Theoretically, such differences could be related to risk of nasopharyngeal cancer in these groups, and this should be explored.

Benign prostatic hyperplasia (BPH) or enlargement is more frequent in Jewish populations including U.S. Ashkenazic Jews in the U.S. than non-Jews, and less prevalent in Japanese and other Orientals than whites (Glynn et al., 1985). The relationship between BPH and subsequent prostatic carcinoma is uncertain (Greenwald, 1982). Jewish populations do not tend to have higher incidence rates for prostatic cancer, and higher rates occur among Chinese both in Shanghai and in the United States.

Physiological characteristics. Higher *serum testosterone* levels in U.S. black than white males may be a factor in the high rates for prostatic cancer in U.S. blacks (see Table 3.6) (Ross et al., 1986). The role of testosterone in prostatic cancer is uncertain, but increased metabolism of testosterone to estrogen in prostatic cancer patients may provide a clue (Level et al., 1985; Meikle et al., 1986). Early-stage or latent prostatic cancers were more common in U.S. blacks than whites at autopsy; many of these cancers were small and apparently lacked the promotional stimuli, perhaps hormonal in nature, required to produce invasive or clinically apparent cancers (Guileyardo et al., 1980). The increasing rates of prostatic cancer in U.S. blacks in recent decades could reflect hormonal stimulation related to dietary changes (see later).

African blacks have lower testosterone levels and lower risk of prostate cancer than U.S. blacks. Thus, genetic factors have been suggested as underlying the U.S. black–white differences in testosterone, since U.S. and African blacks differ genetically (see Chapter 3). Dietary factors, however, require exploration within U.S. blacks (Heshmat et al., 1985) and in explaining U.S. black–white differences in prostate cancer—including the increasing rate among blacks in recent decades (see earlier). Similarly, dietary differences between U.S. and African blacks could be involved in the apparent differences in risk of prostatic cancer.

The higher proportion of estrogen receptor-negative versus -positive breast cancers among U.S. black versus white women found in some studies is apparently not due to differences in age or tumor characteristics, but further studies are needed to determine the explanation for these differences (Stanford et al., 1987). Whatever the underlying mechanism, estrogen receptor-negative cancers are associated with poorer response to therapy and poorer survival; thus black–white differences in receptor status could contribute to differences in breast cancer survival (described earlier).

Genetics

Approaches to the epidemiologic study of the role of genetic differences in explaining population differences in disease rates have been outlined (see Chapter 2). Consistently low rates of Ewing's sarcoma in blacks both in Africa and in the United States suggest the possible role of common underlying genetic factors, although the great genetic heterogeneity within groups in Africa and the genetic differences between U.S. blacks and their ancestral African populations must be recalled (Chapter 3).

The present discussion includes skin pigmentation, blood groups, HLA types, other genetic factors, and results of studies on degree of genetic admixture in relation to disease. Also included is a discussion of the search for genetic heterogeneity in a specific cancer site, as discussed earlier with reference to other disease categories.

Pigmentation. Although genetic factors are involved, the inheritance of human skin and eye color is complex and poorly understood (Byard, 1981). The evolutionary basis for population differences in degree of skin pigmentation, in terms of natural selection, has long intrigued physical anthropologists. The major factor involves selection pressure (albeit weak) related to the protection against skin cancers (both melanoma and nonmelanoma) afforded by dark skin. Other, more speculative hypotheses involve prevention by dark skin of breakdown (photolysis) of light-sensitive vitamins and nutrients (Branda and Eaton, 1978) and protection against infection (Wassermann, 1965; Polednak, 1974, 1987a).

Differences in amount or distribution of melanin in the layers of the skin are a major factor in explaining racial/ethnic differences in risk of skin cancers, including both melanoma and nonmelanoma types. Low rates for melanoma among various black populations are well known (see earlier). The occurrence of melanomas on the soles of the feet in blacks and other groups, however, requires explanation. The frequency of melanomas in various ethnic groups in Bombay, India, appears to be associated with skin color (Jussawalla et al., 1985), although confounding factors should be considered. In India, where lower social class may be associated with darker skin color, biases in detection of melanoma related to SES (i.e., less frequent diagnosis in lower-SES groups) might be involved.

Southern European and Mediterranean countries (e.g., Spain and Malta) generally have lower incidence rates for skin melanoma than northern European countries, and lower rates have been reported in southern than northern Italy, presumably reflecting differences in amount of skin pigmentation (Cristofolini et al., 1987). Within lower-risk countries such as Spain, the well-known age-related increase in risk also occurs, along with the predilection for sun-exposed areas including the lower limbs in females and the trunk in males (Petrelli et al., 1985).

The rarity of melanomas in the uveal tract of the eye in blacks and other more heavily pigmented races such as the Japanese (Hyman et al., 1987) supports the possible role of sunlight in the etiology of these cancers.

Blood groups. Population differences in rates of a variety of infectious and chronic diseases may be related in small part to differences in blood group frequencies as well as to other genetic differences (see HLA-related diseases, discussed below). Blood group A has been associated with *stomach cancer*, but the increased risk is small—about 1.21 for A versus O and 1.04 for B versus O (Mourant et al., 1978). This association has not been found in a case-control study of Japanese (Hirayama, 1986), who have the highest known rates for this cancer (see above), which could simply reflect the difficulty in detecting small excess risks. The contribution of population differences in group A frequency, which is highest in Scandinavia as well as certain Amerindian tribes, to racial/ethnic variation in stomach cancer incidence is probably small, although there are apparently no studies of possible interactions with other risk factors such as diet. Other ABO–cancer associations include *ovarian cancer* and blood group O

(Bjorkholm, 1984) which is common in northwest Europe (Table 3.3) where ovarian cancer is also common (especially in Sweden and Denmark). The relevance of such associations to racial/ethnic differences in cancer rates is obscure because of the overwhelming influence of other risk factors; multivariate analyses are needed.

HLA types. The high rates of nasopharyngeal cancer in southern Chinese have been cited as a possible indication of a genetic factor (Muir, 1971). Dietary habits, however, may be related to degree of Chinese admixture. Although related genetically with southern Chinese, Thailand also shares dietary similarities with China—for example, salted fish (called "plara" in Thailand). The high risk of adenocarcinoma of lung in Chinese females may suggest a genetic factor, but several environmental factors explain at least part of the excess risk (i.e., tuberculosis and passive smoking). Future case-control studies in these areas should include specific genetic factors (e.g., HLA types) along with other risk factors.

The role of HLA genes in susceptibility to cancers, and population comparisons of associations between specific cancer and HLA types, has received attention only recently (Tiwari and Terasaki, 1985). HLA-associated factors may influence susceptibility to nasopharyngeal cancer. High-risk ethnic groups such as Chinese and midrange groups such as Malays show the same HLA-B17 antigen association (Chan et al., 1985). This is a promising area for research, especially for cancers involving infectious agents and host immune responses. Unlike blood group associations, for which mechanisms may be more obscure (e.g., genetic linkage or pleiotropism of blood group genes), the role of HLA genes in immune responses suggests more direct mechanisms whereby differences in genetic constitution could affect disease susceptibility.

HLA associations with AIDS, which includes Kaposi's sarcoma (KS) as one manifestation or clinical criterion, were discussed in Chapter 6. An association between KS and HLA DR5 has been reported in several studies, based on small sample sizes, including a case-control study in Italy (Scorza Smeraldi et al., 1986) (Table 8.16). In a study of endemic (vs. AIDS-related) KS in Central Africa (i.e., eastern Zaire), it was stated that this association could not be confirmed (using the yardstick of statistical significance) in a case control study using controls matched by tribe (Melbye et al., 1987). As shown in Table 8.16, however, the direction of the difference was as expected from other studies. The frequency of DR5 in the controls was similar to that reported for some African populations such as Nigerians (Table 3.4).

Table 8.16 Comparison of Case-Control Studies on the Association Between HLA-DR5 and Kaposi's Sarcoma (KS)

HLA Phenotype	Italy		Central Africa	
	AIDS/KS	Controls	KS	Controls
DR5	5/7 (71%)	36/105 (34%)	8/20 (40%)	6/22 (27%)

Data from Scorza Smeraldi et al. (1986) and Melbye et al. (1987).

We have noted that classical or endemic KS differs from HIV virus-associated KS in certain clinical features. The lack of a statistically significant association with KS and DR5 within Zaire, if not simply a chance finding not reaching the conventional level of "statistical significance," could indicate an etiological difference. Although the pathology and pathogeneis of both forms of KS are uncertain, the association with immunosuppression may not be strong for classical endemic KS, and therefore the association with HLA types may be different. Population differences in the HIV-associated KS, however, could be due in part to differences in HLA frequencies, since the DR5 phenotype is more common in certain African populations, especially in comparison with Asian groups (Table 3.4).

With the flowering of population genetic studies of various polymorphisms in blood groups and serum proteins, other disease associations are emerging. One example concerns alpha-1 antitrypsin or protease inhibitor (Pi) (see Chapter 3). In a case-control study in north Germany, a significant positive association between bladder cancer and the PiZ allele was reported, as shown in other studies of this cancer (as well as certain other cancers) (Benkmann et al., 1987). Isoelectric focusing techniques (Chapter 3) have permitted distinctions in the PiM variants (i.e., M1–M4), and in the north German study M3 was negatively associated with bladder cancer risk. As more population data on frequencies of Pi polymorphisms are reported (Hjalmarrson, 1988), variation between populations can be considered in relation to incidence rates for specific cancers.

Genetic–environmental interactions should be explored with regard to ethnic differences in choriocarcinoma and hydatidiform mole in Zhuang and Mongolians versus the predominant ethnic group (the Han). These latter ethnic groups in China were discussed in Chapter 3. Thus, further studies are needed on genetic factors, such as ABO blood groups and HLA types, along with socioeconomic and dietary variables in these ethnic groups in China.

Family studies of a specific cancer in different populations. Relatively few comparsions have been made across studies of different populations or racial/ethnic groups regarding the strength of the association between family history of a specific cancer and risk of that cancer. Differences between populations in this association could indicate heterogeneity of causation.

The incidence rate of colon cancer in Israel is higher by a factor of about 2.5 among Ashkenazi or European than non-European (i.e., Oriental and Sephardic) Jews. In contrast, the odds ratio of colon cancer is greater for family members of non-Ashkenazi than Ashkenazi colon cancer patients, or prospectively the increase in risk of screening-detected colorectal neoplasia (i.e., tumors) is greater for non-European-origin than European-origin first-degree relatives of colorectal cancer patients. The role of SES differences between the two ethnic categories, however, is uncertain (Rozen et al., 1987). Higher SES in Ashkenazi than non-Ashkenazi groups might explain the higher colorectal cancer rates in the former, but the higher risk of colorectal cancer among non-Ashkenazi than Ashkenazi family history-positive persons is difficult to explain. The relative roles of genetic versus environmental factors (including familial shared environment) may differ between the two groups.

In the Mexican-American population of Texas, at low risk for colorectal cancer relative to Anglos, no evidence for increased risk among relatives of colorectal cancer cases was detected (Weiss et al., 1986). A major question concerns the *expression* of familial risk. In studies using only clinically diagnosed cancers or cancers mentioned on death certificates, *susceptibility* related to family history of cancer is incompletely assessed. In the Mormon population of Utah, extensive surveillance (by proctoscopic examinations) of family members of colorectal cancer cases, in order to detect tumors as yet clinically silent, has shown evidence for strong familiality most consistent (statistically) with a dominant mode of inheritance (Burt et al., 1985). The Mormon population is at intermediate risk of colorectal cancer relative to certain Hispanic groups (with lower risk) and non-Mormon Anglos (with higher risk). Although such surveillance studies are difficult to carry out, comparative studies in other populations would be useful in assessing the relative importance of familial (possibly genetic) factors in different populations. Alternatively, a genetic or biochemical marker for the presence of neoplasm or precursor lesion could be used in such studies, obviating the need for more invasive procedures such as proctoscopy.

The report of an absence of association between breast cancer risk and family history of the disease in a case control study in a southern Italian study (Brignone et al., 1987) but a positive association in a northern Italian study (La Vecchia et al., 1987) requires examination. The possibility that family history of cancer might be concealed for sociocultural reasons in Sicily was mentioned (Brignone et al., 1987), but such an underreporting bias would have to be stronger in cases than in controls in order to produce the lack of association (if one indeed existed); inaccuracies in reporting, or misclassification of family-history status, could obscure a real association. Future studies should involve validation of positive family histories and also at least a sample of ostensibly negative histories.

Studies of degree of racial admixture. The reader should recall, from the discussion of cardiovascular diseases, that confounding of skin color (one characteristic used in assessing racial intermixture) with SES or social status complicates the interpretation of studies. Studies of associations between degree of admixture, however assessed, could also be influenced by confounding variables related to both degree of admixture and the disease under study (see Chapter 1 for explanation of confounding). Petrakis (1971) showed a correlation between estimated degree of genetic admixture, based on gene frequencies, in several U.S. black populations and breast cancer incidence rates. More detailed studies of specific cancers should consider known risk factors in a multivariate approach in case-control studies.

Acute lymphocytic leukemia (ALL) in childhood, less common in U.S. blacks than whites (see above), shows the same associations between HLA and other genetic markers (i.e., factor B or Bf) in both races. This has suggested the possible role of admixture in explaining the higher rates in U.S. blacks than in African blacks (Budowle et al., 1985). Studies on degree of admixture in ALL cases and controls are needed to explore this speculative hypothesis. Other hypotheses would involve exposure to environmental factors involved in the etiology of ALL in the United States that are not found or are rarer in Africa.

Unfortunately, little is known about risk factors for childhood leukemia, aside from ionizing radiation exposure, although associations with chemical exposures have been suggested.

CONCLUSIONS

Ostensibly, worldwide variation is considerable for most cancer sites, and more data are available on racial/ethnic differences within or across countries for cancer than for other diseases. Such variation must be in part real, especially for incidence data based on population-based cancer registries, and implicates the importance of environmental factors, as supported by ecologic studies and (especially) migrant studies. The major known environmental factors are smoking, alcohol, diet, and infectious diseases. Similarly high incidence rates for certain cancers in widely divergent racial/ethnic groups also implicate environmental factors that may be common. An example is nasopharyngeal cancer, where common exposure to Epstein-Barr virus and specific dietary factors (e.g., nitrosamines and salty foods), has been strongly implicated by separate case-control studies in high-risk areas (Poirier et al., 1987).

Differing habits involving smoking and chewing of tobacco products are a major explanation for worldwide variation in several cancer sites. Although the independent effects of SES and sociocultural factors have not been studied, cultural factors probably play a role in variation in rates of tobacco use in such diverse groups as Jewish, other religious groups (e.g., Mormons and Seventh Day Adventists), Indian populations, and various racial/ethnic groups in the Far East. The dissemination of smoking in the Third World and in China will have a major impact on worldwide cancer patterns.

Much of the variation in cancer incidence and mortality rates is related to underlying differences in infectious diseases (Chapter 6), which in turn reflect largely socioeconomic, ecologic, and climatic factors rather than factors directly associated with racial/ethnic groups. Examples are Epstein-Barr virus (and possibly malaria), determined largely ecologic/climatic factors, which strongly influence the distribution of Burkitt's lymphoma, and probably nasopharyngeal cancer. Degree of crowding, reflecting largely SES differences (Chapter 6), is important in transmission of hepatitis B (a major determinant of liver cancer), tuberculosis (involved in lung cancer in some groups), and leprosy (which may be involved in susceptibility to cancers).

Sociocultural factors, however, are also involved in explaining the distribution of these infectious diseases and hence in influencing cancer rates. This also holds for cancers related to the human immunodeficiency viruses and for viruses related to cervical cancer. An important research question, however, is the independent effects of SES and sociocultural factors in determining these differences in risk of infectious diseases and hence in risks of certain cancers. The practical implications of this question concern the planning of public health programs, including education, which may be targeted to certain SES groups and/or cultural groups.

An increasing number of case-control studies of specific cancers are appearing in diverse populations worldwide. This permits comparisons of the relative importance of specific risk factors across racial/ethnic groups. Problems of comparability of data and statistical interpretation are considerable. The question of causal heterogeneity of specific cancers, including genetic heterogeneity, is an interesting one. Planning of cancer control programs, with regard to primary prevention, may need to recognize heterogeneity. The importance of considering histologic type of cancer and differing roles for specific environmental and genetic factors is evident for such cancers as stomach, liver, lung, and nasopharynx. Causal heterogeneity may include differing roles for dietary constituents versus other environmental factors (e.g., infectious agents and alcohol) for the same cancer in different populations.

The expansion of population genetics, with increasing rates of discovery of new polymorphisms, has increased interest in studying associations between specific genetic factors and specific cancers. Study designs may be both descriptive, comparing population frequencies in the associated genetic factors and the cancer site of interest, and analytic, assessing the consistency of specific associations (e.g., between HLA-DR5 and Kaposi's sarcoma) across populations. Genetic heterogeneity for a specific cancer is difficult to demonstrate because of statistical problems, as well as heterogeneity in the disease category itself (e.g., endemic vs. HIV virus-associated KS).

Prospective studies are needed on specific cancers, similar to those on cardiovascular diseases in Japanese in Hawaii and Japan (Chapter 7). The relative rarity of specific cancers would necessitate large sample sizes. Meanwhile useful approaches include studies such as the comparison of incidence rates in different groups in Los Angeles County, including migrants, with rates in the homeland (Shimizu et al., 1987). The latter study points out the potential value of this approach. The complexity of disease patterns, however, also indicates the need for more detailed studies which include information on age at migration and dietary habits through entire lifetimes. A planned prospective study of cancers in the diverse migrant populations of Australia will include dietary information (McMichael and Giles, 1988).

The important linkage between the epidemiology of infectious and chronic diseases is evident for cancers, and the implications for prevention programs are obvious. Worldwide efforts in hepatitis B control, as described in Chapter 6, should have an impact on incidence and mortality rates for primary liver cancer in high-risk populations, although the challenge is great in Africa and Asia. For other major cancers, however, important environmental measures for *primary* prevention in high-risk groups will involve dietary modifications (e.g., for stomach cancer and colorectal cancers), which may require overcoming cultural barriers (e.g., in parts of Japan, where *secondary* prevention through screening has been emphasized), and changes in habits of tobacco and alcohol use that are both indigenous and acquired (through Westernization).

9

Various Chronic Disorders and Other Conditions

This chapter includes a variety of chronic conditions in the following categories: musculoskeletal system and connective tissue; metabolic diseases including diabetes mellitus; nutritional deficiencies; blood disorders; diseases of the digestive, respiratory, and nervous systems; perinatal conditions and birth defects; mental disorders; and accidents, suicides, and homicides. These diseases generally contribute more to morbidity than to mortality; exceptions are perinatal conditions and birth defects, as well as the nonnatural causes of death, which strongly affect life expectancy or years of potential life lost. Diabetes mellitus affects both morbidity and mortality, including increased cardiovascular disease mortality.

These diverse disorders exhibit contrasting patterns in various populations. Chronic musculoskeletal diseases, for example, are becoming more prevalent in Westernized and developed countries as the age distribution of the population is changing (Verbrugge, 1984). In contrast, nutritional deficiencies and related disorders are much more common in developing countries and in regions where both level of development (or SES) and availability of certain nutrients (e.g., in the soil) are low. Also certain conditions originating in the perinatal period accounted (around 1980) for about 8 percent of all deaths in developing countries in the WHO mortality data bank, versus only 1.6 percent in developed countries (Hakulinen et al., 1986). Infant mortality presents a mixed pattern, because certain minority racial/ethnic groups within developed countries have remarkably higher rates. Injury and poisoning, in contrast, show little variation in death rates for countries grouped by level of economic development. Although difficulties in diagnosis and comparability of statistics are great, some mental disorders appear to be equally common in countries differing in level of development.

Our discussion will follow, for the most part, the categories of the *International Statistical Classification of Diseases, Injuries, and Causes of Death* for conditions not discussed in previous chapters. Exceptions to the use of this classification system will be noted.

DISEASES OF THE MUSCULOSKELETAL SYSTEM AND CONNECTIVE TISSUE

Data on incidence and prevalence of bone, joint, and connective tissue diseases in racial/ethnic groups are difficult to obtain. This is due in part to low mortality rates and hence the limited utility of accurate mortality data, and diagnostic difficulties associated with many of these diseases. Thus, special population prevalence surveys are needed for accurate morbidity rate calculations.

Musculoskeletal Disorders

Population differences in musculoskeletal diseases have been reviewed extensively by Kelsey (1982). *Osteoporosis and fractures* show considerable worldwide variation in prevalence and sex ratio, and a few examples will be cited. Highest rates of *hip* fracture occur in the United States and lowest rates in Singapore and, especially, in the South African Bantu (Gallagher et al., 1980). Within the United States black–white differences in hip fracture incidence rates appear to hold only for females (Farmer et al., 1984). Although fracture rates are lower in U.S. blacks than whites in most studies, a review of cases age 60 years or older at a large urban teaching hospital disclosed that blacks had longer hospitalization and greater disability, related in part to concomitant illnesses and delays in surgery (Furstenberg and Mezey, 1987). *Forearm* fracture rates were lower among Chinese and Malays in Singapore than among Swedes in Sweden (Wong, 1965, 1966). Among patients undergoing spinal roentgenography for low pack pain in Texas, Mexican-American (i.e., Spanish-surnamed) women (but not men) had a lower prevalence of *vertebral* fracture than non-Hispanic whites (Bauer and Deyo, 1987).

Data from the U.S. National Health and Nutrition Examination Survey (NHANES), which included a detailed examination of 6,913 adults aged 25–74 years (Chapter 4), showed almost equal prevalence of some *physician-diagnosed* musculoskeletal disorders such as *osteoarthrosis* among "whites" and "all others" (Cunningham and Kelsey, 1984). Whites, however, had higher prevalence rates for *"other arthritis and rheumatism," "synovitis* and *bursitis," "disc disorder,"* and *rheumatoid arthritis.* The Health Interview Survey of 1976, involving *self-reported* data on disease (Bonham, 1978), had shown similar excesses for whites except for *arthritis,* although prevalence rates were actually higher among nonwhites in older age groups. Noteworthy was the higher prevalence of *disability* associated with these musculoskeletal impairments among nonwhites versus whites (Cunningham and Kelsey, 1984).

In an analysis of NHANES I data on 5,193 persons aged 35–74 years, the prevalence of *radiographically defined* osteoarthritis was higher in blacks (especially women) than whites. Controlling for obesity, income, education, and other confounders in a multivariate analysis did not remove the threefold excess in black women (Anderson and Felson, 1988). Hypotheses advanced were black–white differences in occupational stresses, biomechanical factors, and bone mass (see later). The "wear and tear" hypothesis of osteoarthritis was supported by the cross-sectional association between physically demanding occupations and osteoarthritis prevalence after age 54 years. Although black populations have rarely been studied radiographically, the higher prevalence of knee osteoarthritis in Jamaican blacks versus Europeans has been attributed to the habit of walking barefoot on rough roads. Further studies are needed on the role of occupational and other sources of biomechanical stress on specific joints in explaining population differences in osteoarthritis prevalence.

In contrast to U.S. whites, the Inuit (Eskimos) of Canada's Northwest Territories have a low prevalence of osteoarthritis and of rheumatoid arthritis (RA) among men, but a high prevalence of *Reiter's syndrome* (RS) and *anklyosing spondylitis* (AS) (Oen et al., 1986). RS, involving joint symptoms along with inflammation of the urethra (i.e., urethritis) and skin, is associated with chlamydiae and various bacteria (including *Campylobacter*) (see Chapter 6). A specific HLA type (i.e., HLA-B27) influences susceptibility (Thompson and Washington, 1983). AS, also known as rheumatoid spondylitis or Marie-Strumpell disease, is an inflammatory arthritis of the spine occurring mainly in young men and risk is strongly associated with HLA-B27. High frequencies of AS among various Amerindian groups are well known. Many reports of unusual frequencies of rheumatic diseases among North American Indians preceded knowledge of the association between HLA types and these diseases.

Apparent regional or population differences in arthritic diseases may reflect poor understanding of the causes of clinical syndromes. The disease previously known as "Navajo arthritis," defined in 1971, appears to be not a unique disease but a variant of either RS or AS (Rate et al., 1980). Similarly, so-called tropical arthritis in the Pacific including Papua New Guinea in some cases may actually represent arthritis of infectious or immunological origin (Scrimgeour et al., 1987). Infectious agents such as gonorrhea (Chapter 6) may be a major cause of arthritic disorders in Papua New Guinea, although RA also occurs.

RA is a chronic systemic inflammatory disease involving multiple joints, sometimes with nodules in the skin and other organs, probably due to autoimmune responses. Low prevalence rates of RA have been reported among Puerto Ricans, non-European Jews in Jerusalem, and Japanese, but methodologic and observer variation may be involved. In a case-control study of RA in Lebanon, Christian religion was more common in 100 cases than in 100 controls (i.e., 49% vs. 37%), but the difference was reportedly not statistically significant (Darwish and Armenian, 1987).

Juvenile RA or Still's disease appears to vary widely in incidence rate—from about 2.6 per 100,000 per year (U.S.) to 13.9 in Finland. Although based on hospital admissions rather than community surveys, juvenile RA, defined by criteria proposed by the American Rheumatism Association, was clinically similar in Polynesians (including Maori) and non-Polynesians in New Zealand (McGill and Gow, 1987).

Paget's disease of bone (PDB) increases in prevalence with advancing age and involves localized areas of abnormal bone metabolism leading to bizarre overgrowth of bone. Bony overgrowths impinge on nerves and may cause hearing impairment, possibly including that experienced by Beethoven. PDB requires special radiographic surveys for epidemiologic study, and is too rare to be reported frequently in health surveys such as those discussed earlier. Large-scale surveys indicate that PDB prevalence rates are much higher in Great Britain than in parts of Europe and the United States, and in the northern versus the southern United States. This suggests a role for environmental factors such as infectious agents or sunlight exposure.

On the basis of surveys of selected hospitals (Guyer and Chamberlain, 1980) and analysis of hospital admissions in New York State (Polednak, 1987b), there appears to be little difference between U.S. blacks and whites in PDB prevalence. Average length of hospital stay, appeared to be longer in blacks than whites aged 80 years or older (Polednak, 1987b), but this finding requires confirmation in other studies. If true, it fits in with a pattern of greater disability from several musculoskeletal disorders in U.S. blacks versus whites.

Various Connective Tissue Diseases

Epidemiologic study of certain rare connective tissue disorders also requires special large-scale surveys. Connective tissue diseases linked with autoimmune phenomena include *systemic lupus erythematosus* (SLE), *sarcoidosis*, and *scleroderma*. SLE is the prototype for autoimmune-related disorders involving multiple organs and tissues. In SLE, antinuclear antibodies are directed against the host's DNA, leading indirectly to injury to the skin, joints, kidneys, and other organs and tissues. Scleroderma or progressive systemic sclerosis is characterized by excessive fibrosis or collagen deposition throughout the body. Sarcoidosis is another autoimmune disorder, involving granulomas in various organs including the lung.

These diseases are more common in blacks than whites in the United States and certain other countries, but data from Africa are too limited for comparison (Table 9.1). SLE prevalence is also higher among Polynesians in Hawaii and New Zealand, and among Chinese (reviewed by Polednak, 1974, 1987a).

These and other autoimmune-related diseases are associated with HLA genes, which in turn are closely linked with the immune response gene located on the same chromosome (see later). Studies on sarcoidosis among migrants from apparently high-risk areas (e.g., Sweden) and low-risk areas (e.g., Japan) would be useful in exploring the role of environmental factors and the age at which they operate (Bresnitz and Strom, 1983).

Blacks with sarcoidosis also reportedly have more ocular disease, skin involvement, and disability than whites (Bowers, 1963). This difference was confirmed in a hospital study in London that showed more extensive and severe disease in both blacks and Asians than in Caucasians. The high frequency of eye involvement in blacks was also confirmed; hyperglobulinemia and the need for corticosteroid treatment were also more common in blacks (Edmonstone and Wilson, 1985). Differences in sarcoidosis severity among various black and white populations, including South Africans, are summarized in Table 9.2.

Table 9.1 Relative Frequencies of Certain Diseases of Connective Tissue in U.S. Blacks and Whites

Disease	Approximate black/white ratio	Type of data
Systemic lupus erythematosus (SLE)	2–3:1	Prevalence, mortality
Sarcoidosis	10:1	Incidence, mortality
Scleroderma	3:1	Prevalence, mortality

Note: For references see Polednak (1987a).

Table 9.2 Relative Severity (Highest to Lowest) of Manifestations of Sarcoidosis in Black and White Populations

London, England	South Africa
Blacks[a]	Blacks
Asians[b]	"Coloureds"
Whites	Whites

Sources: Benatar (1977), Edmonstone and Wilson (1985); see text.
[a]From the Caribbean or West Africa.
[b]From India and Pakistan

Explanations for Racial/Ethnic Differences

Errors of Measurement, Age, and Socioeconomic Status

As noted earlier, musculoskeletal and connective tissue disorders present difficulties in population comparisons in frequency, because of lack of comparability of diagnoses and the rarity of population surveys. Differences in access to medical care and diagnostic facilities strongly influence self-reported or hospital-based data. National surveys in the United States, however, have provided data on physician-diagnosed musculoskeletal disorders.

In most studies, rheumatoid arthritis (RA) is more prevalent in lower socioeconomic classes. Although RA is not more frequent in U.S. blacks than whites, comparative studies of RA by race within lower-SES groups apparently have not been conducted. Psychological factors and stressful life events may precipitate RA (Darwish and Armenian, 1987), especially in genetically susceptible persons, and the interaction between these factors and SES in each race should be explored. Osteoarthritis increases with age, with increasing "wear and tear" related to physical stress and increasing body weight. Thus, age-specific rates of disease must be compared along with habits of work and leisure activities in different groups.

Body Constitution and Diet

Since some black populations tend to have more bone to begin with, the effects of bone loss with age may be less severe. Also, there is evidence for less bone loss with age in various black populations, and possible differences in parathyroid effects on bone resorption, as reviewed elsewhere (Riggs and Melton, 1986). Such differences in bone density have often been cited to explain lower rates of osteoporosis and bone fractures in various black populations. Differences in bone density may be involved in the low fracture rates in the Bantu and in U.S. black–white differences in osteoporosis and possibly fractures. Bone density has apparently not been studied in Mexican-Americans, in relation to their reduced incidence of hip fracture (Bauer, 1988).

The causation of fractures is complex, however, and osteroporosis is not the only factor. Lower rates of hip fracture in U.S. black than white adults over age 50 years may hold only for females (Farmer et al., 1984). Lower fracture rates in black and Mexican-American females may be related in part to differences in obesity prevalence; that is, increased body fat may be protective owing to an effect of estrogen production in peripheral fat tissue, since estrogens protect against bone loss (see Polednak, 1987c). Anatomical differences in the head of femur, or the neck-shaft angle, between U.S. blacks and whites have been suggested as contributing to lower rates of hip fracture in blacks (Walensky and O'Brien, 1968).

Greater bone density may not hold for all "black" populations, according to studies of metacarpal bone density in Nigeria and South Africa (reviewed by Solomon, 1979). As noted earlier, black populations in Africa are diverse genetically and culturally. Also, qualitative differences in bone architecture may be involved in lower rates of femoral neck fractures in black populations.

Lower forearm fracture rates among Chinese in Singapore versus Sweden may be unexpected, in view of the reduced bone density of some oriental populations, presumed to be genetic in origin (Garn et al., 1969). Among Japanese in Hawaii, bone mineral content of the radius was lower than that in Caucasians (Yano et al., 1984). Body size and environmental factors such as diet and physical activity require examination as explanations, and the role of reduced bone mineral content in increased rates of osteoporosis among Japanese requires further study.

Other population differences in osteoporosis and hip fracture may involve an effect of differential calcium intake on initial bone density attained in adulthood, as suggested by a comparison of two districts in Yugoslavia (Matkovic et al., 1979). Both ancient and modern Eskimo populations of Canada and Alaska show early-adult bone loss, with mineral content lower than that of U.S. whites, possibly due to dietary factors such as low calcium intake. Despite these differences, however, symptomatic fractures may not be common in Eskimos because of large bone size and increased mechanical strength (Harper et al., 1984).

Genetic Factors

A specific HLA type (i.e., HLA-B27) is associated with ankylosing spondylitis (AS) in all populations studied. Populations with low frequency of the B27 allele, such as certain black groups and Japanese, have low prevalence rates for AS, in contrast to Amerindian groups studied. The frequency of HLA-B27 antigen is high among certain Amerindian groups, and the association with AS is demonstrable within these groups. The proportion of AS cases that are B27 positive, however, was lower among Pima Indian females and U.S. blacks than among whites or other groups (see Kelsey, 1982). The association between AS and B27 positivity may be due to linkage between the HLA gene and another gene involved in AS pathogenesis and/or to direct effects of HLA gene products.

An association between HLA-DR4 and rheumatoid arthritis (RA) has been reported in various ethnic groups, and family studies suggest linkage between susceptibility to RA and a gene in the HLA region (Tiwari and Terasaki, 1985). Ostensibly, racial/ethnic groups with high frequencies of the DR4 gene, such as Japanese and Amerindians (Table 3.4), might be expected to be at higher risk of RA. The discovery that an uncommon DR4 genetic variant, DW14, may be involved in the DR4-associated variety of rheumatoid arthritis (Nepom et al.,

1986) should lead to comparative studies of this association across populations. Heterogeneity of disease causation across populations should be explored.

Molecular DNA analyses, including use of RFLPs (Chapter 3), of HLA-D region genes shows that DR4 specificity is shared by different haplotypes and linked DQ loci. In a case-control study of Caucasians in Canada, a specific DQ variant, DQw3.1, was strongly associated with RA risk within DR4-positive persons (Singal et al., 1987). Additional case-control studies are needed in different racial/ethnic groups, again to test for heterogeneity. As further data on the frequency of this specific haplotype become available for various racial/ethnic groups, the relevance to population differences in RA can be explored.

Since HLA-DR4 has been associated with both RA and tuberculosis, it has been suggested that host immune responses to *M. tuberculosis* may be relevant to the pathogenesis of RA (Ottenhoff et al., 1986). The precise role of DR4 is unclear, however, and the hypothesis of heightened host immune response to a mycobacterial antigen in RA pathogenesis requires further exploration (Panayi, 1986).

For the connective tissue disorders discussed earlier, the differential roles of environmental factors, involving exposure to unknown precipitating agents, and possible racial differences in connective tissue responses have yet to be clarified (Polednak, 1987b). A hypothesis has been advanced that an original adaptation to infectious and parasitic diseases in tropical African environments involved connective tissue hyperresponses. These responses are evidenced by the high frequency of keloids or raised scars after traumatic skin injury, and by increased humoral immune responses (i.e., serum immunoglobulin levels). This tendency may in turn predispose to certain autoimmune disorders and connective tissue tumors in certain black populations (see Polednak, 1974, 1987a). Thus a disease constellation or syndrome of disorders might be hypothesized. Further studies are needed to identify specific environmental agents and genetic factors (if any) that might be involved in this syndrome. Racial admixture studies in these connective tissue disorders might be fruitful.

The high prevalence of SLE in Australian aborigines may be related in part to the high frequency of an inherited deficiency in a specific complement component (i.e., C4A) (Ranford et al., 1987). Human complement components of C4 are encoded by two loci which map within the HLA complex (see Chapter 3) on chromosome 6. Inherited deficiency of C4 is a risk factor in SLE. Further studies are needed on the frequency of this genetic factor in populations at higher risk for SLE.

ENDOCRINE, NUTRITIONAL, AND METABOLIC DISEASES

Diabetes Mellitus

Population and Racial/Ethnic Differences

Two types of diabetes mellitus have long been recognized clinically, and more recently in terms of their epidemiologic features. These types, called non-insulin-dependent (or formerly "adult-onset") and insulin-dependent (formerly "juvenile-onset"), differ in average age at onset, clinical features, pathogenesis, genetic risk factors, and associated environmental risk factors.

Population comparisons of the prevalence of *"adult-onset" or non-insulin-dependent diabetes mellitus* (NIDDM) and abnormal glucose tolerance are complicated by diagnostic difficulties. Special tests are needed to confirm clinical diabetes—fasting blood glucose and oral glucose tolerance tests. The reproducibility of results of glucose tolerance tests is a problem (Riccardi et al., 1985). The fasting 2-hour postglucose load tolerance test is regarded as best for detection of frank diabetes, although two high fasting plasma glucose test results are also diagnostic. Compliance with fasting may be a problem is some societies, as shown among Samoan migrants in whom only about 58 percent complied (Pawson and Janes, 1981).

Certain Asian, Pacific and Amerindian populations are at increased risk of NIDDM, on the basis of diagnostic criteria involving 2-hour postload plasma glucose level (Table 9.3) (Kirk et al., 1985). Examples include the Nauru (Fig. 3.2) of Micronesia and Pima Indians, who have the highest recorded prevalence worldwide. On the basis of plasma glucose levels 2 hours after a glucose load, certain Aleut groups (of the Pribiloff Islands) have prevalence rates of "diabetes" (i.e., 200+ mg glucose per 100 ml plasma) approaching those of the Pima Indians of Arizona (Milan, 1980). Differences in definition of diabetes, however, affect comparability of prevalence rates.

Table 9.3 Prevalence of Diabetes Mellitus in Various Adult Populations, Based on Accepted Screening Criteria

Population of racial/ethnic group	Prevalence as percent of population
Pima Indians, U.S.	35.5
Nauruans, Micronesia	30.4
Cherokee, U.S.	29.0
Japanese-American males (Washington State)	20.0
Trinidad Indians (males and females)	20–22
Fiji	
Indians	14.0
Melanesians	7.0
Trinidad, Africans (males and females)	8–15
Polynesian, W. Samoa, urban	7.0
Singapore	
Indian	6.1
Malay	2.4
Chinese	1.6
Tokyo, males	4.5
South African blacks	3.6
Polynesian, Cook Island, rural	2.4
Eskimo, U.S.	1.9
Tanzania, rural	1.1

Revised and updated after Kirk et al. (1985), Zimmet et al. (1982), individual references cited in text and other reports (McLarty, D. G. et al.: Prevalence of diabetes and impaired glucose tolerance in rural Tanzania. *Lancet* 1:871–875, 1989).

Note: Age groups may not be exactly the same for all comparisons, but some prevalence rates have been age standardized (Zimmet et al., 1982).

Mortality from diabetes apparently increased substantially among Nauruans between 1976–81 and 1982–85, probably reflecting the gradual Westernization of this population in recent decades (Schooneveldt et al., 1988). In Nauru, diabetes is the underlying cause of death in 12–17 percent of deaths among men and women and also undoubtedly contributes to cardiovascular disease mortality. In follow-up studies of diabetics in Nauru mortality is 4–4.5 times greater than in nondiabetics and is related to a variety of causes of death (Zimmet et al., 1988). Such changes in mortality are part of a general transition with Westernization, as shown for cardiovascular diseases (Chapter 7) as well as NIDDM, in diverse groups including the Maori and Australian aborigines (Thomson, 1984).

Urban–rural differences are common, as are large ethnic differences in prevalence within a single country—for example, higher rates in Indians than other groups in Fiji and Singapore, and in Maori versus Europeans in New Zealand. Studies in various Pacific populations suggest that the roles of specific risk factors, such as obesity and physical inactivity, may vary across populations so that prevention and control programs should be tailored (King et al., 1984). NIDDM appears to be common in Asian countries including the "ASEAN" group—Singapore, Indonesia, Thailand, Philippines, and Malaysia (Mustaffa, 1984). Urbanization and Westernization in these areas may lead to further increases in the prevalence of NIDDM. Thus, risk of NIDDM is influenced by several environmental factors, as well as by complex interactions with genetic factors (see below).

In Israel conflicting data have been reported on NIDDM prevalence by country-of-origin group, due in part to different screening tests and criteria for diabetes. In a survey of 4,660 workers at a plant 30–65 years of age, overall prevalence of high blood glucose levels after ingestion of 75 g carbohydrate was lower in African and Asian born (i.e., 1.2 percent) than in American and European or Israeli born (i.e., 5–5.5 percent) (Stern et al., 1988), in contrast to previous reports of higher prevalence of "diabetes" in the African or Asian born. Differences in life styles, and associated risk factors such as obesity, in the groups compared in different studies, along with use of different screening tests, may account for these discrepancies in findings. The findings of Stern et al. (1988) need to be corroborated in other samples of Asian-African Jews to determine if diabetes prevalence has indeed remained low despite their long residence (i.e., >20 years) in Israel and changes in diet after migration.

Several racial/ethnic groups in the United States have been studied with regard to prevalence of diabetes or abnormal glucose tolerance, as well as mortality. Proportional mortality ratios for "diabetes," or diabetes deaths as a proportion of all deaths, among foreign-born Chinese in New York City increased with increasing length of residence. This probably reflects acculturation or changes in life style and nutrition leading to increased prevalence of obesity (Gerber, 1984). This may also be true for Japanese-Americans (Nisei, or chiefly U.S. born) in Seattle, as discussed later.

The prevalence of NIDDM is higher among Mexican-Americans than Anglo whites (Weiss et al., 1984); the Amerindian genetic component in Mexican-Americans was noted earlier (Chapter 3). The U.S. Mortality rate from "diabetes mellitus" is higher among blacks than whites at all ages (Table 4.5). Self-reported diabetes mellitus is more frequent in blacks than whites (Table 9.4), and prevalence rates are also higher in blacks on the basis of oral glucose tolerance tests given to samples of adults (without medical history of diabetes) aged 20–74 years as part of NHANES II (in 1976–80) (Kovar et al., 1987). Data from the U.S. NHANES (Chapter 4) indicate slightly higher prevalence rates for abnormal glucose tolerance (i.e., 140–200 mg glucose per 100 ml 2 hours after a glucose load) among blacks in younger adults—that is, females aged 20–44 (14.1 percent in blacks vs. 6.5 percent in whites) (Harris, 1984) (Table 9.4).

An atypical form of NIDDM has been described among black youths, which is different from classical IDDM of youth and is not associated with HLA-DR3 or DR4 (Winter et al., 1987).

Japanese-American men in the Seattle Washington area have an estimated prevalence of 20 percent for NIDDM, which is higher than that for all U.S. males (i.e., about 10 percent) and for males in Tokyo (about 4 percent) (Fujimoto et al., 1987). The prevalence of abnormal (i.e., impaired) glucose tolerance is also high in these Japanese-Americans, who are mainly second-generation, born in the United States. Studies of diet, obesity, and exercise are needed in this group.

There is little information on NIDDM in African populations. A survey in a West African village indicated a very low prevalence despite a high-carbohydrate diet, perhaps because protein consumption was also low, and obesity and physical inactivity were rare in comparison with European populations (Teuscher et al., 1987). Similar findings were reported from rural Tanzania.

The adverse consequences of NIDDM, including retinopathy, appear to be similar in high-risk groups (i.e., Micronesians and Amerindians) versus other groups (King et al., 1983). In Mexican-Americans, however, the incidence of diabetes-related end-stage renal disease is even higher than that predicted from their excess of NIDDM and may reflect other risk factors for renal disease prevalent in Mexican-Americans, including earlier age at onset, greater severity,

Table 9.4 Prevalence of Self-Reported Diabetes and Measured Impaired Glucose Tolerance in U.S. Blacks and Whites

A. Self-reported diabetes (after Gartside et al., 1984)

				Age (years)			
45–65				65+			
White M	Black M	White F	Black F	White M	Black M	White F	Black F
5.2%	6.7%	5.6%	12.3%	9.7%	16.9%	8.9%	8.9%

B. Impaired glucose tolerance[a] (Harris, 1984)

				Age (years)			
	20–44		45–54		55–64		65–74
	White	Black	White	Black	White	Black	White	Black
Males	5.7	10.2	13.8	16.8	15.5	14.1	23.0	15.5
Females	6.5	14.1	14.4	15.7	13.9	12.0	23.3	8.7

[a]From the 1976–80 U.S. Health and Nutrition Examination Survey. Criterion was a fasting venous glucose level of <140 with a level of 140–200 mg/dl 2 h after 75-g oral glucose load.

and poorer control of diabetes (Pugh et al., 1988). In Africa there is little information on systematic follow-up of diabetics. One study from a disease registry in Zimbabwe showed a *low* frequency of gross complications, such as retinopathy and neuropathy, among patients regularly followed (Lutalo and Mabonga, 1985). Those patients followed up, however, were undoubtedly a select group, so generalization of findings is difficult. Adverse effects of alcohol consumption on survival were also reported (Lutalo and Mabonga, 1985).

Insulin-dependent diabetes mellitus (IDDM) appears to be rare in western Africa. It is relatively more common among U.S. than African blacks, and there is increasing evidence that IDDM in U.S. blacks is related to admixture with whites (see later). IDDM is especially rare among various Oriental groups, including the Japanese and probably the Chinese (Hawkins et al., 1987). The specific genetic factors (i.e., HLA types) associated with IDDM also may differ by race (see later). Although information on IDDM prevalence is lacking in South America and much of Asia, the difference between Japan and the United States (i.e., Allegheny County, Pennsylvania) in IDDM prevalence is about 18-fold, and there is an almost 37-fold difference in estimated lifetime risk for Japan versus Finland (Orchard et al., 1986). Thus the degree of worldwide variability in estimates of various measures of risk is comparable to that for NIDDM.

Although IDDM is more frequent in U.S. whites than blacks, the disease appears to be much more malignant among blacks, as reflected also in poor survival (LaPorte et al., 1986). The possible role of autoimmune processes in blacks should be considered (Polednak, 1987a) along with other factors such as those associated with socioeconomic status.

Explanations for Racial/Ethnic Differences

Errors of measurement, age, and socioeconomic status. We have noted the problems involved in comparing results of surveys for "diabetes mellitus" due to differences in screening tests used and definitions of prevalence. Field studies of diabetes in various populations require use of screening tests that are less valid than those involved in standardized criteria, because of unavailability of laboratory facilities and noncompliance with fasting. Age and sex differences in prevalence necessitate either standardization of prevalence rates or use of age-specific rates. Prevalence rates are generally higher in lower-SES groups, but few studies have considered SES differences in comparing prevalence rates in different populations.

Body constitution. SES is related to prevalence of obesity, as noted earlier. The finding of higher prevalence of diabetes and impaired glucose tolerance in young adult U.S. black versus white females is of interest in view of the higher prevalence of obesity among young black versus white women and the association between obesity and NIDDM. In the Second Health and Nutrition Examination Survey (HANES II), the prevalence of self-reported diabetes mellitus was higher in blacks than whites of both sexes except for persons over 65 years of age; black–white differences in the prevalence of overt weight and obesity are greatest in young adults and lowest at older ages. Programs of increased physical activity in young adult black females could be important in obesity prevention and control, but decreasing caloric intake may be a less important objective, because total caloric intake may not be higher in adult female blacks than whites in the United States (Gartside et al., 1984). In contrast, among Zuni Indians, both decreasing caloric intake and increasing exercise level have been effective in controlling the disease in diabetics.

Even after adjustment for increased body fat, especially abdominal fat, prevalence rates in Mexican-Americans for NIDDM are about twice as high as in Anglo whites (Weiss et al., 1984; Haffner et al., 1986a). Thus, Mexican-Americans are similar to other high-risk groups such as Amerindians and Micronesians, who also have more hyperinsulinemia than can be explained by their adiposity (Haffner et al., 1986a, b). Insulin resistance may be a major factor in the pathogenesis of NIDDM in these groups (Kahn, 1986). Both obesity and genetic factors may contribute to insulin resistance, which could lead to oversecretion of insulin by the pancreas and eventual depletion of insulin. Reduced hepatic extraction of insulin and increased secretion of insulin are other proposed models, and prospective epidemiologic studies are needed on these mechanisms. Genetic factors in NIDDM are discussed below.

Whatever the mechanisms involved in the increased risk of NIDDM among certain ethnic groups, the results of the Zuni Diabetes Project show that life style modification including decreased caloric intake and increased aerobic exercise can be effective in secondary prevention (i.e., control of the disease among patients) and perhaps in primary prevention or prevention of disease onset (Leonard et al., 1986). The program of life style change adopted in the Zuni Project may serve as a model for other areas in that cultural factors, including preservation of the heritage of a grueling foot race, were incorporated in the community program which resulted in weight loss and withdrawal from medication for some diabetic participants (Leonard et al., 1987). In other populations, such as U.S. blacks, cultural perceptions of overweight and obesity should be considered; the paucity of cross-cultural comparisons has been noted (Chapter 2).

Genetic factors. Insulin-dependent diabetes mellitus (IDDM) has been associated with genes in the HLA-DR region and specifically with DR4 in both blacks and whites in the United States. The finding of an absence of the DR4 association for IDDM in Nigeria has been fitted into a genetic hypothesis involving different types of IDDM. A "recessive" DR3-associated type requires other determinants in order for disease to occur, and a "dominant" type is associated with DR4 (MacDonald et al., 1986). Further, the occurrence of IDDM in U.S. blacks, as opposed to the reportedly lower prevalence in West African blacks, suggests that the HLA-DR4-associated disease in U.S. blacks may be due to admixture with U.S. whites (MacDonald et al., 1986). Support for this hypothesis is derived from studies in South African blacks, who also do not show the DR associations evident in U.S. blacks and whites, while the Cape "coloureds," who have a significant proportion of Caucasian genes, showed the association with DR4 (Orren et al., 1985). Racial admixture was shown to be a factor in IDDM in U.S. blacks and whites (Reitnauer et al., 1982).

The hypothesis that the DR3-associated form of IDDM requires other genetic factors for expression is supported by findings of an interaction between

DR3 positivity and a specific Gm type (i.e., $Gm^{1,3;5}$) (Tait et al., 1986) in affecting IDDM risk. Gm types of immunoglobulins were mentioned in Chapter 3. In southern Chinese in Hong Kong, not only HLA-DR3 but Aw33 and B17 antigens were increased in frequency among IDDM cases versus controls, and early-onset IDDM (before age 20 years) was associated with both DR3 and DRw9 (Hawkins et al., 1987).

In Japanese the frequency of HLA-DR3 phenotype is low and DR4 is high in normal persons (Table 3.4); the association with IDDM is with DR4 (Svejgaard et al., 1983). The low prevalence of IDDM in Japanese, however, suggests that other factors are involved in etiology of IDDM and other autoimmune diseases (Anon., 1986h). Orchard et al. (1986) also noted that population differences in IDDM prevalence, including low rates in Japan, cannot be adequately explained by differences in HLA types, and suggested that differences in the prevalence of an environmental factor (i.e., an infectious agent) must be involved. The HLA association is complex, however, as shown by more detailed studies of haplotypes. The specific haplotype "DR4, DQw3.2" has been associated with IDDM, in contrast with the DQw3.1 haplotype associated with rheumatoid arthritis (see above). Thus, further studies of this association across various racial/ethnic groups are needed to test for genetic heterogeneity. Undoubtedly population differences in prevalences of both the specific genetic substrate(s) and infectious agents are important.

Risk of non-insulin-dependent diabetes (NIDDM) has not been consistently associated with HLA antigens. This may not be unexpected because most HLA-disease associations involved autoimmune or immune-related diseases (such as IDDM), while the pathogenesis of NIDDM involves other mechanisms. A study in Natal, South Africa, reported an association with HLA-B15 among Indians of northern origin and AW24 among Indians of southern origin (Omar et al., 1985). These findings suggest possible heterogeneity of disease causation, but chance associations cannot be ruled out. Extensive studies in the Pacific suggest a possible association in some populations, but not others, with HLA-Bw61 or Bw22 (Bw56), and also with non-HLA loci in some populations (Serjeantson and Zimmet, 1984). In a study of Spanish NIDDM patients, HLA-Dr5 was increased above expectation and DR3 decreased (though not significantly) (Arnaiz-Villena et al., 1984), while in Trinidad a positive association with B5 was reported (Wilson et al., 1986). The earlier literature was reviewed in Tiwari and Terasaki (1985).

Evidence for a major gene(s) in NIDDM is considerable, though less strong than for IDDM. Evidence for a role for genetic factors includes associations between NIDDM and degree of admixture in Mexican-Americans (Gardner et al., 1984) and in Pacific Islanders (i.e., Nauruans) (Serjeantson and Zimmet, 1984; Zimmet et al., 1986). The percent native American admixture of Mexican-American groups in Texas was estimated from skin color measurements, and comparison with rates for NIDDM suggested that the high rates of NIDDM are largely confined to groups with substantial Amerindian heritage (Gardner et al., 1984). More extensive comparisons across Amerindians and Mexican-American populations in North America also show a correlation between NIDDM prevalence and percentage of Amerindian ancestry (Chakraborty and Weiss, 1986). The relationship between a Gm haplotype marker for Caucasian admixture and prevalence of NIDDM in Pima and Papago Indians (Knowler et al., 1988) is also consistent with this interpretation. These results provide an impetus for further work involving estimates of admixture, especially on the individual versus the group level, and for studies of the specific genetic mechanism involved in the high risk of NIDDM in Amerindian or Amerindian-related groups.

The evidence from many population studies suggests an interaction between genetic susceptibility, probably heterogeneous (i.e., more than one particular locus is involved) and environmental influences related in part to Westernization. Rapid increases in prevalence of NIDDM along with obesity and other diseases of civilization such as peptic ulcer in Amerindians support such a conclusion. It is likely that a gene or genes once adaptive in times of nutritional deprivation are now maladaptive and influence NIDDM susceptibility as suggested by Neel in 1959 (reviewed by Weiss et al., 1984; Zimmet et al., 1986). Neel's "thrifty" gene may not be the same gene in all populations with the putative adaptation to scarce food resources. The search for genetic factors in diabetes mellitus is best approached through family studies, with formal genetic analyses of modes of inheritance, using population-based registries of disease (Orchard et al., 1986). Family studies in Mexican-Americans in the San Antonio Heart Study suggest that the mechanism in this group may involve a gene related to insulin resistance (Haffner et al., 1988).

Hyperuricemia and Gout

The increased prevalence of *hyperuricemia*, or elevated uric acid level in the blood, among Pacific Island populations is well known (Prior, 1981; Kelsey, 1982). Hyperuricemia is found in *both* traditional and Westernized Pacific Island populations, in contrast to findings for various other chronic conditions such as diabetes mellitus, hypertension, and cardiovascular disease. The importance of environmental factors in clinical *gout*, however, is indicated by its rarity among rural versus urban females in Western Samoa (Jackson et al., 1981). Studies among the Marshall Islanders in Micronesia suggest that "hyperuricemia" may not be pathologic, in that clinical gout does not appear to be greatly increased in comparison to the United States (Adams et al., 1984). Thus, Pacific populations may not be uniform in their expression of the sequelae of hyperuricemia. Acculturation is related to hyperuricemia in some studies but not in New Guinea or the Solomon Islands.

Thyroid Disorders

For the autoimmune thyroid disorder, *Graves' disease*, an association with Drw6, an HLA type has been reported among U.S. blacks in contrast with the DR3 association among whites, suggesting immunogenetic heterogeneity in the disease (Sridama et al., 1987). In Singapore, Graves' disease is reportedly more common in Chinese than in the other major racial/ethnic groups. Different racial groups including Japanese and Chinese show different HLA-DR allele associations, suggesting that the autoimmune pathogenesis is somehow related to class II antigens, but the specific mechanisms vary across populations (Rapoport, 1987). Another autoimmune disease, resembling GD, is *Hashimoto's thyroiditis* or "autoimmune thyroiditis," a chronic disease causing goiter in areas where iodine is not insufficient. This autoimmune disease is associated with HLA-DR5 in Caucasians, but with DR9 in Chinese (Wang et al., 1988).

The major effects of *iodine deficiency* include goiter or thyroid gland enlargement, as well as abnormal prenatal neurological development. These conditions have been labeled "iodine deficiency disorders" (IDD) (Hetzel, 1986). Areas of endemic goiter, where thyroid enlargement affects more than 10 percent of the population, due to iodine deficiency include parts of Africa such as Zaire and Zimbabwe (Jenesi et al., 1986), Southeast Asia, South America and the Himalayas. In schoolchildren in the southern highlands of Tanzania, the prevalence of endemic goiter due to iodine deficiency is about 90 percent (Wachter et al., 1986). Iodine supplementation during pregnancy is useful in Tanzania because of prolonged breast feeding (i.e., 3 or more years), which ensures adequate iodine for children (though only until breast feeding is stopped).

In the mountainous areas of northern Nepal, cretinism with mental deficiency and neuromuscular disorders was prevalent before the importation of iodine-rich foods. Interestingly, cretins were "tolerated" in these rural areas and were not considered to be "disabled" but "just a part of daily life" (Achard, 1987). This is another example of the importance of cultural factors in disease perception and treatment.

In Southeast Asia, where soils are often deficient in iodine, an estimated 300 million people are at risk of IDD, about 102 million have goiter, and more than 43 million suffer some mental and physical impairment (Clugston and Bagchi, 1986; Hetzel, 1986). A UNICEF-supported International Council for Control of IDD offers some hope of progress in control. Thus, apparent ethnic differences in IDD reflect geophysical and resultant nutritional factors.

Although endemic goiter is usually the result of iodine deficiency, iodine excess can also be involved—as shown in central China, where iodine-rich water and foods are consumed in villages adjacent to areas of iodine deficiency (Mu et al., 1987). Both excess and deficiency of iodine may lead to borderline hypothyroidism or reduced thyroid functioning.

Nutritionally Related Diseases

Southeast Asia is a high-risk area for eye disease, *corneal xerophthalmia*, which often leads to blindness. One of the major causes of bilateral corneal ulceration is malnutrition or vitamin A deficiency. Perhaps a half million new cases occur each year in pre-school-age children (Sommer et al., 1981). Results of the first population-based study of xerophthalmia in Africa suggest a prevalence of 3.9 percent in children under age 6 years, thus indicating a major public health problem. In some parts of Africa, however, seasonal intake of vitamin A-rich foods may contribute to normal levels of serum beta-carotene in lactating women and thus in the newborn (as in Machakos District, Kenya) (Kusin et al., 1985). As with iodine deficiency (discussed earlier), maternal supplementation may be useful in cultures where breast feeding is prolonged. In Tanzania a 2-year surveillance study showed that antecedent measles was associated with corneal ulceration and vitamin A deficiency was related to bilateral ulceration (Foster et al., 1986).

Thus, the apparent concentration of xerophthalmia in certain regions and ethnic groups is a reflection of nutritional deficiencies and infectious diseases. Evidence from Asia also suggests possible increased general morbidity and mortality due to subclinical vitamin A deficiency (Sommer et al., 1983, 1984), although further studies are needed. Thus, vitamin A supplementation offers the hope of improvement in general health as well as prevention of eye disease and blindness (discussed below).

Primarily of nutritional origin is the high prevalence of *rickets* or defective bone mineralization in Asian (Indian or Pakistani origin) immigrants to the United Kingdom, as noted in Glasgow in 1956 and in more recent surveys. Vitamin D supplementation in Asian children has had an impact, and pregnant women remain a target group for prevention of congenital rickets in their offspring (Goel et al., 1981). Since these Asian immigrants retain their traditional diet long after arrival in the United Kingdom, vitamin supplementation is a short-term solution, but health education, involving dietary changes, is a longer-term solution. The situation is complicated by the possibility that dietary factors other than vitamin D deficiency may be involved in rickets and osteomalacia in these populations (Dunnigan and Robertson, 1980). Osteomalacia is the adult form of childhood rickets.

Nonspecific nutritional disturbances may be responsible for dental *enamel hypoplasias* or deficient enamel thickness. In rural Mexican children, such deficiencies were most common at the age of weaning (2–3 years), while the slightly higher prevalence in females versus males suggests differences in access to resources, including food and medicine, a key issue with regard to sex differences in infant mortality across various cultures.

Iron deficiency anemia, classified with diseases of the blood in the ICD (WHO, 1977), is discussed in the next section.

DISEASES OF BLOOD AND BLOOD-FORMING ORGANS

Genetic disorders involving the blood and blood-forming organs, including hemoglobinopathies and thalassemias, were discussed under genetic diseases (Chapter 5). Genetic blood coagulation disorders, some of which are more frequent among Ashkenazi Jewish and Mediterranean populations, are listed in Table 5.1. Polycythemia vera was mentioned in the discussion of cancers (Chapter 8).

In discussing normal physiological characteristics (Chapter 3, Table 3.6), we noted that black populations tended to have lower hemoglobin concentration (and lower average white blood cell count) (Fulwood et al., 1983) in the blood than white populations. "*Polycythemias*," or disorders involving increased red cell mass, hemoglobin concentration, or hematocrit, tend to be rare, and "*anemias*" tend to be more frequent among black populations. In a community survey of young adults in Bogalusa, Louisiana, black females had the highest prevalence of "anemia" (16 percent) and the lowest prevalence of "polycythemia" (3 percent) (Creasanta et al., 1987). The black–white difference in hemoglobin level in various studies is not explained by socioeconomic factors (e.g., poverty level in the U.S. National Health Survey) (Fulwood et al., 1983), or by diet (i.e., intake of vitamins and iron) (Nicklas et al., 1987b). Differences in frequencies of genetic traits such as thalassemias and hemoglobinopathies (discussed in Chapter 5) also do not appear to be involved.

These findings on hemoglobin concentration have sparked debate over whether or not definitions of "anemia" by hemoglobin level should be different for black versus white children and adults. One argument for a race-specific definition is that some black children may be unnecessarily treated for iron deficiency anemia (Owen and Yanochik-Owen, 1977). On the other hand, use of arbitrary cutoff levels may also misclassify some persons as nonanemic, and population-specific distributions of blood parameters should be used in defining anemia and polycythemia (Cresanta et al., 1987).

A rather speculative hypothesis might be advanced for the lower hemoglobin concentrations in the blood of certain black populations. There is evidence that iron deficiency may protect against malaria in infants and that iron supplementation increases risk of malaria; lower malaria rates were reported in infants who had low hematocrits at birth in Papua New Guinea (Oppenheimer et al., 1986). Thus adaptation to malaria could be an explanation for black–white differences in hemoglobin concentration.

As noted above, black–white differences in hemoglobin level apparently are not explained by the higher prevalence of thalassemias and abnormal hemoglobins in blacks. In fact, hematocrit levels among blacks with sickle cell trait (HbAS), the most common hemoglobin-related condition in the United States, are not lower in comparison with blacks with HbAA (Polednak and Janerich, 1975). In the usually benign condition of true heterozygous beta-thalassemia (Chapter 5), however, a refractory anemia occurs among women during pregnancy (Weatherall and Clegg, 1981). We have noted the common occurrence of beta-thalassemias among Southeast Asians (Chapter 5). Among Southeast Asian (Hmong) refugee mothers in Minnesota, the prevalence of low hematocrit was higher than among white mothers. Although the authors (Erickson et al., 1987) had no data on thalassemias, their possible role was mentioned. The high prevalence of anemia during pregnancy in Liberians was apparently not due to hemoglobinopathies but to low iron intake related to quality of diet and food taboos (Jackson and Jackson, 1987). In northern Nigeria malaria and iron deficiency were the major causes of maternal anemia, with HbSS reportedly ranking fourth; variation in staple foods and hookworm contributed to regional variation in iron deficiency (Fleming, 1987).

Iron deficiency anemia has long been recognized as a nutritional problem among Alaskan native children, and increases in hemoglobin levels after oral iron supplementation indicate that iron deficiency is the main cause. Surveys in several Alaskan native populations indicate high prevalences of low hemoglobin or hematocrit levels greater than 20 percent in children under 5 years of age, in comparison with only about 4 percent in the U.S. Second National Health and Nutrition Examination Survey (Thiele et al., 1988). Reduction in intake of iron-rich traditional foods such as fish and meat, and adoption of nonnative foods of generally lower iron content may be involved. Maternal coffee consumption, and direct feeding of coffee to infants, may contribute to iron deficiency anemia in Costa Rica and other parts of Central America (Munoz et al., 1988).

Hereditary ovalocytosis, although listed in statistical classifications of disease (WHO, 1977) is an apparently benign autosomal-gene-related condition characterized by oval-shaped red blood cells. It is of interest because of evidence for possible resistance to malaria in Southeast Asia and Papua New Guinea (Holt et al., 1981). As with other genetic polymorphisms related to malarial adaptation (Chapter 5), there is evidence for separate mutations in different populations.

DISEASES OF THE DIGESTIVE SYSTEM

Gallbladder Diseases

Gallbladder disease is common in some Amerindian populations, while peptic ulcer has been rare in the past. This may be due to a common factor—that is, gastric hyposecretion in persons with gallstones (Sievers and Fisher, 1981). This propensity toward gallstones in Amerindians has been known since the 1950s (Comess et al., 1967). Gallbladder disease is part of the complex of "disease of civilization," including cardiovascular diseases and diabetes mellitus, that have increased in frequency in Amerindian groups during historical times.

As with these other diseases, a combination of a genetic predisposition and changes in diet may be the explanation (Weiss et al., 1984; Weiss, 1985). Upper-body obesity is a risk factor for self-reported gallbladder disease among Mexican-American women in the San Antonio Heart Study, as previously shown for white women (Haffner et al., 1988). An underlying genetic mechanism is suggested by the finding that the increased risk of both gallbladder disease and diabetes mellitus in southern Texas Mexican-Americans—who are genetically related to Amerindians (see Chapter 3)—cannot be explained entirely by body mass (Hanis et al., 1985). We have noted the high incidence rates for gallbladder cancers, and the strong effect of antecedent gallbladder disease as a risk factor, among Amerindian and Amerindian-related groups (Chapter 8).

In a prospective study of white women in the Kaiser Permanent Medical Care Program in California, risk of cholecysectomy was strongly associated with the highest category of body mass index (i.e., weight/height) in a nonlinear fashion (Petitti and Sidney, 1988). Populations with large proportions of women with large body masses may be at high risk of gallbladder disease and cholecystectomy.

The higher prevalence of cholesterol gallstones in Amerindians and in northern Europe (including Sweden) in contrast to Africa and the Far East, has led to Lowenfels' (1988) theory of an original adaptation to cold climates via storage of excess calories for future needs. This is an expansion of Neel's (1962) "thrifty gene" hypothesis.

Peptic Ulcer

Comparison of incidence and prevalence rates of peptic ulcer across populations and racial/ethnic groups presents the same problems of differences in diagnostic reliability and validity as exist with other chronic diseases. Also "peptic ulcer" includes two distinct forms, gastric or stomach ulcer (GU) and duodenal or small-intestine ulcer (DU), which differ in associated genetic factors and in apparent pathophysiology; increased secretion of pepsin precursors (especially pepsinogen-I) is more important in DU and may be influenced by a dominant trait.

High rates of "peptic ulcer" have been reported in surveys in Norway, the Faroe Islands (Fig. 3.1), Iceland, and Scotland as well as other North Atlantic areas (Bonnevie, 1985; Kaer et al., 1985). Annual incidence rates for GU and DU in the Faroe Island in 1981–83 were very high—2.3 and 1.0 per 1,000 per year, respectively—in comparison with most areas except Scotland and the Arctic areas. In Iceland and other areas, rapid changes in incidence rates for DU indicate the influence of environmental factors.

Two surveys among male factory workers in Japan are noteworthy. The incidence of active and inactive peptic ulcer was reportedly 5 percent or higher per year, and smoking and family history were major risk factors (Araki and Goto, 1985), although psychosocial stress may be another factor. These Japanese studies cannot be compared with other surveys, because in Japan special diagnostic methods, involving radiological and endoscopic examinations, increase the detection rate for ulcers. As noted earlier (Chapter 8), the high incidence of gastric ulcer in Japan has led to gastric screening for cancers; thus, ulcers are also inadvertently detected.

The often reported association between peptic ulcer incidence and smoking has been confirmed in a study in London that involved endoscopic evidence. The dose response relationship between prevalence of ulcer and number of cigarettes smoked was striking (Ainley et al., 1987). Thus differences in smoking rates among ethnic groups and populations are undoubtedly involved in explaining some of the true variation in ulcer incidence and prevalence and (along with other factors) time trends in incidence and severity in different regions.

In recent years attention has turned to the possible role of infectious agents, especially *Campylobacter*-like organisms (see Chapter 6), in gastritis and gastric ulcer (e.g., Hazell and Lee, 1986). The role of variation in frequency of these agents in explaining population and racial/ethnic differences in ulcer is unknown. Evidence strongly suggests that *Campylobacter pylori* is involved in the pathogenesis of the more common of the two varieties of *gastritis* or inflammation of the mucosal lining of the stomach (Barthel et al., 1988) and in duodenal ulcer (also shown in China). There is discussion of treatment with antimicrobials. Population studies of the association between *Campylobacter* infections and gastritis–ulcer should be aided by the development of noninvasive tests for presence of the microorganisms (Graham et al., 1987).

The high rates in Norway, Iceland, and the Faroe Islands may involve "anthropological" affinities, presumably genetic, among these groups (Kaer et al., 1985), but this remains to be demonstrated. The high frequency of blood group O in northwestern Europe (Table 3.3) is noteworthy. Blood group O has long been known to be associated with increased risk of *duodenal ulcer*. Curiously, however, American Indian populations have had low prevalence of peptic ulcer despite a high frequency of group O (Table 3.3) (Sievers and Fisher, 1981). Again, many other factors are involved in the etiology of this disease, and the relative risk for ulcer associated with blood group O is only about 1.4 (Segall, 1981). Recent mapping of the complex of genes controlling the human pepsinogen (enzyme) fractions, and demonstration of polymorphic variation in these genes, should lead to further exploration of the role of population variation in explaining differences in disease rates.

The importance of environmental factors within specific populations previously at lower risk is indicated by apparent recent increases in ulcer prevalence among certain Amerindian groups. Heredity and environment probably interact in a complex fashion in explaining the recent increase in peptic ulcer among off-reservation Indians, in view of the direct association between degree of non-Indian admixture and duodenal ulcer frequency (Sievers and Fisher, 1981).

Chronic Liver Disease and Cirrhosis

We have noted worldwide variation in age-adjusted mortality rates from chronic liver disease and cirrhosis (Table 4.5) and the higher age-specific death rates in U.S. blacks versus whites prior to age 65 years (Table 4.1). Problems in comparability of death certification, however, and the heterogeneous nature of cirrhosis in terms of causal factors, complicate such comparisons. Mortality rates in some studies are higher in lower-socioeconomic groups or areas, as in parts of the United States (Dayal et al., 1986), although the association with education is less clear (Mendeloff and Dunn, 1971). Greater increases in mortality from cirrhosis in U.S. blacks versus whites during the 1950s and 1960s may largely reflect changes in rates of alcoholism (see later). Death rates from chronic liver disease and alcohol-related causes are high among Amerindians and Alaskan natives (Rhoades et al., 1988), and the Indian Health Service has an alcohol-abuse treatment program.

Although much of the worldwide variation in mortality rates for this category may be due to population differences in alcohol consumption, only a proportion of liver cirrhosis is alcoholic cirrhosis (with a higher proportion for males than females in many countries). The remainder of cases are related to hepatitis infections and unknown causes. As with hepatic cancer, chronic liver diseases and cirrhosis are heterogeneous categories in terms of causation.

Nevertheless, countries with high per-capita alcohol consumption, such as France, Portugal, and parts of Eastern Europe, have the highest death rates from cirrhosis (Table 4.5). Mortality rates are high for Chile (Table 4.5), especially for cirrhosis with mention of alcoholism. Italy also ranks high, with death rates especially high in northeastern areas, where alcohol consumption is greater; age-standardized death rates almost doubled in males from 1955 to 1979 (La Vecchia et al., 1986). Regional differences in the proportion of cirrhosis death associated with alcohol consumption are considerable in Italy (Capocaccia and Frachi, 1988). In contrast, an ecologic study in Canada showed that regional differences in mortality rates for cirrhosis in Canada were significantly correlated with pork rather than alcohol consumption (Nanji and French, 1985), and this requires further exploration.

In the United States, time changes in cirrhosis mortality, including a decline since 1973, have not paralleled changes in alcohol consumption. More detailed studies are needed on time changes in racial/ethnic groups in relation to patterns of alcohol consumption as reported in U.S. national surveys. Analytic studies should determine to what extent black–white differences in mortality from cirrhosis are related to differences in alcohol consumption involving SES and/or sociocultural factors, as well as to other causal factors (e.g., previous infectious diseases) and differences in medical care.

Similarly, such studies are needed in other areas with different racial/ethnic groups. One example is Australia, where aboriginal alcoholism is said to be a problem but mortality statistics on cirrhosis are not routinely available for the entire aboriginal population (Thomson, 1984).

Other Digestive Diseases and Disorders

A variety of other diseases of Western civilization—for example, appendicitis, constipation, and irritable bowel syndrome, as well as colon cancer (Chapter 8)—have often been attributed to low fiber intake. This hypothesis developed largely from the work of D.P. Burkitt and colleagues in rural Africa, where these diseases are rare. It is now recognized, however, that many other factors may be more important, including other dietary components (e.g., fat and protein intake), exercise, and mental stress.

Inflammatory bowel disease, comprised mainly of ulcerative colitis and Crohn's disease, which tend to affect different parts of the bowel, shows a remarkable predilection for Jews in North America, but the association is much less striking in other areas including Israel (Calkins and Mendeloff, 1986). This type of disease distribution, as noted elsewhere in this book, presents an opportunity for fruitful exploration into the explanations. The mechanisms for the differential effects of smoking on Crohn's disease and ulcerative colitis risk, for example, might be explored in studies in Jewish groups in various countries or in Jews of different origins or differing in religious practices in the same country. Studies of U.S. Hispanics and Asian groups, as well as religious groups such as Mormons and Seventh Day Adventists, have also been suggested (Calkins and Mendeloff, 1986).

DISEASES OF THE RESPIRATORY SYSTEM (EXCLUDING PNEUMONIAS)

Some diseases of infectious origin, including pneumonias and acute upper respiratory infections, were discussed in Chapter 6. Of main interest here are "*chronic ostructive pulmonary disease and allied conditions,*" or COPD (i.e., codes 490–496 in the ICD) (WHO, 1977). This category includes *bronchitis, emphysema, and asthma.* Emphysema is mainly a morphologic or pathologic diagnosis involving the observation of destruction of the walls of air spaces in the lungs, and clinical assessment requires physiologic testing; both emphysema and chronic bronchitis are part of the same spectrum of diseases. Thus it is clear that comparisons of these two categories across populations are fraught with difficulties. Even the comprehensive category of COPD is subject to differences in clinical interpretation of cases and coding practices, which may influence death rates reported across Europe (Mackenbach et al., 1987).

Ranking of COPD age-adjusted death rates 51 of the 52 countries included in the WHO (1987) data base (not shown in Table 4.5) reveals considerable apparent variation, from 2.3 per 100,000 per year in Malta to 39.9 in Mauritius. Israel, the United States, Canada, and Japan had low rates, while high rates prevailed in Eastern Europe, Denmark, and Italy. Analysis of mortality trends in chronic lung diseases from 1971 to 1980 among males 65 years of age or older indicated some downward trends in selected countries, including New Zealand, Hong Kong, Japan, Chile, Singapore, and Canada, but some countries showed apparent increases related to the change in ICD code in 1979–80. Mauritius, with the highest rates (as noted earlier), and Thailand, with the lowest rates, showed no clear trend over time. Among this same group of older males, mortality rates were positively but "not quite significantly" associated with per capita tobacco sales in 1971 (Melia and Swan, 1986).

U.S. mortality rates for the entire category were higher in 1985 for blacks than whites for ages 15–54 (Table 4.1). As noted earlier by Mason et al. (1981), rates among nonwhites versus whites were higher only for *asthma*. In 1985, mortality rates in blacks versus whites were lower for bronchitis and emphysema, but higher for asthma in all ages before 85 years and in both sexes (Table 9.5).

Higher smoking rates in young adult black males, as mentioned earlier, may be involved in the age pattern for bronchitis and emphysema mortality, with small differences in young adults; the lower level of smoking within black versus white smokers, however, also must be considered. In Philadelphia, neighborhoods with highest death rates for ICD codes 490–496 were predominantly white (Dayal et al., 1986), but age-specific and cause-specific rates (e.g., for asthma alone) were not presented. Among all *hospital discharges* in Maryland between 1979 and 1982, after adjustment for differences in poverty by area, the annual asthma discharge rate was only slightly and not significantly higher in black children (i.e., 2.70 vs. 2.20 per 1,000 per year) (Wissow et al., 1988).

Asthma, involving increased irritability of the tracheobronchial and bronchial spasm, is a complex entity consisting of several types defined by the preci-

Table 9.5 Mortality Rates (per 100,000) for Chronic Obstructive Pulmonary Disease in U.S. Blacks and Whites in 1985

	Age (years)							
	15–24	25–34	35–44	45–54	55–64	65–74	75–84	85+
Bronchitis (ICD 490–491)								
White	0.0	0.0	0.1	0.4	2.0	6.6	14	30
Black	0.1	0.1	0.1	0.5	1.6	2.7	5.8	8.8
Emphysema (492)								
White	0.0	0.0	0.2	2.0	11	33	56	51
Black	0.0	0.1	0.3	2.3	6.7	17	26	28
Asthma (493)								
White male	0.4	0.4	0.6	1.3	2.9	5.0	9.3	12.4
Black male	1.6	1.7	3.2	4.5	7.3	9.5	10.2	7.7
White female	0.4	0.5	0.8	2.0	3.8	5.9	8.7	12.2
Black female	0.9	1.2	2.1	5.1	7.3	9.1	9.8	7.9

Data from *Vital Statistics of the United States* for 1985, published in 1988.

patating agents and the nature of the response. Consideration of apparent black–white differences in asthma illustrates the complexity of interpretation, in that biological differences may have a predominantly environmental explanation. Elevated serum levels of immunoglobulin (i.e., IgE) are characteristic of immediate "hypersensitivity" reactions to foreign antigens and are also found in *allergic* asthma. Certain black populations are known to have higher serum levels of IgE, but the explanation is unclear. In the U.S. HANES survey (phase II), consistent but statistically insignificant excesses in allergic skin test reactivity, reflecting immediate hypersensitivity, were found in black versus white adults (Gergen and Turkeltaub, 1986). In this survey, however, rates of immediate hypersensitivity reaction were positively associated with SES, suggesting greater tolerance to foreign antigens in lower-SES groups due to previous exposures.

The association between asthma *hospitalization* and poverty level in children may reflect increased exposure to environmental agents that exacerbate the allergic response and its consequences or cumulative effects. Controlling for poverty level would thus reduce black–white differences in asthma hospitalization rates. Other types of asthma are provoked by viral infections and do not involve positive skin tests or elevated serum IgE, and controlling for poverty level may also control for prevalence of these previous diseases.

The role of indoor versus outdoor pollution in asthma is unclear. In an interesting review of epidemiologic research on asthma, Gregg (1986) noted higher prevalence rates in Maori versus Europeans in a national survey (i.e., 18.9 vs. 3.4 per 100,000). A remarkable increase in the prevalence of asthma occurred in the eastern highlands of Papua New Guinea, and a further increase from the previously high prevalence of asthma occurred among Polynesian migrants from the Tokelau atoll (Fig. 3.2) to Australia. Mortality rates for COPD are also reportedly high among Australian aborigines, but the quality and completeness of data are open to question (Thomson, 1984).

In New Zealand Mormon versus non-Mormon males have lower death rates for bronchitis and for emphysema (Smith et al., 1985), undoubtedly reflecting differences in smoking rates. Chronic pulmonary diseases are no exception to the general rule for chronic diseases, involving a genetic substrate strongly modulated by environmental influences.

For emphysema family studies showed a hereditary defect involving decreased antitrypsin activity or alpha-1-antitrypsin (AAT) deficiency; AAT is also known as protease inhibitor, or Pi (see Chapter 3). The autosomal-condominant gene locus is polymorphic, and one variant of Pi (i.e., Pi^z) is common in the United States and Europe but rare in other groups studied including some African populations (Summers, 1987). Pi^z is associated with Pi deficiency. This genetic substrate of low-level activity of an enzyme, which inhibits proteinases (mainly elastases), increases susceptibility to emphysema and probably interacts with smoking through a common mechanism of elastic-tissue destruction due to high proteinase activity. In a cross-sectional study of 1,787 white adults without disease in Baltimore, however, "airways obstruction" (defined by pulmonary function tests) was predicted not by an interaction between smoking and the Pi^z allele but by interactions between smoking and other genetically related factors (i.e., blood group A antigen and a family history of lung disease) (Khoury et al., 1986). The complex, multifactorial nature of the causation of emphysema is evident, and the explanation for apparent population differences in death rates requires further study. In prenatal diagnosis of AAT deficiency, which is of practical value because it is associated with both lung disease in adulthood and liver disease in infancy, two RFLP probes in the region of the AAT gene have proved useful in prenatal diagnosis in Britain (Abbott et al., 1987). Further studies using these probes are needed in other populations.

In asthma, a hyperresponsive state, due to genetic or acquired mechanisms, interacts with largely undefined environmental provoking agents. Thus population differences in both aspects of the pathogenesis of these chronic conditions can be involved in determining differences in disease prevalence.

COMPLICATIONS OF PREGNANCY, PERINATAL CONDITIONS, BIRTH DEFECTS, AND RELATED CONDITIONS

In the United States in 1985, *maternal mortality* rates were almost four times higher in blacks than whites (i.e., 20.4 vs. 5.2 per 100,000 live births). Although this disparity is projected to increase by 1990, reduction in maternal mortality rates to 5.0 in blacks and 4.1 in whites is a target for the 1990 Health Objectives for the Nation made by the U.S. Public Health Service (Anon., 1988e). While maternal mortality rates have continued to decline in recent decades in Westernized nations, in developing countries death rates related to pregnancy, delivery, and abortion continue to be high (Stein and Maine, 1986). Part of the decline in developed countries, as shown in Massachusetts (Sachs et al., 1988), is due to a reduction in the prevalence of rheumatic heart disease (and hence a decline in cardiac-related maternal mortality) (see also Chapter 7) as well as control of hypertension during pregnancy and increased use of antibiotics. In contrast, pregnancy-induced hypertension, obstetric hemorrhage, and cardiac diseases are major causes of maternal death in China (Lingmei and Hui, 1988). Thus, maternal mortality provides another example of differential access to medical care as an explanation for racial/ethnic differences in disease and mortality.

Maternal death rates are actually relatively low in China (i.e., about 25–59 per 100,000 live births in urban and rural areas), although not as low as in Japan, where rates have declined in recent years (to about 15). Rates in Massachusetts (cited earlier) are about 10 per 100,000 live births and are comparable to Western and Southern Europe. The highest rates are in Africa, reaching as high as 1,000 in some areas, and in parts of Asia, (except for China, Hong Kong, and Singapore) (i.e., 300–650), while rates in Latin American countries are somewhat lower (i.e., 100–300) (Royston and Lopez, 1987). The author is not aware of any reports of rates by ethnic group in such multiethnic areas as Singapore. Another (albeit less extreme) exception to the Asian pattern of high rates has been the decline in Sri Lanka from about 555 in 1950 to 239 in 1980, perhaps because of a decline in high-parity births. Variation in age at first and last pregnancy across countries and cultures is one factor in explaining variations in maternal mortality rates, since pregnancy at both very young ages (e.g., in Bangladesh) and older ages (i.e., after 30–35 years) increases risk of maternal death. In areas of Bangladesh maternal causes account for a striking 25–45 percent of all deaths among women of reproductive age, versus 1 percent in Japan, the United States, and Hong Kong (Royston and Lopez, 1987). The immensity of the public health challenge is evident from these statistics.

Complications of pregnancy and childbirth are included in a separate major category in the ICD (WHO, 1977). Hydatidiform mole or molar pregnancy in the Far East was mentioned earlier with reference to cancer (i.e., choriocarcinoma) (Chapter 8). Black women tend to have narrower bony pelvises and hence more frequent obstetric problems than whites, at least in the United States. There is evidence that black women with sickle cell trait (HbAS; see Chapter 5) have delivery complications such as pelvic contraction more frequently than other black women, possibly related to linear body build or narrower bony breadths (Hoff et al., 1983). Dystocia or difficult delivery was also reported among mothers of newborns with HbAS (Polednak and Janerich, 1980).

Short maternal height has been associated with risk of difficult delivery and cesarean section, due to cephalopelvic disproportion (i.e., disproportionate size of fetal head in relation to the maternal pelvis) in various populations including Tanzanians (Atken and Walls, 1986). Thus populations or racial/ethnic groups with shorter maternal stature, especially less than 60 inches or 152.4 cm, may be at higher risk of difficult delivery, although maternal body size is also correlated with size (birth weight) of offspring. Such variation in maternal stature is itself poorly understood, but a legacy of poor nutrition in the life of the mother is probably involved.

Perinatal Conditions and Infant Mortality

Conditions originating in the perinatal period are assigned to a separate major category in the ICD (WHO, 1977). Perinatal conditions include hemolytic disease of the fetus or newborn. Population differences in risk of hemolytic diseases of the newborn due to blood group incompatibility are related to population differences in frequencies of Rh and ABO blood group alleles (see Chapter 3 and Table 3.3). These disorders are due to the destruction of fetal red cells by antibodies produced by the mother in response to fetal antigen, as in Rh incompatibility (i.e., Rh− mother and Rh+ fetus) and ABO incompatibility.

In most of Europe the frequency of the Rh-negative genotype—called cde or r, depending on the allelic nomenclature—is around 40 percent, except in the Basques, where it reaches 53 percent (Mourant et al., 1976). In other populations, however, Rh-negative individuals are much less frequent—for example, 0–11 percent in parts of Africa, around 8 percent in Amerindian populations, and 0 percent in southern Chinese (or 0.34% in Shanghai China) (Mourant et al., 1976; Ting, 1981). Data from the United States have long indicated that hemolytic diseases of the newborn are less frequent in nonwhite than white groups, undoubtedly due to the rarity of Rh-negative phenotypes in the former groups. The importance of Rh incompatibility has declined with screening of pregnant women for presence of anti-D antibodies and medical treatment of infants by transfusions of blood in developed countries.

Perinatal conditions include disorders relating to low birth weight and short gestation, as well as specific conditions such as infections and respiratory distress syndrome. The extensive literature on racial differences in birth weight and gestation length will not be reviewed here. A few recent studies will be cited. A study among Southeast Asian refugees in the United States found a lower mean birth weight but a similar proportion of low birth weight among infants of Hmong versus white women (Erickson et al., 1987). Data from the U.S. National Infant Mortality Surveillance project, using linked birth and infant death certificates, confirmed the well-known higher percentage of low-birth-weight births and the higher neonatal mortality risk among blacks versus whites (Anon., 1987a). Neonatal mortality rates for deaths due to congenital anomalies, however, were equal in blacks and whites (see later).

Table 9.6 shows neonatal and postneonatal death rates, per 1,000 live births, in various U.S. racial/ethnic groups in 1984. Rates were higher in blacks than whites for the entire infant period (i.e., < 1 year) as well as during the neonatal and postneonatal periods. Amerindians, Aleuts and Eskimos, who have been shown to differ anthropologically (Chapter 3), have been combined into one group labeled "Indians," with *infant* death rates similar to those for whites. Infant death rates were slightly lower in Chinese and Japanese births, and lowest among Filipinos. The subcategories of neonatal and postneonatal periods in many groups are based on small numbers. Higher *postneonatal* death rates (i.e., from 28 days to less than 1 year of age) in "native Americans," however, have been confirmed by data from the Indian Health Service areas for 1981–83; higher death rates from accidents, pneumonia, and gastroenteritis in native Americans undoubtedly reflect socioeconomic conditions in many Indian communities (Honigfeld and Kaplan, 1987). The Indian Health Service has recognized the need to

Table 9.6 Infant Mortality Rates (Age < 1 Year) by Race or National Origin and Sex, per 1,000 Live Births in United States (1984)

		Type of rate (infant, neonatal and postneonatal)					
		Infant (< 1 Year)		Neonatal (< 28 days)		Postneonatal (28 days to 11 mos.)	
Group	Sex	No.	Rate	No.	Rate	No.	Rate
White	M	15,805	10.5	10,240	6,8	5,565	3.7
	F	11,803	8.3	7,818	5.5	3,985	2.8
Black	M	5,961	19.8	3,811	12.7	2,150	7.1
	F	4,920	16.9	3,191	10.9	1,729	5.9
Indian[a]	M	222	10.6	105	5.0	117	5.6
	F	171	8.3	75	3.6	96	4.7
Chinese	M	51	6.2	36	4.3	15	1.8
	F	35	4.4	21	2.7	14	1.8
Japanese	M	17	3.6	10	2.1	7	1.5
	F	23	5.0	17	3.7	6	1.3
Filipino	M	51	4.9	36	3.5	15	1.4
	F	37	3.9	22	2.3	15	1.6

Source: Vital Statistics of the U.S., 1984 (published 1987).
[a]Includes Aleuts and Eskimos as well as "native Americans" (see Chapter 3).

examine living conditions and access to medical care among Indians, in view of higher postneonatal death rates for sudden infant death syndrome (SIDS; see later) and infectious diseases among native Americans found in data (by birth weight category) from the National Infant Mortality Surveillance project which links birth and death records for infants born alive in 1980 (Vanlandingham et al., 1988). Thus, Native Americans, along with blacks, have been targeted for programs to reduce postneonatal mortality; in contrast to blacks, however, birth weight is not reduced among Indians.

Neonatal death rates in U.S. blacks versus whites have been studied extensively. In a detailed study of neonatal and childhood mortality in Boston, higher neonatal death rates in blacks than whites in 1972–79 persisted among all groups of median incomes based on census tract of residence (Wise et al., 1985). The well-known higher rate of low birth weight among blacks, or difference in birth weight *distribution*, accounted for much of the difference in neonatal mortality. *Within* the lower-birth-weight categories (i.e., 1,500 g and 1,500–2,500 g), however, neonatal mortality was lower in blacks than in whites. Although income differences did not appear to account for racial differences in neonatal mortality in this study, income was crudely assessed as in many other studies discussed in this book. Median income of the census tract of residence is a group (vs. individual) variable, and does not adequately characterize the SES of individuals.

Briefly, the same association between low birth weight and infant mortality exists within blacks and whites, but blacks have a different distribution of birth weights. As noted in Chapter 1, this type of pattern is quite common in racial/ethnic differences in disease. Thus, increasing the birth weight of black infants would remove some but not all of black–white disparity in infant mortality rates. Other interventions must be devised to reduce infant mortality among blacks, including non-low-birth-weight subgroups. In the National Infant Mortality Surveillance Project, postneonatal mortality rates were about twice as high in black as in white infants, and the overall excess in infant mortality was related not only to the larger proportion of low-birth-weight infants among blacks but also to higher postneonatal death rates among black versus white infants of normal gestation and birth weight (Sappenfield et al., 1987).

As in the United States as a whole, *postneonatal* death rates in Boston were also higher in blacks than white, including deaths from respiratory disease (primarily bronchopneumonia) (Wise et al., 1985). In the United States in 1984, infections and sudden infant death syndrome also showed higher death rates in blacks than in whites (Anon., 1987a). Again, death rates from congenital anomalies, however, were only slightly higher in blacks.

Reduction in infant mortality rates among U.S. blacks is a major public health objective, and improvements could be achieved through increased maternal health services (Anon., 1987a). Controlling for adequacy of prenatal care in categories defined by month of initiation of available prenatal care and number of prenatal visits, however, black–white differences in birth weight and neonatal mortality persisted in North and South Carolina (Alexander and Cornely, 1987). Again, mortality rates were higher in black than white infants of higher birth weight even within each level of prenatal care. Nevertheless, programs to reduce the frequency of low birth weight among blacks should be developed. In North

Carolina a program of patient and hospital staff education regarding preterm labor and its treatment resulted in a reduction in very low birthweight births in blacks (Covington et al., 1988).

Improvements in prenatal care, both in quantity and quality, should result in improvements in infant mortality in U.S. minority groups. In New York City, Puerto Ricans had the highest rates for lack of prenatal care, according to vital statistics data (Anon., 1987i). Puerto Rican "Hispanic" maternal risk profiles resembled those of blacks, while non-Puerto Rican Hispanic mothers were better educated and less likely to have out-of-wedlock births. In the 1979 and 1982 Youth Cohort of the National Longitudinal Survey of Labor Market Experience, the majority of first births among Puerto Ricans and blacks were out of wedlock, while Mexican-origin women tended to have first births within marriage (Darabi and Ortiz, 1987). Again the heterogeneity of "Hispanic" groups is evident in cultural and social patterns. Noteworthy is the observation that women in Puerto Rico are more likely to receive prenatal care than Puerto Rican mothers in New York City, suggesting that SES rather than culturally influenced personal habits are important.

A key issue is the proper measurement of adequacy of prenatal care in terms of effectiveness of educational messages and aspects of the maternal–fetal environment that may differ even after controlling for SES and (at least crudely) adequacy of prenatal care.

Other groups showing increased rates of low birth weight and infant mortality include the Australian aborigines (Thomson, 1984), but detailed studies of aborigines and nonaborigines apparently have not been carried out.

Worldwide, total death rates from all causes (Table 4.5) are influenced by infant mortality rates, in that the high total death rates for developing countries such as Guatemala are due in part to high infant mortality rates representing infectious diseases and malnutrition (and hence, low birth weight). The WHO compiles statistics on infant mortality rates (per 1,000 live births) and in 1985 the highest rates were in parts of Africa (as high as 186 in Sierra Leone, 179 in Senegal, and 132 in Somalia), parts of the Americas (e.g., 110 in Bolivia, 57 in Guatemala, and 88 in Peru, versus 11 in the United States), parts of Asia (e.g., 190 in Afghanistan, 138 in Yemen, 132 in Nepal, 122 in Bangladesh, 108 in Pakistan, 106 in India, and 76 in Indonesia), and the Western Pacific (e.g., 87 in Papua New Guinea). Rates were relatively low in China (33) but lowest in Hong Kong (11) and Japan (7), while parts of Europe also had low rates (e.g., 6–7 in various Scandinavian countries and 7 in Switzerland).

Infant mortality rates are influenced by maternal nutrition during pregnancy, and reductions in rates have been shown in Guatemala after food supplementation to mothers reduced the prevalence of low birth weight (Martorell, 1980). It is well known that breast milk protects against infant infection by providing immunoglobulins and promoting beneficial bacterial growth, while weaning exposes infants to contaminated food; the occurrence of another pregnancy in the same mother is a major risk factor for malnutrition in the previous infant. In southern Africa, breastfeeding is commonly practiced and is of long duration (i.e., at least to the age of 6 months) in the majority, but subsequent malnutrition contributes to the infant mortality rates of about 50–200 per 1,000 live births in South African nonwhites (Griesel and Richter, 1987).

In the United States lower SES groups, including blacks and Hispanics, have lower rates of breastfeeding than whites; in choosing to bottle-feed their infants Hispanic (i.e., Mexican-American) women are reportedly influenced by the need to return to work and by feelings of embarrassment (Young and Kaufman, 1988). In Texas, however, individual prenatal counseling programs were effective in increasing breastfeeding among both Mexican-American and black women. The impact of such programs on infant mortality has apparently not been assessed.

There is considerable interest in time changes in the extent and duration of breastfeeding in various populations and subgroups, because of the implications for infant health and mortality. Widespread declines in breastfeeding have occurred in recent years in some developing countries, but trends are variable, with some countries showing marked declines (e.g., Taiwan) and others showing little or no change (e.g., Thailand) (Popkin et al., 1989). In the Philippines a 5 percent decline in the proportion of infants ever breast fed was found between 1973 and 1983, with no change in duration of breastfeeding. In contrast, increases in duration of breastfeeding occurred in Jakarta, Indonesia, between 1976 and 1983 (Joesoef et al., 1989). In contrast to developed countries such as the United States where highly educated women have increased breastfeeding practices, the increase in breastfeeding duration began among less educated women in Jakarta, and an increase in initiation of breastfeeding was also observed among less educated women in Malaysia (with cultural and religious values similar to Indonesia). Social and medical anthropologists should become increasingly involved in examining the factors influencing changes in breastfeeding habits and in planning intervention programs.

It should be recalled, however, that breastfeeding is only one factor involved in infant health and survival, because sanitation and nutrition after weaning also have an impact. In the Malay Peninsula, for example, breastfeeding increased most among Indians but infant mortality rates declined more among Malays and Chinese between 1970 and 1982, perhaps indicating the need for improved weaning practices and nutritional improvements among Indians (Haaga, 1986).

Sudden infant death syndrome (SIDS) is reportedly more frequent among U.S. blacks than among Hispanic and Anglo whites. Differences in income, education, and birth weight apparently do not account for most of the black–white difference in SIDS in Chicago (Black et al. 1986). High incidence rates (i.e., one in 170 infants) for SIDS, as yet unexplained, also occur among Alaskan natives (Adams, 1985, 1986) and the "native Americans" as a group (as noted above). Apparent regional variation in SIDS rates among Amerindians groups may reflect SES differences and variation in tribal living conditions or maternal and perinatal factors (Honigfeld and Kaplan, 1987), but such explanations are speculative at present. The reportedly low rate of SIDS, or "cot death," in Hong Kong (Davies, 1986) and the suggested role of cultural factors related to sleeping habits have been questioned by Swift (1986), who noted underreporting in England among religious groups who avoid necropsy. Further cross-cultural comparisons of where infants sleep and with whom, along with data on parental smoking, may provide insights into population differences in SIDS (McKenna, 1986).

Variation in mucosal thickness in the upper airways has been suggested as a possible explanation for differences in rates of SIDS—for example, the higher incidence in the Maori of New Zealand (Guilleminault et al., 1986). Further studies are needed on anthropometric characteristics of the upper airways, such as cephalometric measurements in various ethnic groups, in relation to SIDS risk.

Birth Defects

Reliable data on the frequency of birth defects in various racial/ethnic groups are limited because of difficulties in obtaining such data without costly surveys. Routine vital statistics, even where available, are of limited value for most major defects. The best epidemiologic data are from prospective studies in which clinical ascertainment of defects is extensive and follow-up is long-term so that internal defects and those not diagnosed at birth can be detected systematically. The U.S. Collaborative Perinatal Project (USCPP) was the most comprehensive population study of birth defects. This project involved a large cohort of women and standardized examinations of offspring until 5 years of age (Heinonen et al., 1977). Table 9.7 shows some selected findings from this project, indicating lower rates of certain defects among black than white infants, as shown in other studies (reviewed by Polednak, 1986c).

Neural tube defects (NTDs), including anencephaly and spina bifida, comprise a range of defects related to lack of closure of the neural tube; severity varies from an asymptomatic defect in a single vertebra to anencephaly or absence of the brain. NTDS are less common in U.S. blacks than in whites, as also shown for other black as well as Mongoloid populations (Leck, 1984; Polednak, 1986c).

Table 9.7 Rates of Selected Birth Defects in Black and White Live Births, from the U.S. Collaborative Perinatal Project (Heinonen et al., 1977)

Birth weight (g)	Defect	White	Black	Ratio W/B
	Central nervous system			
< 1,999		41.9	18.3	2.3
2,000–2,999		8.3	5.3	1.6
3,000+		3.5	2.8	1.3
	Hypospadias			
< 2,000		27.6	13.3	2.1
2,000–2,499		14.1	13.5	1.0
2,500+		7.2	5.9	1.2
	Respiratory			
< 1,499		64.4	18.3	3.5
1,500–1,999		27.8	16.5	1.7
2,000–2,499		11.7	5.3	2.2
2,500+		3.4	2.6	1.3

Rates are per 1,000 live births. Birth weight categories were as reported by Heinonen et al. (1977); see Polednak (1986c).

The popularly held belief that all major malformations among "primitive" or prehistoric populations were eliminated by infanticide has been challenged by the discovery of the skeletal remains of a young adult aboriginal female from Australia with congenital meningocoele (i.e., spina bifida with the meninges extending into a sac covered with skin) (Webb and Thorne, 1985). Interestingly, there has recently been debate over the severity and need for treatment among a subgroup of patients with myelomeningocele, an NTD involving the meninges (or coverings of the spinal cord), spinal cord, and spinal nerves. Some survivors may not have severe intellectual impairment, but most do have severe physical handicaps (Rickwood, 1985). Pediatricians sometimes are unduly pessimistic about the prognosis, and this affects decisions about treatment (Siperstein et al., 1988).

Although reporting of NTDs on birth certificates is more complete than that for many other defects, a classic study of ethnic differences in the prevalence of NTDs in Boston (Naggan and MacMahon, 1967) involved hospital data rather than birth certificates. High rates were shown in offspring of parents of Irish ancestry, and low rates in offspring of Jewish mothers. The high rates among persons of Irish ancestry have been corroborated. In a cooperative study of congenital anomalies in registries in 16 regions of Europe involving some 767,000 births in 1980–83, the highest rates for NTDs (i.e., 40 per 10,000 births) were found in Dublin and Belfast (along with Glasgow) (De Wals et al., 1987). Thus the high-risk groups include most of the United Kingdom, although Liverpool and Galway were apparent exceptions, while rates in Continental Europe ranged from six to 13 per 10,000 births. The reasons for these differences are unknown, although declining rates in the United Kingdom implicate environmental factors. The multifactorial model, with both genetic (i.e., polygenes) and environmental factors influencing fetal growth rates, may be appropriate, as in oral clefts (see later).

The finding of equal infant and neonatal death rates for congenital malformations in U.S. blacks and whites, and equal infant death rates within low-birth-weight groups, is noteworthy. Prenatal development may differ among racial groups and may influence susceptibility to certain birth defects. A hypothesis involving differences in rates of prenatal development has been advanced to explain lower rates of certain defects (including NTDs) among U.S. blacks versus whites (Polednak, 1986c), since the former are more advanced skeletally (at least at later ages of gestation). An alternative hypothesis for the nearly equal infant mortality rates for congenital anomalies in black and white infants and lower death rates for these causes within low-birth-weight blacks vs. whites, involves a differential magnitude in the shift in the birthweight distribution for all black births vs. those with congenital anomalies, but direct evidence is lacking (Berry et al., 1987). Further studies are needed to explore these hypotheses—preferably, cohort studies of birth defect rates in relation to prenatal measurements such as ultrasonically estimated skeletal dimensions and examination of birth weight distributions in black fetuses with and without malformations.

In contrast to neural tube defects, certain "Mongoloid" populations reportedly have higher rates of *oral clefts* (i.e., cleft lip with or without cleft palate). An interesting study in an Amerindian population (Mayans) in Mexico did not suggest an unusual frequency of oral clefts, but the partial non-Amerindian ancestry of the group and the need for further studies including degree of racial admixture were noted (Weiss et al., 1987).

In reviewing the geographic distribution of cleft lip, with or without cleft palate, and neural tube defects, Leck (1984) observed that consistent racial differences across environments suggested genetic factors but modulation of neural tube defect risk by environmental influences (as in a multifactorial model) is also suggested by migrant studies. Again demonstrating the importance of family studies (Chapter 2), Chung et al. (1986) showed that data on 627 Japanese families were most consistent with a multifactorial model alone, while in 2,998 Danish nuclear families, the best model incorporated both a major gene and a multifactorial component. This is an apparent example of genetic heterogeneity of disease, at least within the limits of the procedure of best-fitting models in segregation analysis.

Chung et al. (1986) had previously shown that prenatal growth factors, reflected in palatal size and shape, may play a role in the multifactorial model, and racial differences in these growth rates may help to explain the high rates of oral clefts in some oriental populations. In Hawaii various Mongoloid populations—including Japanese, Chinese, Koreans, and Filipinos (see Chapter 3)— tended to have wider palates than Caucasians, which may increase the risk of lack of palatal closure (i.e., cleft palate).

In multifactorial models of disease and other characteristics, apparently "sporadic" cases without a family history of the condition may still share a polygenic background with "familial" cases. Several studies have suggested that *asymmetry* for certain bilateral characterstics, including anthropometric features of the face, may be involved in oral clefts. A methodology involving asymmetry in dermatoglyphics and dental measurements has been developed for studies of sporadic cases, and further follow-up of relatives of these cases should prove informative (Crawford and Sofaer, 1987); that is, higher recurrences in families with various asymmetries could suggest a genetic predisposition involving growth factors.

"*Clubfoot*" is a heterogeneous group of disorders showing higher prevalence rates in Polynesians than Caucasians and lowest rates in Mongoloid groups in Hawaii. Family studies using segregation analysis are in progress in Hawaiian and Caucasian populations to examine genetic heterogeneity involving major genes and/or multifactorial inheritance (Wang et al., 1988). This study plan, therefore, is similar to that shown to be useful for oral clefts in Japanese versus Caucasians (as noted above).

"*Congenital*" *dislocation of the hip* (CDH) appears to be less frequent in certain black versus white populations, but more frequent in various Amerindian groups since prehistoric times. Although a study of hospital data in Louisiana suggested that CDH may be more common in blacks than previously believed, the estimated prevalence was still more than three times greater in whites (Burke et al., 1985).

Lapps reportedly tend to have a shallow or dysplastic acetabulum (i.e., socket for the head of the femur) in the pelvic bone and a high frequency of congenital hip disorders (see Milan, 1980). In contrast, studies in Africa suggest that the greater depth of the acetabulum in certain black populations may explain their low rates of congenital hip dislocation, as reported also in the United States (Burke et al., 1985). The explanation for higher rates of congenital hip disorders in American Indians is under debate. The often quoted statement that infant swaddling practices contribute to CDH in populations such as Amerindians, who use cradleboards, has been questioned, in part because of the occurrence of hip dislocations in early neonatal periods prior to cradleboard use (Sievers and Fisher, 1981).

We have noted that certain populations have relatively high levels of *consanguineous marriages*, resulting in inbred offspring. Studies of the effect of level of inbreeding on disease risk provide clues regarding genetic factors in disease in some populations. Recent studies have attempted to control for confounding factors associated with level of inbreeding, such as SES (i.e., occupation of father) and sibship size, in assessing effects on reproductive outcomes. In a case control study among the Old Order Amish of Pennsylvania, close inbreeding was a significant risk factor for prereproductive mortality (i.e., death prior to age 20 years) due to congenital malformations and perinatal problems. That is, the mean level of inbreeding in the offspring was higher for cases (i.e., deaths before age 20 due to all causes and to congenital malformations specifically) than for controls who were Amish but had survived to age 20 years (Khoury et al., 1987). The high inbreeding levels in Old Order Amish due to marriages of second cousins or closer relatives resulted in a high proportion of prereproductive deaths attributable to inbreeding in populations with a long history of consanguineous marriages, such as those in southern India. Some studies have shown higher inbreeding coefficients in children with genetic defects versus normal newborns (Bittle et al., 1986), while others have shown no apparent effects on rates of malformations or infant mortality (Rao, 1984) *within* these groups.

Certain *chromosomal anomalies* are of interest with regard to mental retardation (as discussed below) and other clinical effects. *Down syndrome* (DS), both trisomy (i.e., an extra chromosome 21) and chromosomal translocation varieties, is of interest for a variety of clinical and epidemiologic reasons—for example, its association with increased risk of childhood leukemia and senile dementia or neurological disorders with a genetic basis (see later). DS prevalence is about one in 800 live births in most populations. In the British Columbia study of over 1 million live births followed to age 25 years, DS occurred in 1.2 per 1,000 births and comprised the vast majority of known disorders of autosomal chromosomes (Baird et al., 1988).

Racial/ethnic variation in DS prevalence has not been extensively studied. In the U.S. National Perinatal Collaborative Study, mentioned above, the risk of DS was comparable in blacks and whites (i.e., 29 of 24,030, or 1.21 vs. 30 of 22,811 or 1.32 per 1,000 live births). The only suggestive difference, based on small numbers of DS cases, was the high rate for maternal ages of 40+ years among blacks (Heinonen et al., 1977).

Studies using birth certificates are subject to errors of both under- and overreporting (i.e., false positives), which could vary by racial/ethnic group. Relative to European Caucasians, rates at birth are reportedly lower in Taiwanese but similar in Japanese, and highest in Israel. As observed by Hook (1981), the reportedly high rate of DS in non-European versus European Jews in Israel may be confounded by the lower SES level of the former group, and appropriate analyses have not been conducted.

Among 730 pregnancies in the South Birmingham Health District in 1974–82, the recorded prevalence of DS at birth was lower among Asian immigrants (three of 507 infants) than among Europeans (3/196, excluding one trisomy 21 mosaic) (Rogers, 1986). If this difference is not due to biased reporting or chance, it could reflect higher spontaneous abortion rates among DS fetuses in Asians, a difference in maternal age (i.e., younger maternal age in Asians than Europeans), or other factors. Further studies using DS rates specific for single years of maternal age are in progress.

The strong influence of maternal age on DS prevalence has enabled prediction of DS prevalence in a population on the basis of the maternal age distribution, along with rates of amniocentesis and resulting abortion rates (Kiely, 1987). Thus, additional studies are needed comparing populations to examine differences in the maternal age effect and to explore differences in DS rates independent of (i.e., after controlling for) differences in maternal age. The effect of paternal age independent of maternal age on DS is controversial, but population differences in paternal exposures to environmental agents could be important (Polednak and Janerich, 1983). A suggested negative association between maternal smoking and DS in black (but not white) live births, in USCPP (described earlier), requires confirmation (Hook and Cross, 1988) with larger samples.

Fragile X syndrome (FXS) or *Martin-Bell syndrome*, an X-linked mutation associated with a "fragile site," or unstainable gap on the chromosome and with mental retardation, was not discussed in Chapter 5. A relatively high mutation rate has been reported for this locus, and the disorder occurs in about one in 2,000-2,500 mentally-retarded Caucasian males. No large racial differences in prevalence of FXS were reported in Hawaii (Jacobs et al., 1986), and its frequency among mentally retarded males in Japan was similar to that reported for Caucasian populations (Arinami et al., 1986). The discovery of suitable linked RFLPs would facilitate studies of possible genetic heterogeneity among populations (see Chapter 5).

DISEASES OF THE NERVOUS SYSTEM AND SENSE ORGANS

Neurologic Diseases

A general overview of the epidemiology neurologic and eye disorders, including some discussion of racial/ethnic differences, may be found in Poskanzer (1981). Some selected topics will be discussed here. Despite their infectious origin, bacterial meningitis and meningitis due to other organisms (see Chapter 6) are included with diseases of the nervous system in the ICD (WHO, 1977). Also included in this ICD category are cerebral degenerative diseases such as lipidoses, due to single-gene factors (Chapter 5).

A single-gene disorder, due to an autosomal-dominant gene, classified with diseases of the nervous system is *Huntington's disease* (HD), which was not discussed in Chapter 5. HD is also called Huntington's "chorea" because of symptoms involving choreiform movements. The disease is of great interest because of variability in age at onset and the prospects for prevention through genetic counseling. A survey of HD reported similar prevalence in blacks and whites but evidence for earlier age at onset, and hence clinically more severe disease, among blacks (Folstein et al., 1987). The linkage method of prenatal diagnosis is appropriate for this disorder, in which the basic gene defect is presently unknown. The mapping of an RFLP linked (though not closely) to the HD gene on the short arm of chromosome 4 has been of assistance in genetic counseling (McKusick, 1988) and should be useful in comparative studies across populations.

For many other diseases of the nervous system, some role for genetic factors has also been implicated, but there may be multiple genes and/or strong gene–environment interactions involved in their pathogenesis.

As with many other chronic diseases discussed earlier, comparisons of incidence and prevalence rates across countries and/or racial/ethnic groups are hampered by numerous problems regarding completeness of ascertainment and comparability of diagnoses. Mortality statistics are influenced by both prevalence of disease and survival of patients with the disease.

A pilot study of neurological disorders, including Parkinson's disease, in the Parsis of Bombay (Bharucha et al., 1987) is noteworthy in showing that trained lay health workers can be instrumental in obtaining useful information on the prevalence of neurological disorders in developing countries with few neurologists. Bharucha et al. (1987) also advocate simultaneous case-control studies to identify risk factors as a prelude to prevention programs. Also, prevalence ratios of specific neurologic disorders can be compared across different developing countries, providing possible leads for further investigation of apparent differences.

Slow-Virus Diseases of the Nervous System

In addition to various types of meningitis (Chapter 6), "infectious" or inflammatory diseases include viral encephalitis disorders, among which are diseases due to "slow viruses." The most colorful of these is *kuru*. Kuru is cross-classified under both viral diseases and diseases of the nervous system in the ICD (WHO, 1977). Although resembling other slow-viral diseases with long latent periods between infection and clinical disease, characterized by "spongy" changes in the gray matter of various brain areas, kuru is found only in the Fore tribe of the eastern highlands of Papua New Guinea, where it has declined concomitantly with reported "cannibalistic" rites. Considerable debate has ensued regarding the existence of cannibalism versus possible transmission via other animals eaten. The present generation of Fore people reportedly have little recollection of or concern about kuru (Cooke, 1986).

Jacob-Creutzfeldt disease is also called "subacute spongiform encephalopathy" because of spongiform changes in the gray matter, or "transmissible agent dementia" due to its transmissibility (like kuru) from human to primates. Incidence is reportedly high in European and North African (including Libyan) immigrants in Israel and among Tunisian Jewish immigrants to France, with evidence for strong familial clustering (Cathala et al., 1985). In Benghazi, Libya, only one hospitalized case was reported between 1982 and 1986 in a population of over 500,000, which does not suggest an unusually high incidence of *hospitalized* cases, but further studies are needed in North Africa (Radhakirishnan and Mousa, 1988).

Subacute sclerosing panencephalitis (SSPE) is of interest because of its association with measles infection in early childhood, and its diagnosis on the basis of personality changes and characteristic "bursts" in the electroencephalogram. Measles, common in developing countries (Chapter 6) such as Pakistan, contributes to SSPE prevalence (Kondo et al., 1988). Measles vaccination programs in Pakistan, like those in the United States in the 1960s, should reduce the incidence rate for SSPE. Incidence rates are difficult to estimate in different countries because of the lack of adequate surveys and reliance on hospital or clinic data, but the estimated prevalence in Karachi Pakistan may be 8–13 per million, versus <0.5 (e.g., in the U.S. and Japan) to 2.0 in other developed countries (Kondo et al., 1988). SSPE thus provides another example of a "chronic" disease whose distribution is largely explained by the distribution of an infectious disease involved in its etiology.

Degenerative Diseases

"Degenerative" diseases of the nervous system are classified according to the anatomical structures involved (i.e., the cerebrum or "higher" areas vs. lower areas). Thus Parkinson's disease and Huntington's disease involve the basal ganglia and mesencephalon or extrapyramidal system, while motor neuron diseases involve the motor system or pyramidal system. For both groups of disorders, several distinct subgroups exist, with different causal factors, which complicates comparisons of rates. In addition to genetic disorders previously discussed (Chapter 5), "cerebral degenerations" include Alzheimer's disease (see later).

Parkinson's syndrome (PS). The epidemiology of PS is complicated by the recognition of subcategories, although most cases are "idiopathic" or of unknown cause (also called "paralysis agitans"). Other cases, in declining numbers, are related to the 1914–18 influenza epidemics and are called "postencephalitic" PS, while "toxic" (i.e., drug- or chemical-related) and "vascular" subgroups are also recognized. Variation in severity of PS, as with most other chronic diseases, results in variation in reliability and comparability of studies based on hospital series, while neurologic surveys may vary in the criteria used.

In a survey of all hospitalized cases in Baltimore, prevalence rates for PS were significantly lower in blacks than whites during 1967-69 (Kessler, 1972). Only 39 percent of PS hospital cases who died had PS mentioned on the death certificate. Using numbers of deaths reported in the United States for 1984 (Table 9.8), death rates (calculated by the author) for PS were lower in blacks than whites after age 54 years. If these differences are real, hypotheses involve infectious agents, with protection in lower-SES groups due to early exposure when clinical effects are benign and biological differences related to degree of pigmentation. Loss of pigment in certain parts of the brain (i.e., the substantia nigra of the midbrain) in PS has suggested the latter hypothesis, but the relation (if any)

Table 9.8 Mortality Rates (per 100,000) from Parkinson's Disease and Multiple Sclerosis in the United States for Blacks and Whites in 1985

	Age (years)									
	45–54		55–64		65–74		75–84		85+	
	No.	Rate	No.	Rate	No.	Rate	No.	Rate	No.	Rate
Parkinson's disease										
White male	6	0.06	93	1.0	698	10.4	1,411	47.4	533	76.7
Black male	5	0.46	6	0.7	30	4.8	40	15.6	13	20.0
W/B ratio	0.13		1.6		2.1		3.0		3.8	
White female	10	0.10	58	0.6	394	4.6	1,121	22.2	595	33.5
Black female	0	0.00	1	0.1	25	3.0	28	6.7	12	8.6
W/B ratio	—		6.2		1.6		3.3		3.9	
Multiple sclerosis										
White male	109	1.1	136	1.5	117	1.7	46	1.6	7	1.0
Black male	12	1.1	10	1.1	6	1.0	3	1.2	0	0.0
W/B ratio	1.0		1.4		1.7		1.3		—	
White female	183	1.8	238	2.3	184	2.2	82	1.6	14	0.8
Black female	24	1.8	20	1.8	7	0.8	2	0.5	0	0.0
W/B ratio	1.0		1.3		2.8		3.2		—	

Data calculated from numbers in *Vital Statistics of the United States* for 1985, published in 1988.

between skin and brain pigmentation is apparently still uncertain. Other risk factors in PS include certain drugs and environmental contaminants as well as cerebrovascular disease, which should be considered in future case-control studies of blacks and whites.

Although Parkinsonism patients in Bulgaria receive treatment free of charge, reports of large proportions of cases of mild severity in such areas (i.e., Sofia) based on registered patients at clinics and hospital neurology departments (Chalmanov, 1986) are subject to unknown biases.

Micronesians, especially the Chamorros of the Marianas Islands of Guam (Fig. 3.2 and Chapter 3) and Rota, and some genetically related groups in Japan (in the Kii peninsula) and the Philippines have unusually high rates of *amyotrophic lateral sclerosis* (ALS) and a clinical variant known as *Parkinsonism-dementia*. ALS is classified under "motor neuron disease" (MND), one category in a larger group of diseases of cells in the anterior horn of the spinal cord. These foci of unusual risk have long been of interest in the search for clues to the causation of these disorders.

MND is also reportedly common in surveys in the middle part of Finland (i.e., incidence rate estimated at 2.4 per 100,000 per year), and lower in Benghazi Libya (i.e., 0.89 per 100,000) and other parts of Europe, but the comparability of such data is uncertain (Radhakrishnan et al., 1986). A rather high crude annual incidence rate of about 2.0 per 100,000 (or 2.4 adjusted to the 1970 U.S. population), for example, has been reported in careful population studies in Rochester, Minnesota, from 1925 through 1984 (Yoshida et al., 1986).

With the exception of the isolated areas of high risk, early surveys of the literature had suggested a rather uniform worldwide incidence of ALS of about one per 100,000 per year (Kurland, 1957). In view of the findings from Minnesota, a range of 1–2 per 100,000 may be more accurate. A recent study in England, involving both death records and hospital records validated by surveys of physicians, found a crude incidence rate (in 1981) of 2.2 per 100,000 and a mortality rate of 2.2 and suggested that mortality data can be used to assess incidence patterns (Qizilbash and Bates, 1987) for this progressive, fatal disease. When both parts of the death certificate are considered, clinical diagnoses made during life are almost always recorded on the certificate. Routine vital statistics, however, usually include only the single "underlying" cause of death and not contributory conditions. Additional studies in various populations should involve examination of all diseases and conditions recorded on death certificates.

The etiology of ALS remains enigmatic. Studies of Filipino migrants to Guam suggest that causal factors operate in adult life and long latency periods may be involved. The environmental factors have not been identified (Garruto et al., 1981), but dietary factors (i.e., plant toxins) have been suggested for these disorders. The calcium deficiency hypothesis for ALS has not been supported by recent studies, and the two disorders common in Guam may be distinct etiologically, because changes in incidence have not been similar (Reed et al., 1987). A specific agent implicated is the neurotoxic seed of the cycad tree, which is used for food and medicines, and cultural changes may have reduced both exposure to this agent and risk of neurological disease (Spencer et al., 1987a). Formal epidemiologic (i.e., case-control) studies of these specific exposures are needed. An animal model involving macaques showed that feeding an amino acid found in the cycad seed resulted in clinical and pathologic features of the disease (Spencer et al., 1987b).

In areas other than Guam, different etiologic factors may operate. Ecologic and descriptive studies of poliomyelitis and MND in England and Wales have suggested an hypothesis of a causal association (Martyn et al., 1988), which should be explored. Delayed effects of previous infection are probably involved in many neurologic disorders, as discussed in this chapter.

Genetic susceptibility to ALS has been suggested by studies of genetic relationships and admixture among various Pacific populations, including data on HLA frequencies. ALS tends to occur in genetically related populations—for example, Chamorros living on various islands in Micronesia, and certain local groups of Japanese and Filipinos (Benfante et al., 1979). Thus some role for genetic factors is probable. This role may involve susceptibility to the toxic effects of certain endogenous and exogenous amino acids.

Alzheimer's disease (AD). AD is one type of "senile dementia." Prevalence rates of AD are different to compare across populations because of differences in diagnostic criteria and methods of case ascertainment. Since prevalence depends on incidence and duration, longitudinal or prospective studies are of particular value in delineating the natural history of AD and in assessing its effects on mortality independent of age. In blacks, dementia due to multiple infarcts related to complications of hyptertension must be distinguished from AD, but the Baltimore Longitudinal Study of Aging was too small and selected to consider black–white differences in AD (Sayetta, 1986). A prevalence study in a southern California retirement community was also limited to whites (Pfeffer et al., 1987).

The growing proportion of elderly persons of diverse racial/ethnic groups in the U.S. population and the availability of an oligonucleotide genetic probe for an abnormal protein (i.e., amyloid beta protein) encoded by a gene located on chromosome 21 near the gene for the familial type of AD (McKusick, 1988) suggest that interest in population differences in AD and its causes will increase. An additional impetus for research is evidence of similarities in the neurologic disturbance in Down's syndrome (discussed earlier) and Alzheimer's disease. The neurologic features of DS may be due in part to a gene (on chromosome 21) that encodes part of a calcium-binding protein called S100 protein that is involved in the functioning of the central nervous system (Allore et al., 1988). Whether or not the ostensibly "nonfamilial" varieties of AD involve genes on chromosome 21, and/or interactions with environmental agents that influence CNS functioning, remains to be explored. Epidemiologic studies are needed on exposure to aluminum, and individual differences in its possible effects on neurotransmitter defects (Birchall and Chappell, 1988) in different populations.

Multiple Sclerosis

Multiple sclerosis (MS), first described by Charcot in 1868, is classified with demyelinating diseases of the nervous system, which involve loss of myelin sheaths of axons. The strong association between latitude and the incidence and prevalence of MS was mentioned in Chapter 1, as a problem in distinguishing racial/ethnic or population differences from larger-scale graduations by geography. Prevalence is higher in the temperate, higher latitudes of both the northern and southern hemispheres than in equatorial regions.

Mortality rates in 1985 were slightly lower in U.S. blacks than whites (Table 9.8), but the author is unaware of any studies separating the effects of latitude (i.e., higher concentration of blacks in southern or lower-risk areas) from other factors in this difference.

In a case-control study within the United States, the association with latitude was shown to be independent of various climatic factors including air pollution index, concentrations of minerals in groundwater, and annual solar radiation (Norman et al., 1983). Therefore, within this population at least, some other environmental factor associated with latitude must be involved. In Bulgaria, however, rates were associated with temperature and amount of sunshine (Kalafatova, 1987). An ecologic study has suggested that diffused solar radiation may be a factor, when the large geographic variation in this variable is considered by international comparisons, in influencing hospital admissions and hence in some aspect of the natural history of MS (Laborde et al., 1988). As with other diseases, studies within countries may not detect associations because of the smaller amount of variation in the putative factor (see Chapter 1). As always, methodologic issues complicate the interpretation of associations reported from different countries. In a population-based study of MS in northern Colorado, using multiple sources of ascertainment, MS service organizations as well as neurology practices were an important source of data for estimating prevalence (Nelson et al., 1986). Thus, studies using one or a few sources for data may underestimate MS rates, and regional differences could be obscured.

Until about 30 years ago, MS was stated to be "rare" in Japan. Careful checks of medical records and reexamination of patients in Kumamoto Prefecture (on Kyushu Island) disclosed seven cases or a prevalence of 1.3 per 100,000 in 1976-82, which was higher than previous reports from Japan, possibly reflecting improvements in diagnosis and therapy (and hence survival for enumeration in prevalence studies). This rate was still lower than that reported from Western countries (Araki et al., 1987).

Studies of migrants from both high-risk and low-risk areas to low-risk areas have implicated an important *environmental* determinant (probably an infection) *early* in life (i.e., before age 15 years) and another factor operating later in life (Haile et al., 1983). This pattern contrasts with that for ALS, described above. On the basis of estimation of population denominators and case records at hospitals and clinics, children of West Indian immigrants (a low-risk group) born in the United Kingdom had high incidence and prevalence rates of "probable" MS, similar to those of Northern Ireland and the Irish Republic (Elian and Dean, 1986). Again, environmental factors are strongly implicated by these data, although accuracy of estimation of rates is open to question.

The occurrence of epidemics of MS, as in the Faroe Islands and nearby Iceland, implicates an infectious and/or toxic environmental agents, although the existence of true epidemics has been questioned (Poser, 1987; Poser and Hibberd, 1987). The hypothesis involving canine distemper virus is controversial. An unusually high prevalence of MS has been reported in Key West, Florida, a tropical area—even higher than that observed in the Faroe Islands. Cases have included migrants to Key West, prior to age 16 years, as well as native-born cases (Roman and Sheremata, 1988). A small case-control study in Key West found that cases more often resided in Key West at age 18 than controls and more often had a previous "viral infection" (Helmick et al., 1988).

The ubiquitous chronic-disease model of genetic susceptibility interacting with key environmental exposures appears to hold for MS. The genetics of MS remain obscure, aside from associations with HLA types and possible linkage with a gene in the HLA region of chromosome 6. Genetic heterogeneity has been suggested by comparison of HLA associations in different racial/ethnic groups (Spielman and Nathanson, 1982), but small samples sizes were involved in Japan and Israel. Poser (1987a, b) has suggested that the geographic distribution is correlated with predominance of "Germanic-origin" groups, but the theory of genetic factors introduced by "Viking invasions" has been questioned (Plaut, 1987). Although Spielman and Nathanson (1982) favored a dominant mode of inheritance on the basis of family studies, or a modified dominant mode involving a double dose of a putative allele, family studies in the high-risk area of the Orkney Islands (United Kingdom) suggested that multifactorial inheritance was more likely (Roberts et al., 1979).

A common problem in family studies, as noted with reference to colon cancer and precursor lesions as markers for susceptibility (Burt et al., 1985), is the absence of a marker for susceptibility to MS versus reliance on overt disease that varies widely in severity. Thus exploration of genetic modes of inheritance is difficult and problematic. A biochemical or physiologic marker of preclinical MS or MS susceptibility would be useful in family studies and in population comparisons.

Migraine

It is worthwhile to recognize negative reports of lack of racial/ethnic differences in disease for several reasons including the fact that biased reporting of positive studies may occur, as well as practical reasons related to clinical decisions. Several surveys, including the U.S. National Health Survey, found only a slight and not statistically significant difference in prevalence of migraine (or frequent and severe headaches) between blacks and whites (Linet and Stewart, 1984). A recent survey in Guangxi, China, involving screening examinations, has reported a prevalence of 3,170 per 100,000 (age-adjusted to the 1960 U.S. population) during 1984 and confirmed the higher prevalence in females (Yao and Huang, 1988) reported in other countries. This prevalence rate is similar to that reported in surveys in Western countries (see Poskanzer, 1981).

Muscular Dystrophies (MD)

The muscular dystrophies are a diverse group of diseases, including several varieties due to different genes. "Hereditary progressive muscular dystrophies" were the most common (i.e., 77 per million) X-linked disorders among the genetic diseases found in the large British Columbia study of over 1.2 million births followed to age 25 years (Baird et al., 1988). Both the Becker (BMD) and Duchenne (DMD) forms of MD are X-linked recessive disorders, the latter being more common, and there is strong evidence that these two disorders are allelic (i.e., they represent the effects of alternative forms of gene deletions at the same locus) (Hart et al., 1987).

Polymorphic markers of RFLPs, linked to DMD and BMD and useful in carrier detection and prenatal diagnosis (see Chapter 5), appear to be of similar value in Finnish (Lindlof et al., 1987) and other European populations studied, but the occurrence of new mutations complicates predictions. Clinically, DMD was reportedly similar in Caucasian, "negroid," and "Mongoloid" (i.e., predominantly Amerindian) patients in Brazil (Bortolini and Zatz, 1987).

Autosomal-dominant myotonic dystrophy, the first human disease for which linkage with a genetic marker (i.e., the ABH blood group secretor locus or Se and the blood group Lutheran) (Greiner et al., 1988), does not appear to have been studied extensively in different populations.

Conclusion

This section has considered a wide range of disorders including some related to single-gene defects, others that are heterogeneous but include familial forms (e.g., Alzheimer's disease), and a larger group probably involving complex interactions between genetic susceptibility and environmental influences. Population differences for many of these diseases have not been adequately studied, due in part to methodological difficulties related to incompleteness of ascertainment of cases. Foci of high risk for certain disorders appear to reflect environmental factors, but an interaction with genetic susceptibility has not been ruled out (e.g., for motor neuron diseases and MS). Differential exposure to infectious agents, often early in life in certain social classes (and hence, racial/ethnic groups) or geographic areas, has been implicated in a variety of neurologic disorders. With regard to neurologic diseases with either known or suspected genetic components in causation (i.e., Huntington's disease, or HD; and Parkinson's syndrome, or PS), racial admixture studies offer potential for helping to elucidate the roles of modifying genes that affect expression of HD and genes involved in the multifactorial disease PS. Family studies are also important, but the identification of a preclinical or other marker of MS *susceptibility* would be useful. The recent demonstration of expression of HLA-DR glycoprotein in brain cells of patients with MS, PS, HD, and other degenerative diseases, in comparison with normal brains (McGeer et al., 1988), offers promise.

Eye Diseases

As with infectious diseases (Chapter 6), the main demarcation for blindness rates is between developing versus developed countries, and not distinct population or racial/ethnic boundaries. Most of the burden of the estimated worldwide blindness prevalence of at least 28 million, the great majority of whom live in developing countries, is due to infectious disease (i.e., trachoma) (Chapter 6), cataracts, and vitamin A deficiency (i.e., xerophthalmia) (discussed earlier). Although reliable data on blindness are not available from many developing countries, some 45 countries have implemented blindness prevention programs, and simplified methodologies are being developed for use in data collection for blindness registries as part of the World Health Organization's goal of health for all by the year 2000 (Thylefors, 1987).

Trachoma varies considerably in frequency and severity within a country, reflecting behavioral and environmental factors, and the importance of grading severity in order to target areas for intervention has been recognized (Taylor et al., 1987; Thylefors, 1987). As for other diseases such as neurological disorders, involvement of local auxiliary health personnel is important in collecting such data in developing countries such as Tanzania. Large-scale field surveys in Australian aborigines indicated a very high prevalence of trachoma, including severe forms with scarring, in contrast to nonaborigines (Thomson, 1984), thus identifying another population in need of intervention programs.

Glaucomas

The discussion of glaucomas is complicated by the existence of several varieties, etiologically distinct, and subgroups within each variety, as well as the lack of standardized clinical criteria for definitions. Ocular hypertension and visual field loss, the latter due to "cupping" or excavation of the optic disc, may occur independently of each other in primary open-angle glaucoma (POAG) or chronic glaucoma; secondary OAG is related to other known causes including injuries. POAG presumably involves a reduction in outflow of fluid from the anterior chamber of the eye, which may be manifested in increased intraocular pressure. In open-angle glaucoma, the anatomical relationships within the anterior chamber of the eye are not distorted. In angle closure glaucoma, sudden increases in pressure and mechanical obstruction of outflow channels result in closure of the angle or contact of the iris with the adjacent tissues.

The estimated proportion of blindness or low vision caused by glaucomas varies from 2–4 percent in Gambia, Nepal, and Saudi Arabia to 15 percent in Malawi (Thylefors, 1987). The higher prevalence of POAG black populations is well known (Leske, 1983) (Table 9.9). A role for racial differences in intraocular and systemic hypertension is possible, but further studies are needed. The disease also has an earlier onset and more rapid course in U.S. blacks. In a small case-control study of glaucoma (with visual field loss) in blacks and whites in Baltimore, diabetes showed the strongest association with risk of the disease (i.e., odds ratio = 2.80) (Katz and Sommer, 1988); diabetes was a risk factor in each race. Thus, black–white differences in diabetes prevalence (see earlier) is one explanation for black–white differences in glaucoma. A pilot study of POAG in Barbados suggests that prevalence is apparently high; consideration is being given to intraocular and systemic blood pressure, diabetes, and other risk factors (Leske, 1987). In contrast to Africans, raised intraocular pressure and glaucoma were rare in the Solomon Islanders (Friedlaender et al., 1987).

Primary *angle closure* glaucoma is reportedly more common in certain Eskimo groups in Greenland and Canada, and the ratio of angle closure to POAG is also high in Japan and Southeast Asia (Nixon and Phelps, 1986). In blacks, angle closure glaucoma tends to be more serious and insidious. Explanations for these differences are unknown; suggestions for genetic factors require exploration.

Results of studies on genetic markers in POAG, including blood groups serum proteins, and HLA types (David and Trevor, 1980; Tiwari and Terasaki, 1985), have been conflicting. A reported slight excess in G6PD deficiency among blacks in South Africa (David and Trevor, 1980) requires confirmation. Studies of degree of racial admixture could prove rewarding. In Australia various types of glaucomas and normal controls among patients at an eye research unit were analyzed separately with regard to blood groups (Brooks and Gillies, 1988). Although some statistically significant differences were reported, mainly regarding ABH secretor phenotypes and not ABO groups (see Chapter 3), a large number of comparisons were made, and further studies are needed to confirm these findings before speculating on their significance regarding population differences in glaucomas.

Cataracts

Cataracts or lens opacities are classified on the basis of their location—for example, "cortical" for the cortical layers, "nuclear" for the central nucleus of the lens, and "subcapsular" or beneath the anterior or posterior capsule of the lens. On the basis of data from the first U.S. National Health and Nutrition Examination Survey (1971–72), which involved actual examination of lenses, certain types of cataract (i.e., nuclear and cortical, but not posterior subcapsular) are more common in blacks than whites (Table 9.9) (Hiller et al., 1986). The explanation is unknown, but racial differences in such risk factors as sunlight exposure, diabetes mellitus, and hypertension could be involved, although the latter two factors are associated mainly with the posterior subcapsular variety.

Table 9.9 Prevalence of Selected Eye Diseases in
U.S. Blacks and Whites

Disease	Black–White Ratio
Cortical cataract	3.5
Nuclear cataract	1.8
Glaucoma blindness	8.0

Sources: Hiller et al. (1986); Leske (1983). See text for discussion.

In Nepal a nationwide cross-sectional survey has confirmed the high prevalence of cataracts, as also reported in the Punjab plains of India (Mitchell and
Lepkowski, 1986). Again, sunlight exposure may be a factor, especially in males,
and dietary factors were also suggested, but further studies are needed.

MENTAL DISORDERS

Problems of incomplete ascertainment of cases and comparability of diagnostic
procedures, common to epidemiologic studies of all chronic diseases, are especially crucial in the interpretation of apparent population differences in the
prevalence and manifestations of mental disorders. This topic requires separate
and extensive review, and only selected research issues will be reviewed here.
Recent issues include the possible role of genetic factors in explaining racial/
ethnic differences in alcohol metabolism and alcoholism—for example, the low
rates in Japanese and other orientals as opposed to Caucasians and Amerindians
(Anon., 1985e). An area of research interest for many years has been the role of
socioeconomic and psychosocial factors in black–white differences in mental
disorders. More recently, U.S. Hispanics versus Anglos have been studied with
regard to the prevalence of psychiatric symptoms and disorders, and the roles of
socioeconomic and psychosocial factors (e.g., acculturation) have been considered. These issues will be discussed briefly.

Depression and Other Disorders

The literature on the prevalence of *manic-depressive disorders* in Africa is inconclusive, due in part to the lack of reliable data based on community surveys versus
hospital statistics, which are subject to various selection biases. There is an
impression that *depression* is common in some parts of Africa and that only
about one in four seeks psychiatric help (Ovuga, 1985). Hospital-based studies
provide conflicting data on the relative frequency of affective disorders; for
example, depression is more common than mania in Zambia, but the reverse
pattern has been reported in Kenya (Acuda and Ovuga, 1985). Some of these
differences may reflect sociocultural patterns affecting admission to hospital,
especially with regard to tolerance of manic behavior, as also suggested for U.S.
Hispanics (Markides and Coreil, 1986). Wide cross-cultural variation in prevalence of affective disorders receiving treatment, versus untreated cases, may

reflect differences in the status of depressed persons or "ethnocentric" conceptions of depression (Marsella, 1980). Community surveys of adults in Uganda also suggest a high prevalence of affective disorders in comparison with European and Australian surveys (WHO; 1973; Regier et al., 1988), so that hospitalization or treatment-related factors may not be the only explanation.

Consideration of the relative frequency of psychiatric disorders in U.S. blacks and whites has a long history, reviewed by Fischer (1969) with reference to the myth that blacks had higher rates than whites. In the northeastern United States a survey of more than 400,000 hospital admissions in a multistate system, using data centralized at the Rockland Research Institute (Orangeburg, New York), corroborated previous reports that the incidence of manic-depressive illness in the treated population is lower in blacks than in whites (Marquez et al., 1985). The diagnosis of manic-depressive illness appeared to be increasing in frequency among blacks, but the authors questioned whether hospital statistics reflect true prevalence and noted the need for community-based epidemiologic studies.

Although awareness of the occurrence of mania in U.S. blacks may be increasing, the diagnosis is still being missed. Also, blacks tend infrequently to use community mental health centers located in predominantly white areas, and are more often referred out of such centers (Mayo, 1974). Well-known inaccuracies in diagnoses of psychiatric disorders due to sociocultural distance between clinician and patient should also be mentioned.

Community surveys of mental disorder in five areas of the United States have involved oversampling of blacks ($N = 4,287$ or 23 percent and Hispanics ($N = 1,433$ or 8 percent), but racial/ethnic comparisons had not yet been reported (Regier et al., 1988). Kessler and Neighbors (1986) analyzed results of eight epidemiologic surveys of black–white differences in *psychological distress* in relation to social class, and found racial differences to be particularly pronounced among persons with low incomes. That is, an interaction between social class and race was apparent, suggesting that factors related to race, and not social class alone, were involved. Explanations are uncertain, but factors related to frustrated aspirations for upward social mobility, stress associated with goal striving, or discrimination and lack of resources for coping with stress could be important.

Surveys within the U.S. black population are providing useful information on factors that may precipitate or ameliorate psychologic distress or disorder. In a community survey of depressive symptoms in a black community in Alabama, using a random sample of households and obtaining a 68 percent response rate, education and income had no independent effect, but sociocultural processes involving stressors and support systems were judged important (Dressler and Badger, 1985). Significant variation in the importance of gender and marital status was observed across communities or regions, suggesting cultural diversity within the "black community" in the United States. The extent of sex differences in depression, for example, differed between the North and the South, and differences in the role of black women in the family were suggested as a factor (Dressler and Badger, 1985).

Data from the National Survey of Black Americans, involving a representative sample of 2,107 adults, indicated negative associations between socioeconomic status indicators and "psychologic distress" as assessed by a symptom checklist (Neighbors, 1986). An important interaction effect between (low) SES and an experience of economic crisis on risk of psychologic distress appeared to emerge. These data are useful in planning prevention programs and treatment strategies among black communities. One tentative conclusion would be that low-income blacks are at high risk for psychological distress, possibly related to acute crises, and that inadequate social support mechanisms both in the family and in the community may be a major factor. This may be considered a general model for stress amelioration that also applies to the mental health of immigrant groups, where cultivation of social networks or support systems may be crucial (Kuo and Tsai, 1986).

In U.S. Hispanic communities, the role of social support systems in amelio-rating psychiatric symptomatology is unclear, but level of acculturation appears to influence prevalence of depressive symptoms among Mexican-Americans in California as shown by the higher prevalence in Spanish-speaking than English-speaking groups (Vega et al., 1984). In the Mexican-American population in San Antonio, Texas, within two of the three generations studied, prevalence rates for depressive symptoms were lower than those reported for other studies (i.e., of whites and blacks) (Mendes de Leon and Markides, 1988).

Another group of growing interest in the United States is the Southeast Asian refugees (discussed earlier), and prevention of mental disorders through understanding of acculturation stresses has been advocated (Westermeyer, 1987). In a small case-control study of Hmong refugees with major depression, postmi-gration factors appeared to be important, including a supporting sponsor and a stable residence during the first few years after migration (Westermeyer, 1988).

In Kuwait, an area undergoing rapid Westernization related to petroleum wealth, interparental conflict between traditional and "liberal" or Western atti-tudes was related to frequency of reported psychiatric symptoms in these parents. Large interparental age differences, reflecting traditional polygynous practices, apparently contributed to parental conflicts among Kuwaiti natives (El-Islam et al., 1988). Thus acculturation or rapid culture changes may influence self-re-ported psychological impairment.

Intriguing data are emerging on depression in the People's Republic of China, including a suggestion that depressive symptoms may be common in Chinese medical patients (Yang et al., 1987). Kleinman's (1986) study of 100 consecutive mental patients at Hunan Medical College showed that the majority (i.e., 87) could be diagnosed as having a major depressive disorder on the basis of standard diagnostic criteria. "Neurasthenia," or psychologic distress involving physical complaints, is the more acceptable diagnosis in China, and "somatiza-tion" of stress may occur in that sociopolitical environment. Similar observations on somatization of depression in Japan and Taiwan had been made by Kleinman and others (Marsella, 1980).

We shall not review here the extensive and fascinating literature on transcul-tural psychiatry and culture-specific manifestations of psychiatric disorders, for which there is considerable evidence. The reader is referred to classic works by Opler (1959) and more recent compendia (Kleinman, 1985; Simons, 1985), as well as the literature in medical anthropology (e.g., Harwood, 1981; Chrisman and

Maretzki, 1982). Although there is evidence that similar kinds of abnormal behavior are recognized in different cultures, with similar rates for such disorders as schizophrenia (Murphy, 1976), local cultural factors also may influence expression of disturbed behavior. Precipitating events may vary. Among Australian aborigines, fear of sorcery is commonplace and contributes to acute depression (Watson, 1984), thus recalling the classic work of Walter B. Cannon (1942) on "voodoo death" induced by the power of suggestion. To cite one example of a "culture-bound" syndrome, "koro" has long been recognized historically in the Far East among Chinese-origin males in Southeast Asia (Ackerknecht, 1982), involving fear of retraction or shrinkage of the penis. Although epidemics of koro have been limited to Southeast Asia, sporadic cases have been reported in the Western hemisphere, including a case in an Ashkenazic Jewish male in Israel who emigrated from Rumania at age 6 and proved to have a brain tumor, suggesting the need for neurologic investigation of such sporadic cases (Durst and Rosca-Rebaudengo, 1988).

There is debate regarding the relative severity or chronicity of schizophenia in indigenous tropical peoples versus Western cultures (Murphy and Raman, 1971; Murphy, 1976), as well as the interpretation of "culture-bound" syndromes.

Schizophrenia is another chronic disease that is recognized as involving an interaction between genetic factors, as shown through studies of twins and adopted children of schizophrenics, and environmental influences, but both aspects are poorly understood. Regarding the environmental component, the theory of "ethnic density," which predicts a negative correlation between disease incidence and the size of a particular ethnic or immigrant group, has some support from studies in New York City, but a recent analysis in England found no correlation between hospital admissions among specific immigrant groups and their proportions of the total population (Cochrane and Bal, 1988). Within the Irish immigrants, however, rates of hospitalization were higher in areas where few Irish-born persons live versus other areas with higher concentrations; the latter may be a statistical artifact, because many comparisons were made, or may represent a mechanism of maladaptation as suggested by alcoholism rates.

Recent discoveries of genes (both X linked and autosomal dominant) involved in various manic-depressive and depressive disorders will provide a basis for population comparisons of the frequencies of these genes and their roles in population differences in disease prevalence. Also potentially aiding international comparisons of mental disorders will be the development and field testing of a new version of the section "Mental, Behavioral and Developmental Disorders" in the 10th revision of the *International Classification of Diseases* (ICD). More than 190 centers in 55 countries will participate, including Hunan in China, Moscow, Japan, India, New Zealand, Nigeria, Cuba, and parts of Europe (Sartorius et al., 1988).

Alcoholism

Cross-cultural and racial/ethnic differences in alcoholism have been reviewed extensively elsewhere (Babor, 1986; Heath, 1987). Alcoholism, as with many other chronic disorders, involves a complex interaction of important sociocultural factors and some probable contribution of genetically related metabolic factors involving liver alcohol enzyme (i.e., dehydrogenase or ALDH) activity or enzymic variation. Population genetic differences in alcohol dehydrogenases (ADH) related to several human ADH gene loci, involving enzyme electrophoretic and kinetic studies, have been reviewed by Smith (1986). Atypical ADH alleles have been described in Oriental populations, including Japanese, Chinese, and other Orientals in Hawaii. An atypical aldehyde dehydrogenase gene $(ALDH_2^2)$ is frequent in Japanese but absent in Caucasians, and the resultant enzyme deficiency has been implicated in "alcohol flushing" reactions which may lead to avoidance of alcohol in Japanese (but not in Eskimos and Amerindians) (Omenn, 1988). Such genetic variation in ALDH loci may be involved in the complex etiology of alcoholism (Anon., 1985e), but the paramount importance of sociocultural factors including cultural attitudes is also apparent.

Cross-cultural studies of alcoholics in France, Canada, and the United States suggest differences in concepts of and attitudes about alcoholism, regarding its causation and effects (Babor et al., 1986). In the United States, although alcohol consumption has increased among black adults in recent decades as reflected in cirrhosis mortality (see earlier), overall use is lower in black than in white teenagers, and multivariate analyses of national survey data in 1974 from students in grades 7–12 showed differential exposure to drinking models or peers among abstinent blacks versus whites (Harford, 1986). Heavy drinking versus abstention may be more common among certain U.S. black than white populations (especially males), as also shown in the frequency of heavy drinking among black male controls in case-control studies of cancer (Chapter 8). Further studies are needed on factors, including SES and sociocultural differences, involved in patterns of alcohol consumption among black versus white young adults, as also suggested by differences in the role of alcohol in homicide rates (see later).

The problem of alcoholism is evident in groups that have undergone acculturation, even for long periods of time, such as Australian aborigines (Thomson, 1984) and Amerindians. The extent of alcoholism in certain native American groups is evidenced by the high prevalence of fetal alcohol syndrome—an average of one in 633 live births in American Indians and as high as one in 100 births in some tribes (Honigfeld and Kaplan, 1987). The cultural traditions of certain tribes (e.g., Navajo, Pueblos, Apaches, and Utes) may contribute to tribal differences in alcoholism (Honigfeld and Kaplan, 1987), but these "traditions" may reflect acculturation effects. In another part of the world, a traditional native drink (i.e., kava) of the Pacific Islands has been introduced into Australian aboriginal groups in Arnhem Land in recent years. Kava was involved in ritual and social functions in the Pacific (e.g., Fiji, Vanuatu, and Tonga), as described by Captain Cook in the 1760s (Anon., 1988f). The need for educational programs regarding the harmful effects of kava among aboriginals has been recognized.

Mental Retardation (MR)

Methodologic issues in the epidemiology of MR and results of population surveys have been reviewed by Kiely (1987). As with other chronic disorders that vary in severity, comprehensive surveys are required for accurate data on prevalence (especially for mild mental retardation). Surveys in Sweden suggest lower prevalence rates (i.e., about 3.7–3.8 per 1,000 population of children) for mild mental retardation than other surveys. One survey in northern Sweden involved a population with Swedes, Lapps, and Finns (reviewed by Kiely, 1987), and it would be interesting to assess differences among these culturally and racially diverse groups.

Down syndrome (DS) is the most frequent cause of mental retardation, comprising perhaps almost a third of cases of severe MR in some populations (Kiely, 1987). Another important cause of MR, probably second in frequency to DS, is the fragile X syndrome (see earlier). Other causes of MR are PKU (Chapter 5), birth defects (e.g., neural tube defects), and perinatal problems (see earlier). The frequency of the fragile X syndrome among mentally retarded males is reportedly similar for Japanese and Caucasians (Arinami et al., 1987). As yet, no racial/ethnic variation among retarded males has been reported for the prevalence of fragile X syndrome in Greece and other parts of Europe, North America, Australia, and Japan (Mavrou et al., 1988). Although fragile X syndrome is X linked, heterozygous females also have a risk of moderate to severe MR, including Japanese.

ACCIDENTS, INJURIES, HOMICIDE, AND SUICIDE

Death rates related to *motor vehicle accidents* and deaths due to *injuries* will be discussed only briefly. Worldwide variation in *reported* death rates for motor vehicle accidents is evident in Table 4.5 and is related in part to level of economic development—for example, rates are lowest in Guatemala and Chile. In Guatemala, for example, death rates from injuries are relatively high, while rates for motor vehicle accidents are low. In the United States, incidence and mortality rates for accidents and injuries, including moving-vehicle accidents, are positively associated with SES (Iskrant and Joliet, 1968). Iskrant and Joliet's (1968) observations have been supported by more recent data on deaths due to injury among blacks and whites in 1984 (Gulaid et al., 1988). Nonwhites (i.e., blacks) in the United States, including children in Boston (Wise et al., 1985), have higher rates for deaths related to fire, drowning and motor vehicle accidents to pedestrians. SES differences are a major factor in these racial differences.

Accidents in children and young adults have been recognized as a major global problem by WHO, which has recently developed a program for accident prevention and a 1986 report (Manciaux and Romer, 1986) summarized methodologic issues as well as comparisons in broad geographic areas. Rapid increases in motor vehicle ownership in developing countries has resulted in increasing death rates from accidents, as shown in Mexico, Thailand, Venezuela, and Chile (although absolute rates are still relatively low).

Homicides and suicides will also be discussed briefly. U.S. black young adults in several age groups had higher death rates than whites for homicides, but not for suicides, in 1985 (Table 4.1). For homicides in 1980, rates for Hispanics were intermediate, and rates for Anglos were lowest (Anon., 1985c). U.S. white males aged 15–24 years have shown a greater increase in suicide rates from 1970 to 1980 than blacks and others, and white males aged 20–24 years have the highest suicide rates.

As shown for psychiatric disorders (discussed earlier), SES has a major effect in that high homicide rates characterize the lowest SES areas. Combining homicides, suicides, and accidents reveals no clear associations with SES in ecologic studies (e.g., in Philadelphia; Dayal et al. 1986) because of the contrasting epidemiologic patterns of these causes of death in relation to SES.

In the U.S. southwestern states, homicide rates were about 2.5–3.0 times higher in Hispanics (i.e., Mexican-Americans), while suicide rates were more than 50 percent lower than those for Anglo whites (Smith et al., 1986). In Los Angeles in 1970–79, blacks were 5.6 times and Hispanics 2.3 times more likely than whites to be homicide victims. High blood alcohol levels were more common in black and Hispanic than Anglo homicide victims in Los Angeles (Anon., 1986g). In Erie County, New York, black victims also had more alcohol in their blood and were younger than white victims; personal disputes were more common among blacks (Welte and Abel, 1986). Further work is needed to separate the roles of sociocultural factors (if any) and socioeconomic factors in explaining these racial/ethnic differences.

Recorded suicide rates are high in Hungary (i.e., 35.2 per 100,000 per year), Suriname, and parts of Scandinavia (i.e., Denmark and Finland) (Table 4.5). Sri Lanka, for which data on suicide death rates were not reported by WHO (Table 4.5), also has a high recorded death rate (i.e., 29.0 per 100,000), and ingestion of readily available pesticides is involved in a large proportion of these deaths (Berger, 1988). Speculative explanations for this apparently high rate include civil strife between Sinhalese and Tamils, who are genetically related (see Chapter 3), economic problems, and the stresses of Westernization, but immediate public health efforts could involve restrictions in the availability of pesticides; such efforts would present a challenge, in view of the widespread use of pesticides in farming (Berger, 1988). Pesticide ingestion is also the main method of suicide among Indians in Malaysia, where estimated suicide rates are much higher for Indians than for Chinese, Malays, or others (mainly aboriginals). Maniam (1988) has suggested that an "ambivalent" attitude including the condoning of suicide under certain circumstances (e.g., in suttee or by ascetics) among Hindus might be a factor in the high suicide rates among Tamil-speaking Indians in Malaysia (and Indians elsewhere), but evidence is lacking. Accidental poisoning, due to exposure to neurotoxic chemical contaminants during the ritual of menarche in Sri Lanka, is mentioned below.

Worldwide variation in suicide rates (Table 4.5) has often been regarded as misleading, for methodologic reasons, and unworthy of discussion. Other analyses using undetermined deaths and accidental poisonings along with suicides, however, suggest that the relative *ranking* of countries in international comparisons may not be greatly affected by the unreliability of official statistics on suicide (Kliewer and Ward, 1988).

Officially reported suicide rates for Spain, for example, have been historically uniformly low in comparison with the average for Europe or other countries (see Table 4.5), and explanations involving close social and family networks have been offered. Examination by "blind" reviewers of all unnatural deaths occurring in 1982 in Valencia, Spain, however, resulted in rates far higher than those reported officially; the behavior of the local magistrate regarding inquest was an important factor in suicide reporting (Asencio et al., 1988). A similar discrepancy from officially reported suicide rates in Ireland (see Table 4.5) has also been reported (Clarke-Finnegan and Fahy, 1983). These studies suggest that the absolute levels of reported suicides are higher than reported, but studies across countries are needed to determine if relative rankings would be greatly affected by more complete ascertainment of suicides.

The Valencia study (Asencio et al., 1988) also showed that, in agreement with some other studies, suicide rates were higher among "immigrants" (undefined) than the home population (by a factor of almost 2). In a study of 25 immigrant groups in Canada, based on mortality statistics, Spaniards had the lowest rates among males, and Finns the highest. For all foreign-born groups combined, the age-specific suicide rates were lower than those for the native-born Canadians for males but higher for females. The suicide rates in immigrants appeared to depend on an interaction between attitudes developed in the country of origin and those adopted in the new country (Kliewer and Ward, 1988). As with other studies of migrants (Chapter 2), age at migration is probably an important factor, in this case relevant to attitudes about suicide and other sociocultural factors, but relevant data were not available for Canada. Factors contributing to racial/ethnic differences in suicide rates and risk factors for suicide are undoubtedly complex and include religious and cultural attitudes.

There are few studies of suicide in U.S. Hispanics, including Mexican-Americans. On the basis of death records, suicide rates (1960-80) in Bexar County (San Antonio), Texas, were lower in Mexican-Americans than Anglos, and the rate of increase over time was greater in the latter (Hoppe and Martin, 1986). Problems with these data include evidence for underreporting of suicides, especially among Mexican-Americans, and inaccuracies in both numerator (i.e., in Hispanic identification) and denominator (i.e., undernumeration of Hispanics), although the latter errors would result in overestimation of death rates.

Suicide rates may not be increasing in Hopi Indian youths in the American Southwest, and recognition of the influence of traditional attitudes regarding social disapproval of behaviors such as marriage between persons of different tribes or socioeconomic levels may be more important than consideration of acculturation (Levy and Kuntz, 1987). In other groups undergoing rapid cultural change or acculturation, however, factors related to the acculturation process (including social support systems) may be important.

Accidental poisonings will be mentioned briefly. In the "E" or external cause coding system of the ICD (WHO, 1977), accidental poisonings are classified according to the nature of the agent. Minimata disease was first reported in Japan in 1956, related to methylmercury contamination of fish by discharges from a chemical plant. Community-based studies have shown increased death rates for liver cancer, chronic liver disease, and cerebral hemorrhage (Tamashiro et al., 1986). Outbreaks of illness including skin disorders (called "yusho") occurred in Japan in 1968 as a result of mass poisonings from cooking oil contaminated with chlorinated hydrocarbons (i.e., polychlorinated biphenyls, or PCBs), and in Taiwan in 1979. The legacy of past exposures to PCBs in Taiwan includes the birth of children of small size to mothers whose body tissues retain the chemical (Rogan et al., 1988). In Korea accidental poisoning due to carbon monoxide from domestic fuel burning in heating and cooking indicates the need for epidemiologic studies of factors contributing to the thousands of recorded deaths (Kim, 1985). As a more esoteric example related to cultural practices, girls attaining menarche in Sri Lanka are exposed to the neurotoxic chemical tricresyl phosphate through the practice of eating raw eggs with contaminated oil (Senanayake and Jeyaratnam, 1981). These few examples must suffice.

CONCLUSIONS

The wide range of disorders discussed in this chapter share common problems regarding completeness of ascertainment and comparability in medical diagnoses as well as in coding. For these chronic disorders population differences in prevalence rates are influenced by differences in incidence and duration, while differences in mortality rates for many diseases may also reflect differences in treatment. Socioeconomic and sociocultural factors influence the ascertainment of many of these disease and (for mental disorders) the clinical expression.

Many of these disorders also have a genetic substrate, in some instances involving a single gene, but in most cases multiple genes that interact with environmental influences such as specific dietary constituents, infectious and toxic agents (including smoking), psychosocial factors and obesity. This pattern holds for peptic ulcer, gallbladder diseases, chronic lung diseases, Parkinson's disease and other neurologic disorders, diabetes mellitus, schizophrenia, and alcoholism. Racial/ethnic differences in the frequency of these disorders largely reflect differences in the environmental component of these multifactorial diseases, but genetic heterogeneity across populations also exists (e.g., for diabetes mellitus), and racial/ethnic differences in frequencies of certain genes and genetic polymorphisms are also involved in differences in diseases ranging from rheumatoid arthritis subtypes to chronic lung diseases and even behavioral disorders such as depression and alcoholism.

10

Summary and Conclusions

RACIAL/ETHNIC GROUPS REVISITED: THEIR VALUE IN EPIDEMIOLOGY AND PUBLIC HEALTH

Genetically the overlap between racial groups has been emphasized by recent research. In our evolutionary history, small, fortuitous variations due to random events and geographic isolation were subjected to natural selection in the process of adaptation to diseases and other aspects of the environment. As Livingstone has observed, it is difficult to determine how much of current genetic variation is related to adaptations to disease, partly because the history of specific diseases such as malaria is usually uncertain. We have noted, however, that malaria and other previously known infectious diseases, as well as newer diseases, will continue to operate as agents of natural selection. Also involved in natural selection are genetic polymorphisms that influence susceptibility or resistance to chronic diseases, and there must be a balance between selective forces operating on the same genetic systems (e.g., specific HLA types). The continued discovery of polymorphisms, including those involved loci unrelated to gene products, also suggests that some of human genetic variation does not represent the influence of natural selection but rather the operation of other mechanisms including gene flow, migration, and random mutation. Arguments regarding "selectionist" as opposed to "neuralist" schools of emphasis in population genetics need not concern us here.

While new polymorphisms continue to be described at a rapid pace, associations between these polymorphisms and specific diseases also continue to be suggested. Some associations may be supported by further research, while others may prove to be chance findings. In some instances associations between specific diseases and a particular genetic polymorphism (e.g., an HLA type) may not hold across all racial/ethnic groups studied and, if statistical problems can be adequately addressed, may represent genetic heterogeneity in the disease under study (e.g., diabetes mellitus). Genetic heterogeneity is one form of causal heterogeneity, which indicates that different pathways of causation for (ostensibly) the same clinical disease may exist. In the case of diseases due to single gene defects, genetic heterogeneity among populations has important implications for genetic counseling.

Recent research has shown greater genetic heterogeneity within versus between major racial groups. While emphasizing the genetic overlap between major racial groups, research in population genetics has also shown some differences in gene frequencies, as demonstrated in the use of specific polymorphic "markers" which are more or less restricted to populations of common ancestry. This expansion of research in population genetics has implications for understanding of the distribution of diseases among racial/ethnic groups, and this potential has recently been recognized.

Both long-term and short-term human adaptation involve predominantly cultural and sociocultural rather than genetic mechanisms, as shown in studies of groups undergoing acculturation as the result of migration or cultural contact. Acculturation and migration may result in biological as well as sociocultural changes in the groups involved, and the biological plasticity of human populations has been shown both in anthropometric studies and in epidemiologic studies of disease.

Groups that differ little genetically may differ in socioculturally related habits. European populations, as we have noted, differ little in genetic characteristics. In parts of France, however, the highest recorded incidence rates of esophageal cancer (in males) are related to traditionally high levels of alcohol consumption, which starts in childhood. Dietary habits relevant to disease may vary greatly within large geographic areas such as China and Japan, with few major racial groups, and these differences represent socioeconomic and sociocultural factors that require further study. Complicating such interpretations of regional differences in disease is the genetic heterogeneity within populations, sometimes reflected in clinal patterns of geographic gradations in frequencies of specific genes. Analytic epidemiologic studies of specific groups, including genetic, socioeconomic and sociocultural variables, are needed to explore these complexities.

Sometimes the main value of racial/ethnic groups in public health is related to their strong associations with SES and/or *perceived* cultural or biological differences reflecting in large part the prejudices of the dominant group(s). The subtle effects of discrimination, with its psychodynamic and psychosocial processes, are also probably involved in the explanation for racial/ethnic differences in specific diseases such as hypertension and depression. Whatever the explanations for racial/ethnic differences in disease rates or prognosis of disease, epidemiologic data can be used in planning public health programs targeted to high-risk groups. Optimally such intervention programs can recognize and take advantage of cultural variation and utilize local community leaders, as demonstrated in programs involving diabetes mellitus in Zuni Indians.

BIOLOGICAL ANTHROPOLOGY AND EPIDEMIOLOGY

We have pointed out some of the difficulties with the use of racial/ethnic group as a variable in epidemiologic studies. Racial/ethnic groups are kaleidoscopic entities when viewed in the long term. Great overlap in frequencies of genetic characteristics generally exists among major racial groups, and heterogeneity within groups is greater. Within-group genetic variation depends on complex influences of founder populations, migrations, marriage patterns, and other factors. Ethnic groups may differ in sociocultural factors, but these patterns may change rapidly, as shown in various migrant groups.

The overwhelming importance of socioeconomic factors has been emphasized for both infectious and chronic diseases, along with ecologic differences for infectious diseases. Sociocultural factors have also been shown to be important. Of lesser importance, but of major interest with regard to the interface between biological anthropology and epidemiology, are biological differences. Some of these biological differences are secondary, because they reflect underlying differences in socioeconomic or sociocultural factors, while others may be influenced by genetic factors. It is clear that the causation of most diseases is complex and that the explanations for social/ethnic differences in disease rates also involve complex interactions between socioeconomic/sociocultural and biologic/genetic factors.

The expanding data base on population genetics, or differences in frequencies of polymorphic genetic markers, offers promise of eventual integration with epidemiologic approaches through descriptive and analytical studies. The demonstration of many clines or geographic gradients in phenotypic and genotypic traits suggests that the use of racial/ethnic groupings will eventually prove obsolete. Meanwhile, methods such as estimation of degree of genetic intermixture as a factor in risk of disease, and interpopulation comparisons of genetic (e.g., HLA) associations with specific disease, continue to provide valuable clues regarding causation.

Disentangling socioeconomic and sociocultural factors, along with investigating genetic influences through studies of polymorphisms, in disease causation and progression should involve collaboration between social and biological anthropologists as part of larger teams of investigators in epidemiologic studies (Figure 1.1). Continuing challenges are evident for many chronic diseases—such as diabetes mellitus, cardiovascular diseases, and cancers—which involve complex interactions among risk factors. For infectious diseases similar complex interactions are involved, as in the ever-present diseases such as tuberculosis and in diseases that are new (such as AIDS-related disorders) or change over time, as well as across populations, in mode of transmission (e.g., hepatitis B).

Some of the contributions of biological or biomedical anthropology to epidemiology, which are relevant to the investigation of racial/ethnic differences in disease, are summarized in Table 10.1. The importance of these contributions should be apparent from this book, but will be emphasized in the next section.

REVIEW OF MAJOR THEMES

A review of some major themes that have emerged from our consideration of racial/ethnic differences in disease may help to consolidate the reader's thinking, perhaps through review of material presented in the chapters indicated along with each theme.

Prominence of Infectious Diseases
and Infectious Agents in Disease

The prominence of infectious diseases as a force in natural selection, via differential mortality, is evident in their effects on frequencies of genetic markers (Chapter 3) in heterozygotes and the concomitant burden of genetic disease in homozygotes (Chapter 5). In modern populations infectious diseases are still prominent in developing countries as major causes of death. In both developing and developed countries, infectious diseases of major importance include hepatitis B, especially in certain high-risk groups, and AIDS-related diseases (Chapter 6). In addition, infectious agents are causal factors in chronic diseases including certain cancers—for example, cervical, nasopharynx, liver, and lymphomas and sarcomas (Chapter 8).

Poverty and Disease

The overwhelming importance of socioeconomic status (SES) factors in explaining racial/ethnic differences in incidence and mortality rates for many diseases has been emphasized in this book, for both infectious and chronic diseases. It is important to control for SES as closely as possible in comparisons of disease rates across racial/ethnic groups, as shown for studies of U.S. black–white differences in cardiovascular diseases (Chapter 7) and cancers (Chapter 8). The effects of poverty go beyond variables of personal risk factors or medical-care services, and suggest the influence of a broad range of environmental factors including differential exposure to crowding, psychosocial stress, and noxious environmental agents. A legacy of poverty may continue to influence such variables as clinical

Table 10.1 Some Contributions of Biological (Biomedical) Anthropology to Epidemiology

Anthropological method or approach	Applications
Use of surnames in definition of groups—e.g., "Hispanics"	Define culturally distinct groups for studies of disease
Racial admixture estimation	Broad delineation of possible role of genetic factors in a specific disease
Population genetics: polymorphisms in blood groups, serum proteins, DNA material	Associations with various diseases through descriptive and analytical studies

Anthropometry
  Weight/height indices
  Anatomical distribution of fat (skinfolds, circumferences)
	Epidemiologic studies of "fat" in relation to disease risk, using case-control and cohort designs, and surveys of malnutrition.

Migrant studies, beginning with Franz Boas, on growth and anthropometric characteristics	Migrant studies of disease and understanding of environmental and genetic factors
Biocultural approaches to biology and behavior in populations, including racial/ethnic groups	Biocultural approaches to disease causation in studies of acculturation and disease, or changes in disease frequency over time (i.e., secular trends)

stage at diagnosis of cancer in certain migrant groups (e.g., Caribbean women residing in New York City) (Chapter 8).

Evidence has also emerged for interactions between SES, especially low SES, and other risk factors. Studies on various diseases, including cardiovascular diseases and depression, in the United States suggest that low-income black populations may be at especially high risk (Chapter 9).

Acculturation and Disease

In various societies the complexity of the effects of "acculturation" processes on disease risk is also becoming apparent through migrant studies. Further studies are needed on ethnic differences in health practices and disease involving use of available indices of acculturation, as among U.S. Hispanic groups. The need for the development of better indices of acculturation in various ethnic groups is also recognized. In some ethnic groups, rapid acculturation may preclude meaningful studies of these processes and their effects on dietary and other habits, while in other groups acculturation may be less rapid and therefore subject to scrutiny.

The literature on human ecology and medical anthropology includes a controversy regarding the effects of acculturation on health. Using data from the central highlands of New Guinea, Dennett and Connell (1988) have marshaled evidence against the "widespread tradition" in human ecology/anthropology that acculturation results in reduction in health, nutritional status, and homeostatic ecologic adaptations. This "tradition" is rather a straw man. The opposing effects of acculturation have long been recognized, as evident in the Solomon Islands studies described by Damon in the late 1960s and early 1970s (summarized in Damon, 1977). Damon showed the similarities between disease pattern in the Solomon Islands, with the prominence of infectious diseases, to that found in the United States in the early part of this century and also showed the different disease patterns of unacculturated versus acculturated or Westernized groups. These contrasts involve life expectancy in birth and the relative importance of certain infectious diseases versus chronic diseases (or "diseases of civilization"). The shift in fertility, life expectancy at birth, and causes of death is part of the "demographic transition" (of demographers) and the "epidemiologic transition" (of epidemiologists and public health workers) described with industrialization in Western countries as well as in developing countries (Olshansky and Ault, 1986).

It is clear from studies in numerous populations undergoing various rates of acculturation that the disease pattern changes over time and at varying rates, depending on the length of time that acculturation has occurred and numerous other factors such as the degree of segregation of the previously unacculturated group (especially with regard to quality of medical care). In Australian aborigines, for example, although some improvement in infant mortality and control of infectious diseases (such as leprosy) has occurred in recent years, the disease pattern involves both a transition to "degenerative diseases" (Thomson, 1984) and a legacy of diseases reflecting preacculturation factors. In aborigines and in other groups that have undergone long periods of acculturation and Westernization, such as South Africans, the inadequacy of data on health is still evident. With economic changes such as mining in South Africa (WHO, 1984) and in the

Nauruans of the Pacific (Schooneveldt et al., 1988), "modernization" has involved increases in risks of certain chronic diseases. Even in such long-standing minority groups as U.S. blacks, recent changes in mortality from cardiovascular diseases probably reflect in part the continuing process of acculturation (Chapter 7). In developing countries the indirect effects of contacts with Western countries include increases in cigarette smoking and alcohol consumption, with resulting changes in disease patterns.

The double-edged sword of acculturation is evident in the decline in infectious diseases, after long contact, but increase in blood pressure and certain cardiovascular diseases (except those of infectious origin such as rheumatic heart disease), and certain cancers (Figure 10.1). In some instances previous genetic adaptations to food scarcity in various populations may have been disrupted by dietary changes with acculturation and Westernization and (theoretically) resulted in increased rates of chronic diseases such as diabetes mellitus (Chapter 9). Also well documented are rather rapid changes in body weight with acculturation and migration in such diverse groups as Tokelau Islanders, Nauruans, and Asians (i.e., from the Indian subcontinent).

The first step toward alleviation of these disparities in health status between immigrants or minority groups and the majority or dominant group is their documentation through descriptive epidemiologic studies. Analytic studies can then evaluate the roles of SES-related factors and sociocultural differences affecting risk and prognosis of disease which can be useful in planning public health programs. In the United States the importance of these studies has been increasingly recognized, as evidenced for example by "topics in minority health" (in governmental health agency publications) (see Chapter 4) and programs targeting specific racial/ethnic groups with regard to diverse diseases as AIDS, tuberculosis, hypertension, and certain cancers. At the very least, the need for more detailed studies has been recognized with regard to such important issues as black–white disparities in infant mortality rates (Chapter 9).

Intensive epidemiologic studies of migration and acculturation in such multiethnic areas as Australia (McMichael and Giles, 1988) and in diverse groups in the United States (such as different "Hispanic" populations) will allow quantification of rates of acculturation and their effects on health through a complex pattern of changes in cultural factors (especially diet).

Importance of Population Differences in Diet

In developing countries and in low-SES groups in developed countries, malnutrition or undernutrition interacts with exposure to infectious agents in influencing susceptibility to infectious diseases and their sequelae. In addition to expanded sanitation and immunization programs, improved nutrition is needed in these populations (Chapter 6).

Population or racial/ethnic differences in some cancers and cardiovascular diseases are apparently related largely to differences in intake of specific dietary constituents such as total fats or specific types of fats, vitamins, fiber, and sodium. Other habits of importance include smoking and alcohol, which also affect nutrient metabolism. The complexity of interactions between these dietary con-

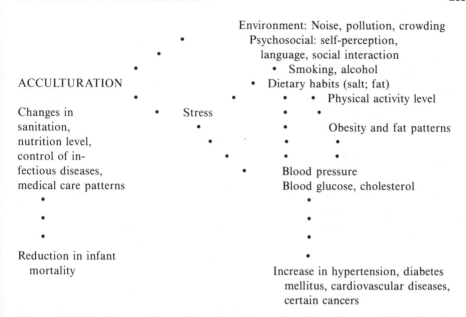

Figure 10.1 The diverse effects of acculturation on health, and potential mechanisms.

stituents and drugs is also apparent. Much work remains to be done to clarify these interactions and to assess the independent influences of population differences in physical activity, in order to develop appropriate intervention programs in these populations. Preliminary studies in high-risk groups, such as diet and culturally tailored exercise intervention regarding diabetes mellitus among the Zuni Indians, offer promise of extension and tailoring to needs of other populations.

Biological anthropologists are concerned with the effects of both undernutrition and overnutrition on health, as well as with the assessment of nutritional status through anthropometric measurements. The study of human adaptation involves consideration of dietary patterns and their variation (Damon, 1975) (Table 10.1).

Again, migrant studies (Table 10.1) have contributed greatly to our understanding of the importance of changes in diet in explaining changes (or lack of change) in body size and in disease rates, especially for cardiovascular diseases (Chapter 7) and cancers (Chapter 8). In cancers, for example, migrant studies have shown the importance of exposures (presumably dietary) early in life in influencing risk of stomach cancer, while dietary factors later in life may be more important in explaining risk of colorectal cancers.

Disease Syndromes or Constellations

Certain complexes of diseases are more frequent in racial/ethnic groups. Examples are diabetes mellitus and gallbladder diseases in Amerindian and Amerindian-related groups, and certain autoimmune disorders and connective tissue diseases in some black populations (Chapter 9). Speculative hypotheses have been advanced involving effects of putative genes that were once adaptive under previous environmental conditions, interacting with present environmental influences. Other patterns of disease in a population or a small number of populations may represent common underlying environmental factors such as specific dietary constituents that influence the risk of multiple diseases, including several cancer sites (e.g., nitrosamines and risk of several cancers).

Causal Homogeneity versus Heterogeneity of Disease

For many diseases the major risk factors are largely consistent in effect, and often in strength, across racial/ethnic groups. The risk profiles are similar. A few examples are IHD in U.S. blacks and whites and in Japanese in both Japan and Hawaii, and certain cancers (e.g., smoking and alcohol as risk factors for certain cancers in both blacks and whites). The relative frequency of the same risk factor, however, may vary with racial/ethnic group and thus explain differences in disease rates in these groups.

Some specific risk factors may vary in importance in populations, suggesting heterogeneity in causation of a specific disease. The methodologic difficulties in comparisons of findings of studies across populations, however, are considerable (Chapter 1). Studies of risk factors for certain specific diseases across racial/ethnic groups have provided evidence for heterogeneity in causation—for example, for diabetes mellitus. Heterogeneity may be genetic, as shown by different HLA associations, or may involve differential roles of such factors as obesity and exercise.

Integration of Data from Population Genetics with Epidemiology

The recent expansion of population genetics has resulted in a growing list of polymorphisms in a range of genetic markers including blood groups, serum proteins, HLA types and other systems as well as direct comparisons of variation in the genetic material itself (i.e., restriction fragment length polymorphisms) (Chapter 3). These data are being integrated into analyses of population differences in diseases, including both descriptive and analytic (especially case-control) studies. As noted at the outset of this chapter, recent increases have occurred both in the pace of discovery of genetic polymorphisms and in the attempt to understand their significance (if any) in terms of adaptation to diseases in the past and/or present.

Role of Racial Admixture Studies

Another application of population genetics concerns the estimation of degree of racial admixture using genetic markers along with previously established methods using anthropometric characteristics (Table 10.1). Thus method has proved to be useful in the general assessment of possible genetic influences in disease, especially in diabetes mellitus. More detailed studies can then be planned to identify specific genetic factors involved. Additional applications of this methodology to specific diseases appear to be in order, and some specific suggestions have been given throughout this text.

Prospects for Elimination of Racial/Ethnic Differences in Prognosis of Chronic Diseases

There is increasing recognition of the importance of socioeconomic status (SES)-related factors, and possibly sociocultural influences, in determining clinical stage at diagnosis of cancers. Further studies are needed to determine how such SES-related and sociocultural factors operate—for example, through delay in diagnosis, medical care access, and nutritional factors. Studies of racial/ethnic differences in cancer survival rates, mainly in the U.S. population, have involved SES-related factors and to a lesser extent sociocultural differences, as well as differences in body constitution whose explanations are uncertain (Chapter 8). Improved medical care probably accounts for improvements in outcome of U.S. black patients with hypertension (Chapter 7), but further improvements are needed in order to reduce the disparities in mortality rates between blacks and whites. Disparities in treatment are also apparent for other racial/ethnic groups including U.S. Hispanic populations with regard to the sequelae of diabetes mellitus and hypertension, reflecting sociocultural factors as well as SES differences. Again, targeted educational progress for patients and physicians, along with increased availability of medical care, may be beneficial.

EXPLANATIONS FOR DIFFERENCES IN DISEASE RATES

The study of disease associations with such host factors as racial/ethnic groups, which are not alterable, are nevertheless important because they provide directions for studies that define causal factors that can be modified (MacMahon and Pugh, 1970). These modifiable factors include changes in diet, exercise, and other habits. Associations between racial/ethnic group and such chronic diseases as hypertension and diabetes mellitus, for example, have led to recognition of the need for primary and secondary prevention programs targeted to these groups, even though the precise mechanisms underlying these associations are unclear or debated.

Racial/ethnic differences in infectious diseases are clearly due largely to factors subject to modification. These factors include nutritional deficiencies and poor host immune status, as well as poor sanitation and certain cultural practices. Population differences in infectious diseases such as hepatitis B include racial/ethnic variation in risk and modes of transmission, reflecting SES and sociocultural differences. Epidemiologic study of AIDS and HIV-related diseases have supported the same conclusion, especially regarding cross-cultural differences in sexual habits, but further studies are needed. Numerous examples of the "bridge" between infectious and chronic diseases (Comstock, 1986) have been discussed for cancers (Chapter 8) and various other chronic diseases (Chapter 9).

Regarding the major chronic diseases, risk of hypertension, cerebrovascular diseases, and ischemic heart disease (IHD) varies considerably among countries and racial/ethnic groups, and these differences demand adequate explanation. In cardiovascular diseases differences in dietary habits affecting cholesterol fractions (high vs. low density) and sodium/potassium ratios, perhaps modulated by genetic differences that may themselves reflect past adaptations to diet, have emerged as most important. Population differences and time changes in smoking and alcohol habits are also important. This also holds for various cancers.

Population differences in risk of hypertension and cerebrovascular diseases may be due in part to differences in salt intake. Differences between various black versus white populations in hypertension risk, however, may involve differences in metabolism of sodium. Studies of U.S. blacks and various migrant groups, such as Samoans and Bahamians, suggest that complex interactions among risk factors for hypertension—including social stress, diet, and physical activity—are involved in such high-risk groups. Additional studies of degree of racial admixture in relation to hypertension are needed to examine the hypothesis that genetic differences play some role in black–white differences in hypertension. Most promising, however, has been recent interest in variation in catecholamine excretion patterns in various populations that differ by degree of acculturation and urbanization. This work promises to further increase collaboration between behavioral scientists dealing with stress and social support, anthropologists interested in sociocultural processes and acculturation, and biomedical anthropologists concerned with the role of biological variation in disease.

Great worldwide variation has also been observed for cancer rates. Some of this variation includes racial/ethnic groups, often in the same country (e.g., Singapore and Malaysia, and U.S. racial/ethnic groups). Much of this variation is unexplained, but the roles of dietary factors, personal habits, and differential exposure to infectious agents are becoming increasingly understood.

The importance of environmental factors in colorectal cancers has been shown by studies of various migrant groups. More research is needed to delineate the roles of specific types of fiber (vegetable vs. cereal) and their interaction with other dietary constituents such as fat, calcium, and vitamins in specific populations and possible differences across populations. For gastric cancers many countries have shown remarkable declines in incidence and mortality rates, but some interesting apparent variations in this general pattern require exploration. Also requiring more intensive study are the explanations for retention of high risk of stomach cancer among certain migrant populations. For hepatic cancers the role of hepatitis B carrier status as a risk factor has been demonstrated by cohort studies, but the strength of the association varies across racial/ethnic groups. Other risk factors that may be involved are smoking, alcohol, and dietary factors, which may also vary across populations.

The promising area of research on HLA associations with cancers and other diseases has also implicated possible genetic factors, perhaps interacting with infectious agents as well as other aspects of the host, in explaining population differences in rates of certain cancers. Examples of cancer types under study with regard to HLA types are Kaposi's sarcoma and nasopharyngeal cancer. Population differences in other chronic diseases (Chapter 9) involve different interactions between infectious agents, dietary factors, and a genetic substrate (including HLA types in some diseases).

PROGNOSIS OF CHRONIC DISEASES

The elimination of racial/ethnic differences in prognosis of diseases, mentioned earlier, requires recognition of the underlying factors contributing to disparities in clinical stage or severity of disease at diagnosis. Clinicians and public health agencies can then plan strategies for improving prognosis. Socioeconomic (SES) and sociocultural factors appear to be most important in racial/ethnic differences in cancer survival. These factors may operate through psychosocial mechanisms, such as fear or disease and increased delay in seeking medical attention, as well as through host mechanisms such as nutritional effects on resistance to disease progression or response to therapy. These interactions may be involved in the prognosis of patients with various cancers. The relative importance of specific factors appears to vary with the cancer site.

Differences in stage at diagnosis of breast cancer may largely explain survival differences shown for U.S. blacks versus whites, Seventh Day Adventists versus others, and Japanese versus whites in the United States. Cultural factors such as attitudes toward cancer, dietary factors, and biological factors, however, are poorly understood and require further study.

Improved treatment of hypertension among U.S. blacks, overcoming the effects of socioeconomic differences, may lead to continuing reductions in black–white differences in mortality from hypertension. Awareness of the higher rates of coronary heart disease among U.S. blacks is increasing, and much of this excess appears to be due to known and potentially modifiable risk factors such as obesity, hypertension, and smoking. As awareness increases among physicians and public health officials, through the aid of increasing numbers of publications on the epidemiology of chronic diseases in racial/ethnic groups, targeted intervention programs should also increase in number and effectiveness.

OTHER CLINICAL APPLICATIONS

Our main focus in this book has been on the description and explanation of associations between racial/ethnic group and disease, with the ultimate goal of application to prevention programs. In clinical practice recognition of diversity in disease risk by racial/ethnic group among patients can be helpful in diagnosis and in planning of both prevention and treatment strategies. For this purpose Table 10.2 presents a summary of diseases with relatively high or low prevalence, organized by racial/ethnic group. The reference category is undefined but generally represents the average of known prevalence or mortality rates, or the best available data, and varies in quality. Each of these differences is established through several studies, and most represent either differences adjusted for age or

Table 10.2 Summary of Racial and Ethnic Differences in Various Disorders

Group	High frequency	Low frequency
Jews		
Ashkenazic Jews	Diabetes mellitus	Alcoholism
	Hypercholesterolemia	Pyloric stenosis
	Ulcerative colitis/regional	Tuberculosis
	enteritis (North America only)	Lung cancer
	Prostatic hyperplasia	Breast cancer
	Polycythemia vera	Cervical cancer
	Leukemia	
	Hodgkin's disease	
	Kaposi's sarcoma	
	Pancreatic cancer	
	Brain cancer	
Sephardic Jews	Brain cancer	Tuberculosis
	Esophageal cancer	Rheumatoid arthritis
	Lymphatic leukemia (females)	
	Lymphosarcoma	
	Gallbladder cancer	
Europeans (selected groups)		
French	Esophageal cancer	Coronary or ischemic heart
	Cirrhosis of liver	disease (IHD)
	Pharyngeal cancer	
	Oral cancer	
	Bladder cancer	
	Testicular cancer	
Belgians	Motor vehicle deaths	
	IHD Bladder cancer	
	Lung cancer	
Czechs	Colorectal cancer	
	Gallbladder cancer	
	Stroke	
	IHD	
Poles	Stomach cancer	Stroke
	Bile duct and gallbladder cancers	
Russians	Stomach cancer	
	Esophageal cancer	
	Esophagitis	
	Tuberculosis	
	Stroke	
	IHD (Siberia)	
Irish (Ireland)	Major CNS malformations	
	Schizophrenia	
	Stroke (N. Ireland)	
	IHD	
Finns	IHD	Breast cancer
	Stroke	Colorectal cancer
	Multiple sclerosis	
	Esophageal cancer (females)	
	IDDM	
	Suicide	
Icelanders	Glaucoma	Cardiovascular (except
	Peptic ulcer	IHD)
	Thyroid cancer	Infant mortality rate
	Kidney cancer	Chronic liver disease
	Breast cancer	

Table 10.2 (*continued*)

Group	High frequency	Low frequency
Lapps	Congenital hip disorders	IHD
Norwegians	Breast cancer	
	Ovarian cancer	
	Peptic ulcer	
Danish	Rectal cancer	Cirrhosis of liver
	Pancreatic cancer	Oropharynx cancer
	Ovarian cancer	Stroke
	Chronic lung disease	
Middle Easterners		
Iranians	Esophageal cancer (north, north-west)	
	Bladder cancer (Caspian, south)	
	Liver cancer (Kurds and Turkish-speaking)	
	Stomach cancer	
Kuwaitis	Rheumatic heart disease	HIV virus seropositivity
	Nasopharyngeal cancer	Suicide
	Motor vehicle deaths	Cervical cancer
		Stomach cancer
		Colon cancer
		Penile cancer
Saudi Arabians	Lymphoma, GI tract	
Egyptians	Hodgkin's disease, childhood	
Asians		
Chinese (in various countries)	Trophoblastic disease	Chronic lymphatic leukemia
	Neurasthenia (China)	
	Koro (S.E. Asia)	Brain cancer
	SLE	Colorectal cancers (China)
	Oral clefts	Melanoma of skin
	Nasopharyngeal cancer	Breast cancer
	Hepatic cancer	Prostatic cancer
	Grave's disease (Singapore)	Prostatic hyperplasia
	Gastric cancer (Shanghai; Singapore)	Hemolytic disease of new-born
	Lung cancer (Singapore)	Sudden infant death syndrome (Hong Kong)
	Esophageal cancer	Diabetes mellitus, type 1 (IDDM)
	Hepatitis B	IHD (Beijing; U.S.)
	Colorectal Cancer (California)	
Thais	Leprosy	Chronic lung disease
	Hepatitis B	
	Malaria	
	Trichinosis	
	Diabetes mellitus (NIDDM)	
	Nasopharyngeal cancer	
	Hepatic and biliary cancers	
	Cancer of hypopharynx/larynx	
U.S. Immigrants from SE Asia	Tuberculosis	
	Leprosy	
	Hepatitis	
	Malaria; trichinosis	

Table 10.2 (continued)

Group	High frequency	Low frequency
Japanese	Cerebrovascular disease	IHD
	Cleft lip/palate	Congenital hip disorders
	Hepatitis B	Chronic lung disease
	HTLV-I infection (S. Japan)	Acne
	Trophoblastic disease	Otosclerosis
	Gastric cancer	Chronic lymphatic
	Adult T-cell lymphoma (Japan)	leukemia
	Choriocarcinoma	Prostatic cancer
	Gallbladder cancer	Prostatic hyperplasia
	Primary open-angle glaucoma	Breast cancer (Japan)
		Multiple myeloma
		Hodgkin's disease
		Lung cancer
		Melanoma of skin
		Ocular melanoma
		Diabetes mellitus, type 1 (IDDM)
		Diabetes mellitus, type 2 (NIDDM)
Koreans (Korea, Japan)	Stomach cancer	
	Cirrhosis of liver	
	Penile cancer (U.S.)	
Indians	Rheumatic heart disease	Multiple myeloma
	IHD (India, and migrants)	Breast cancer (Hindus)
	Diabetes mellitus (NIDDM)	Cancer of uterus
	Tuberculosis	Gastric cancer
	Tuberculous meningitis	Colorectal cancer
	Vitamin D deficiency disorders (ricketts)	Lung cancer
		Stroke (Sri Lanka)
	Cataracts (Punjab)	IHD (Sri Lanka)
	Cholera (Ganges; Bangladesh)	
	Suicide	
	Cervical cancer	
	Oral cancer	
	Cataract (Punjab plains)	
Malays (including those in Singapore)	Ovarian cancer	Lung cancer
	Female lung cancer	Pancreatic cancer
	NIDDM	Stomach cancer
		Colon cancer
		Breast cancer
		Cervical cancer
Pacific Islanders		
Filipinos	Oral clefts	Cerebrovascular disease
	Hyperuricemia (U.S.)	IHD (U.S.)
	Hypertension (Calif.)	Bladder cancer (U.S.)
	NIDDM	
	Thyroid cancer (Hawaii; California)	
	Oral cancer	
Polynesians (Hawaii, etc.)	Rheumatic heart disease (Rarotonga; Fr. Polynesia)	Stomach cancer
		Lung cancer
	Clubfoot	
	SLE	
	Coronary heart disease	

Table 10.2 (*continued*)

Group	High frequency	Low frequency
	Hepatitis B (New Zealand)	
	Diabetes (NIDDM)	
	Breast cancer	
	Ovarian cancer (New Zealand)	
	Myeloid leukemia (New Zealand)	
	Liver cancer (New Zealand)	
	Pancreatic cancer	
	Lymphosarcoma	
	Thyroid cancer	
	Myeloid leukemia (males)	
Maori, New Zealand	Rheumatic heart disease	Colorectal cancer
	IHD	Melanoma of skin
	Otitis media	Ocular melanoma
	SIDS	Gallbladder cancer
	Multiple myeloma	
	Myeloid leukemia (males)	
	Pancreatic cancer	
	Gastric cancer	
	Cervical cancer	
	Stomach cancer	
	Uterine cancer	
	Breast cancer	
	Lung cancer (females)	
	Hepatitis B carriers	
Micronesians	Diabetes (NIDDM)	
	Hepatitis B	
	Hyperuricemia (but not clinical gout)	
	Parkinsonism-dementia/ALS (in Chamorros)	
Melanesians	Yaws	Hypertension (some areas)
	Otitis media	IHD (some areas)
	Pneumococcal disease	
	Malaria	
	Burkitt's lymphoma	
	Kaposi's sarcoma	
	Liver cancer	
	Penile cancer (Lowlands, New Guinea)	
	Oral cancer (Papua New Guinea)	
	Kuru (Fore people) (in past)	
	Tropical arthritis	
Indonesians	Cholera	
	Oral cancer	
	Nasopharyngeal cancer	
	NIDDM	
Australian aborigines (inadequate data)	Chronic lung disease	
	Alcoholism	
	Leprosy	
	Trachoma	
	Otitis media	
	Rheumatic heart disease	
Blacks		
U.S. and/or African	Asthma (U.S.)	Psoriasis
	AIDS, HIV-2	Gallstones
	Tuberculosis	Multiple sclerosis

Table 10.2 *(continued)*

Group	High frequency	Low frequency
	Leprosy (Africa)	Barrett's esophagus
	Pneumococcal meningitis	Parkinson's disease (U.S.)
	Sexually transmitted diseases	Congenital hip disorders
	Yaws (Africa)	Major CNS malformations
	Ainhum (Africa, South America)	Osteoporosis and hip frac-
	Xerophthalmia (Africa)	tures (U.S.; Bantu)
	Sarcoidosis (U.S.)	Temporal arteritis
	Scleroderma (U.S.)	Renovascular disease
	Keloids	Polycythemia vera
	SLE (U.S.)	Xerophthalmia (Africa)
	Polydactyly	Poliomyelitis (Africa)
	Hypertension	Measles (Africa)
	Glaucoma (open angle)	Malaria (Africa)
	Cataracts	Bladder cancer
	SIDS	Malignant melanoma
	Chronic liver disease (U.S.)	(skin, eye)
	Cervical cancer	Testicular cancer
	Lung cancer (males)	Acute lymphocytic leuke-
	Esophageal cancer	mia
	Prostatic cancer	Hodgkin's disease
	Stomach cancer	Ewing's sarcoma (U.S.,
	Multiple myeloma	Africa)
	Hepatic cancer (Africa)	Colorectal cancer (Africa)
	Orbito-ocular cancers (Africa)	Rectal cancer (U.S.)
	Leiomyosarcoma	Breast cancer (after age 40)
	Kaposi's sarcoma (Africa)	Suicide (U.S.)
	Burkitt's lymphoma (Africa)	
	Adult T-cell lymphoma	
	(Caribbean; U.S.)	
	Chorionepithelioma (Africa)	
	Affective disorders (Africa)	
	Homicides (U.S.)	
Caribbean	HTLV-I and leukemia	IHD (some areas)
	Yaws	Osteoarthritis (Jamaica)
	Stroke (Trinidad)	
	Tuberculosis (Haiti)	
	Infectious diseases	
	Penile cancer (Jamaica; Haiti)	
Amerindians	Plague (Southwestern U.S.)	Duodenal ulcer
	Otitis media	Melanoma of skin
	Tuberculosis	Lung cancer
	Congenital hip disorders	Hodgkin's disease (males)
	SIDS	Colon cancer (South and
	Alcoholism	Central America)
	Chronic liver disease	Hypertension (isolated
	Gallbladder disease	South American groups)
	Diabetes (NIDDM)	
	Rheumatoid arthritis	
	Chorioepithelioma	
	Kidney cancer (Canada)	
	Gallbladder/bile duct cancer	
	Cervical cancer (Colombia,	
	Central America, Chile)	

Table 10.2 (continued)

Group	High frequency	Low frequency
	Stomach cancer (South and Central America)	
	Primary open-angle glaucoma	
Eskimo (Inuit) groups (and Aleuts)	Iron deficiency anemia	IHD
	Bacterial meningitis	Prostate cancer
	Hepatitis B	Breast cancer
	SIDS (Alaska)	Leukemia (males)
	Salivary gland tumors	Lymphomas (males)
	Esophageal cancers (Alaska)	Osteoarthritis
	Nasopharyngeal cancer	
	Liver cancer	
	Kidney cancer (females)	
	Glaucoma (angle-closure type)	
	Reiter's syndrome	
Puerto Ricans (Puerto Rico and U.S.)	Cervical cancer	Rheumatoid arthritis
	Gastric cancer	Breast cancer
	Esophageal cancer	Lung cancer
	Chronic liver disease	Colorectal cancer
		IHD
Hispanic, U.S. Southwest	AIDS	Suicide
	Measles	IHD
	Tuberculosis	Melanoma of skin
	Infectious and parasitic diseases	Lung cancer
	Diabetes (NIDDM)	Breast cancer
	Cervical cancer	Colorectal cancer
	Gastric cancer	Fractures
	Biliary tract cancer	
	Leukemia, childhood	
	Homicide	
Mormons (U.S.)		IHD
		Total cancers
		Colorectal cancer
		Pancreatic cancer
		Breast cancer
		Cervical cancer
		Ovarian cancer
Hutterites (U.S., Canada)	Stomach cancer (males)	Total cancer
	Leukemia (males)	Cervical cancer
		Lung cancer (males)
Seventh Day Adventists (U.S., Netherlands)		IHD
		Colorectal cancer
Gypsies (U.S.)	Diabetes mellitus	
	Occlusive cardiovascular disease	
	Hypertension	

Abbreviations: IHD, ischemic heart disease; NIDDM, non-insulin-dependent diabetes mellitus; IDDM, insulin-dependent diabetes mellitus; AIDS, acquired immunedeficiency syndrome; ALS, amyotrophic lateral sclerosis; SLE, systemic lupus erythematosus; SIDS, sudden infant death syndrome; HIV, human immunodeficiency virus.

Adapted and expanded from Damon, 1964, 1971, 1977; McKusick, 1967, 1983; Muir and Nectoux, 1982; Muir et al., 1987; Norio, 1981; Rothschild, 1981; Weatherall and Clegg, 1981; Seligsohn et al., 1982; Waterhouse et al., 1982; Howe, 1986, but largely based on various other individual references. See list of references at end of the book.

results of comparisons of age-specific rates. These details cannot be given in the table, but the reader may refer to other tables and discussions in the text for documentation for some of these patterns.

As is evident in this book, many racial/ethnic groups can be recognized, including various migrant groups, and this summary table cannot deal with all of these groups. This also holds for the subtleties of changes in disease, sometimes rapid, in migrants, and with acculturation and urbanization.

Applications of knowledge of racial/ethnic differences in disease for clinicians relate to decisions about possible diagnostic tests and avoidance of unnecessary tests (e.g., in investigating fevers and anemias) on the basis of racial/ethnic differences in disease risk. *Fever with abdominal pain and leukocytosis*, for example, may have different implications for a patient who is of Northern European background (i.e., suggesting a surgical condition like appendicitis or cholecystitis), or Mediterranean background (i.e., familial Mediterranean fever or other genetically related conditions), or of black (African) background (i.e., possible sickling crisis) (Damon, 1971). Patients may be spared needless surgery, such as laparotomies (McKusick, 1983), if the physician is aware of racial/ethnic differences in disease. The occurrence of a number of cases of familial Mediterranean fever in the large Ashkenazic Jewish population of the United States emphasizes the need for this awareness.

Although a specific diagnostic test has been developed for familial Mediterranean fever or FMF (Barakat et al., 1984), ethnic background should be obtained during medical history taking in order to alert the physician regarding the need for such tests. The occurrence of meningitis in FMF, albeit rare, also should be recognized by clinicians (Schwabe and Monroe, 1988). As another example, tuberculous meningitis should be considered in the differential diagnosis of any patient of Asian (Indian–Pakistani) origin with persistent febrile illness, in order to prevent possible disability or death (Swart et al., 1981). Other groups at risk include blacks and Hispanics. Rapid diagnosis of tuberculous meningitis is possible through the use of cerebrospinal fluid samples (Krambovitis et al., 1984), but the clinician must be alert to the possibility of this diagnosis.

Numerous case histories have been reported of physicians who were unaware of the possibility of beta-thalassemia among migrants from high-risk areas, resulting in misdiagnoses (e.g., as leukemia, anemias, or malabsorption) and such unnecessary treatment as appendectomy (Weatherall and Clegg, 1981). The increasing migration of various groups (such as Southeast Asians) at risk of beta-thalassemias (alone or in combination with hemoglobin E), emphasizes the need for physician awareness.

Among blacks certain symptoms, such as abdominal pain and severe anemia, may suggest systemic lupus erythematosus (SLE)—as shown in a recent case history of a 19-year-old woman seen at a major U.S. hospital (Anon., 1987f). Diagnostic differentiation from various vascular diseases with pulmonary hemorrhage is difficult without serologic assays and biopsy. Noteworthy is the fact that this patient had symptoms for at least 2 weeks prior to diagnosis but presented at a hospital emergency room only 3 days prior to death. We have noted the impact of SES factors in medical care and the greater use of emergency rooms for primary medical care among blacks (Chapter 9). Although SLE is a rare disease, it is significantly more common among black females (Polednak, 1987a), and consideration might be given to developing public as well as physician education programs. SLE is also of interest because of reports of its development in adolescent black girls with sickle cell disease (HbSS) (Katsanis et al., 1987). As Katsanis et al. (1987) observe, it cannot be concluded that SLE is more prevalent in patients with sickle hemoglobinopathies, and prospective epidemiologic studies would be needed to determine if sickle cell disease predisposes to SLE. As we have noted, both of these conditions are more common among blacks. More important, Katsanis et al. (1987) noted that diagnosis of SLE was delayed, because new symptoms were attributed to the underlying sickle cell disease, and that early recognition of other diseases is important in order to initiate appropriate therapy and prevent complications.

In contrast to misdiagnoses based on lack of awareness of racial/ethnic group as a risk factor, clinical oversight may occur with regard to diseases not "expected" to be found in a racial group. In Africa, some diseases may not be recognized clinically, because they are believed to be "rare"; examples include certain autoimmune diseases and cancers (Polednak, 1987a).

As noted earlier, recognition of racial/ethnic differences in prognosis of various diseases due to socioeconomic and sociocultural factors would hopefully lead to interventions such as patient education. This education could be aimed at increasing knowledge and reducing fear regarding specific cancers. Intervention may include control of obesity, for certain cardiovascular diseases and cancers, as well as possible selective nutritional supplementation in the secondary prevention of certain cancers. Recognition of the needs of black patients for hypertension treatment, especially for the prevention of sequelae such as kidney disorders, is another example. The need for more medical school education on hypertension management is becoming increasingly recognized (Moser et al., 1985). Primary-care physicians may need to learn to apply techniques such as goal setting and spouse or community group involvement in the treatment of overweight.

EPILOGUE

Human biological and sociocultural variation is the focus of anthropological inquiry, including subdisciplines of anthropology such as medical anthropology and biomedical anthropology. Multidisciplinary studies involving these anthropological specialties and epidemiology should increase in the future. Both diversity and similarity across populations need to be recognized, whether one is dealing with sociocultural characteristics, biological characteristics, or risk of disease.

In physical anthropology, genetic differences between major races are smaller than the degree of genetic heterogeneity within racial groups. This limited interracial variation, however, has been demonstrated by population genetic studies of various genetic markers, and ethnic groups also show some genetic as well as cultural differences. The relevance of this genetic variation to disease patterns requires further examination as the amount of information on genetic polymorphisms increases. Along with their anthropological relevance, cross-cultural studies of human behavior, including complex behaviors related to dietary habits, sexual and reproductive behaviors and reactions to the stresses of acculturation and migration, are important from an epidemiologic perspective.

The variability or plasticity in human biological development and in disease patterns *within* groups has also been amply demonstrated by migrant studies in anthropology and epidemiology. Such changes in disease, and thus presumably in the underlying sociocultural factors such as diet, may be rapid. The opportunity to study acculturation in "isolated" populations is vanishingly small, but the processes of migration, acculturation, and urbanization continue and provide opportunities for collaborative research efforts in such diverse groups as South American Indians, Melanesians, and Polynesians.

Part of effective preventive medicine involves recognition of modifiable factors involved in disease causation or progression. This recognition may be aided by the results of studies that consider racial/ethnic group, which may provide clues to more specific and modifiable risk factors and better prediction of outcome. The explanation of population differences in rates of disease, which sometimes follow racial/ethnic lines of demarcation, will require attention to multiple potential differences including sociocultural and biological factors. Also required will be a shared foundation in basic epidemiologic methods of study design and interpretation, as persons with a specific disease may involve similar factors, but consideration of these differences requires examination of interactions between patients and health providers. Thus we return to the integration of disciplines (Fig. 1.1) needed for a full understanding of variation in disease risk and outcome. The relevance of applied anthropology, both "social" and "biological," to public health problems is becoming increasingly evident.

While physical anthropologists compile data on genetic polymorphisms in different populations and debate the geographical location(s) and mechanisms involved in the evolution of modern humans, social anthropologists consider the extent of cross-cultural variation in human behavior. Philosophers as diverse as Teilhard de Chardin and Albert Schweitzer have emphasized the need for recognizing the similarities but respecting the differences between individuals and groups. Schweitzer's world view included recognition of the suffering shared by all forms of life and the human moral imperative also shared with regard to its alleviation. Increased social responsibility, including alleviation of the burden of disease and suffering existing or threatened by technological change, may be the ultimate common denominator between these philosophical traditions and applied anthropology, medicine, and public health.

References

Aaby, P., Bukh, J., Lisse, I. M., et al.: Overcrowding and intensive exposure as determinants of measles mortality. *Am. J. Epidemiol.* 120:49–63, 1984.

Aaby, P., Bukh, J., Lisse, J., et al.: Severe measles in Sunderland, 1885. A European–African comparison and causes of severe infection. *Int. J. Epidemiol.* 15:101–107, 1986.

Abbott, C. M., McMahon, C. J., Kelsey, G. D., et al.: a1-Antitrypsin-related gene (ATR) for prenatal diagnosis. *Lancet* 1:1425–1426, 1987.

Abraham, S., Carroll, M. D., Dresser, C. M., et al.: Dietary intake findings United States, 1971–74. Data from the National Health Survey. Series 111, No. 20. DHEW Publication No. (HRA) 77-1647. Hyattsville, MD, National Center for Health Statistics, 1977.

Achard, T.: Aspects of iodine deficiency in Nepal. *Trop. Doctor* 17:5–7, 1987.

Ackerknecht, E. H.: *A Short History of Medicine.* Revised edition. Baltimore, Johns Hopkins, 1982.

Acquaye, J. K., Omer, A., Geneshagurn, K., Sejeny, S. A., and Hoffman, A. V.: Non-benign sickle cell anemia in western Saudi Arabia. *Br. J. Haematol.* 60:99–108, 1985.

Acuda, S. W., and Ovuga, E. B. L.: Psychiatric disorders in General Provincial Hospital in Kenya. *East Afr. Med. J.* 62:229–235, 1985.

Adalsteinsson, S.: Possible changes in the frequency of the human ABO blood groups in Iceland due to smallpox epidemic selection. *Ann. Hum. Genet.* 49:275–281, 1985.

Adams, L. L., LaPorte, R. E., Matthews, K. A., et al.: Blood pressure determinants in a middle class black population: The University of Pittsburgh experience. *Prev. Med.* 15:232–243, 1986.

Adams, M. M.: The descriptive epidemiology of sudden infant deaths among natives and whites in Alaska. *Am. J. Epidemiol.* 122:637–643, 1985.

Adams, M. M.: The author replies. *Am. J. Epidemiol.* 124:492–493, 1986.

Adams, W. H., Harper, J. A., Heotis, P. M., and Jamner, A. H.: Hyperuricemia in the inhabitants of the Marshall Islands. *Arthritis Rheum.* 27:712–716, 1984.

Aday, L. A., Chiu, G. Y., and Anderson, R.: Methodological issues in health care surveys of the Spanish heritage population. *Am. J. Public Health* 70:367–374, 1980.

Adekeye, E. O., Kwamin, F., and Ord, R. A.: Serious consequences with ovulectomy performed by a "native doctor." *Trop. Doctor* 14:160–161, 1984.

Ainley, C. C., Forgacs, I. C., Keeling, P. W. N., et al.: Outpatient endoscopic survey of smoking and peptic ulcer. *Gut* 27:648–651, 1987.

Aitken, I. W., and Walls, B.: Maternal height and cephalopelvic disproportion in Sierra Leone. *Trop. Doctor* 16:132–134, 1986.

Akbari, M. T., Papiha, S. S., Roberts, D. F., and Farhud, D. D.: Genetic differentiation among Iranian Christian communities. *Am J. Hum. Genet.* 38:84–98, 1986.

Akinkugbe, O. O.: World epidemiology of hyptertension in blacks. In Hall, W. D., Saunders, E., and Shulman, N. B. (eds.), *Hypertension in Blacks: Epidemiology, Pathophysiology and Treatment.* Chicago, Year Book, 1985, pp. 3–16.

Akoglu, T., Ozer, F. L., and Akoglu, E.: The coincidence of glucose-6-phosphate dehydrogenase deficiency and hemoglobin S in Cukurkova Province, Turkey. *Am. J. Epidemiol.* 123:677–680, 1986.

Alba, R. D.: The twilight of ethnicity among American Catholics of European ancestry. *Ann. Am. Acad. Polit. Soc. Sci.* 454:86–97, 1981.

Albanses, D., Jones, D. Y., Schatzkin, A., et al.: Adult stature and risk of cancer. *Cancer Res.* 48:1658–1662, 1988.

Alderson, M.: *International Mortality Statistics.* New York, Facts on File, 1981.

Alexander, G. R., and Cornely, D. A.: Racial disparities in pregnancy outcomes: The role of prenatal care utilization and maternal risk status. *Am. J. Prev. Med.* 3:254–261, 1987.

Allison, H. E.: *Benedict de Spinoza: An Introduction*, revised edition. New Haven, CT, Yale University Press, 1987.

Allore, R., O'Hanlon, D., Price, R., et al.: Gene encoding the B subunit of S100 protein is on chromosome 21: Implications for Down syndrome. *Science* 239:1311–1313, 1988.

Alter, M., Zhang, Z. X., Sobel, E., et al.: Standardized incidence ratios of stroke: A worldwide view. *Neuroepidemiology* 5:148–158, 1986.

Andersen, R. M., Giachello, A. L., and Aday, L. A.: Access of Hispanics to health care and cuts in services: A state-of-the-art review. *Public Health Rep.* 101:238–252, 1986.

Anderson, J. J., and Felson, D. T.: Factors associated with osteoarthritis of the knee in the first National Health and Nutrition Examination Survey (HANES I). *Am. J. Epidemiol.* 128:179–189, 1988.

Angastiniotis, M. A., and Hadjiminas, M. G.: Prevention of thalassemia in Cyprus. *Lancet* 1:369–371, 1981.

Anon.: Spinal cord compression in thalassemia. *Lancet* 1:664–665, 1982.

Anon.: Eskimo diets and diseases. *Lancet* 1:1139–1141, 1983a.

Anon.: International effort against malaria. *Lancet* 2:322–323, 1983b.

Anon.: Hepatitis programme. *Lancet* 2:350, 1983c.

Anon.: Cancer as a global problem. *Bull. Pan Am. Health Organ.* 18:291–293, 1984a.

Anon.: Cancer in the third world. *Lancet* 1:1136, 1984b.

Anon.: Leprosy in the Americas. *Bull. Pan Am. Health Organ.* 18:182–188, 1984c.

Anon.: Third world smoking—the new slave trade. *Lancet* 1:23–24, 1984c.

Anon.: Annual report, 1984. *MMWR*, 1984d.

Anon.: Functioning of the international health regulations. *Bull. Pan Am. Health Organ.* 19:88–95, 1985a.

Anon.: Coronary heart disease in the American black population. *Lancet* 1:148, 1985b.

Anon.: Homicide among young black males—United States, 1970–1982. *MMWR* 34:629–633, 1985c.

Anon.: Ethnic differences in survival following diagnosis of breast cancer—Hawaii. *MMWR* 34:646–648, 1985d.

Anon.: Inborn alcoholism? *Lancet* 2:1427–1428, 1985e.

Anon.: Pain-relief in sickle cell crises. *Lancet* 2:320, 1986a.

Anon.: Penicillin prophylaxis for babies with sickle-cell disease. *Lancet* 2:1432–1433, 1986b.

Anon.: Tuberculosis—United States, 1985. *MMWR* 35:699–703, 1986c.

Anon.: Acquired immunodeficiency syndrome (AIDS) among blacks and Hispanics—United States. *MMWR* 35:655–666, 1986d.

Anon.: Yellow fever in Africa. *Lancet* 2:1315–1316, 1986e.

Anon.: Need for malaria prophylaxis by travelers to areas with chloroquine-resistant *Plasmodium falciparum. MMWR* 35:21–22, 27, 1986f.

Anon.: Homicide—Los Angeles, 1970–1979. *MMWR* 45:61–65, 1986g.

Anon.: Genetic probes for immunological diseases. *Lancet* 1:1071–1072, 1986h.

Anon.: Premature mortality in the United States. *MMWR* 35 (Suppl.), 1986i.

Anon.: Current estimates from the National Health Interview Survey, United States, 1983. Data from the National Health Survey, Series 10, No. 154, Hyattsville, MD, 1986j.

Anon.: Infant mortality among Black Americans. *MMWR* 36:1–10, 1987a.

Anon.: Tuberculosis in minorities—United States. *MMWR* 36:77–80, 1987b.

Anon.: Tuberculosis in blacks—United States. *MMWR* 36:212–220, 1987c.

Anon.: Early syphilis—Broward County, Florida. *MMWR* 36:221–223, 1987d.

Anon.: Cigarette smoking in the United States, 1986. *MMWR* 36:581–585, 1987e.

Anon.: Anemia, abdominal pain, and death in a 19-year-old woman. *Am. J. Med.* 83:93–100, 1987f.

Anon.: Hepatocellular cancer: Differences between high and low incidence regions. *Lancet* 2:1183–1184, 1987g.

Anon.: Nutritional status of minority children—United States, 1986. *MMWR* 36:366–369, 1987h.

Anon.: Childbearing patterns among Puerto Rican Hispanics in New York City and Puerto Rico. *MMWR* 36:34–41, 1987i.

Anon.: Meningococcal vaccination for pilgrims to Saudi Arabia. *Lancet* 1:1469, 1988a.

Anon.: Six deaths from measles. *Lancet* 1:1451, 1988b.

Anon.: Fish oil. *Lancet* 1:1081–1082, 1988c.

Anon.: Provisional estimates from the national health interview survey supplement on cancer control—United States, January–March 1987. *MMWR* 37:417–425, 1988d.

Anon.: Progress toward achieving the 1990 objectives for pregnancy and infant health. *MMWR* 37:406–413, 1988e.

Anon.: Kava. *Lancet* 2:258–259, 1988f.

Aoki, E., Tominaga, S., Hirayama, T., and Hirota, Y.: *Cancer Prevention in Developing Countries.* Nagoya, Japan, University of Nagoya Press, 1982.

Araki, S., and Goto, Y.: Peptic ulcer in male factory workers: A survey of prevalence, incidence, and aetiological factors. *J. Epidemiol. Commun. Health* 39:82–85, 1985.

Araki, S., Uchino, M., and Kumamoto, T.: Prevalence studies of multiple sclerosis, myasthenia gravis, and myopathies in Kumamoto district, Japan. *Neuroepidemiology* 6:120–129, 1987.

Arinami, T., Kondo, I., Nakajima, S., et al.: Frequency of the fragile X syndrome in institutionalized mentally retarded females in Japan. *Hum. Genet.* 76:344–347, 1987.

Armenian, H. K., and Sha'ar, K. H.: Epidemiologic observations in familiar paroxysmal polyserositis. *Epidemiol. Rev.* 8:106–116, 1986.

Armstrong, B. K., Margetts, B. M., Masarei, J. R. I., and Hopkins, S. M.: Coronary risk factors in Italian migrants to Australia. *Am. J. Epidemiol.* 118:651–658, 1983.

Armstrong, R. W.: South east Asia. In Howe, G. M. (ed.), *Global Geocancerology.* Edinburgh, Churchill Livingstone, 1986, pp. 272–279.

Arnaiz-Villena, A., Regueiro, J. R., Nieto-Cuartero, J. A., et al.: HLA and complement (C4 and Bf) allotypes in type I and type II Spanish diabetics. In Baba, S., Gould, M. K., and Zimmet, P. (eds.), *Diabetes Mellitus: Recent Knowledge on Aetiology, Complications and Treatment.* New York, Academic Press, 1984, pp. 39–48.

Arrand, J. R., Mackett, M., and Littler, E.: Epstein Barr virus and the molecular biology of nasopharyngeal carcinoma. *Br. J. Cancer* 57:233–234, 1988.

Arthur, M. J. P., Hall, A. J., and Wright, T.: Hepatitis B, hepatocellular carcinoma and strategies for prevention. *Lancet* 1:607–610, 1984.

Asencio, A. P., Gomez-Beneyto, M., and Llopis, V.: Epidemiology of suicide in Valencia. *Soc. Psychiatry Psychiat. Epidemiol.* 23:57–59, 1988.

Aulehla-Scholz, C., Vorgerd, M., Sautter, E., et al.: Phenylketonuria: Distribution of DNA diagnostic patterns in German families. *Hum. Genet.* 78:353–355, 1988.

Austin, H., Cole, P., and Wynder, E.: Breast cancer in black American women. *Int. J. Cancer* 24:541–544, 1979.

Austin, M. A., and Kraus, R. M.: Genetic control of low-density-lipoprotein subclasses. *Lancet* 2:592–595, 1986.

Avigad, S., Cohen, R. E., Woo, S. L. C., et al.: A specific deletion within the phenylalanine hydroxylase₁ gene is common to most Yemenite Jewish phenylketonuria patients. *Am. J. Hum. Genet.* 41:A607, 1987.

Ayuthya, W. I. N.: Current epidemiological status of cancer in Thailand. In Aoki, K., et al. (eds.), *Cancer Prevention in Developing Countries.* Nagoya, Japan, University of Nagoya Press, 1982, pp. 91–105.

Azevedo, E. S., Fortuna, C. M. M., Silva, K. M. C., et al.: Spread and diversity of human populations in Bahia, Brazil. *Hum. Biol.* 54:329–341, 1982.

Babor, T. F. (ed.): Alcohol and Culture: Comparative Perspectives from Europe and America. *Ann. N.Y. Acad. Sci.* 472, 1986.

Babor, T. F., Hellesbrock, M., Radouco-Thomas, S., et al.: Concepts of alcoholism among American, French-Canadian and French alcoholics. *Ann. N.Y. Acad. Sci.* 472:98–109, 1986.

Bain, R. P., Greenberg, R. S., and Whitaker, J. P.: Racial differences in survival of women with breast cancer. *J. Chron. Dis.* 39:631–642, 1986.

Baird, D. D., Tyroler, H. A., Heiss, G., Chambless, L. E., and Hames, C. G.: Menopausal change in serum cholesterol. Black/white differences in Evans County, Georgia. *Am. J. Epidemiol.* 122:982–993, 1985.

Baird, P. A., Anderson, T. W., Newcombe, H. B., et al.: Genetic disorders in children and young adults: A population study. *Am. J. Hum. Genet.* 42:677–693, 1988.

Baker, P. T.: The biological race concept as a research tool. *Am. J. Phys. Anthropol.* 27:21–26, 1967.

Baker, P. T., Hanna, J. M., and Baker, T. S. (eds.): *The Changing Samoans: Behavior and Health in Transition.* New York, Oxford University Press, 1986.

Balgir, R. S.: Serogenetic studies in gypsy Sikligars of northwestern India. *Hum. Biol.* 58:171–187, 1986.

Baquet, C. R., Ringen, K., Pollack, E. S., et al.: Cancer among blacks and other minorities: Statistical profiles. National Cancer Institute NIH Publication No. 86-2785, Bethesda, MD, 1986.

Barnes, D. M.: Strategies for an AIDS vaccine. *Science* 233:1149–1153, 1986.

Barakat, M., El-Khawad, A. O., Gumaa, K. A., El-Sobki, N. I., and Fenech, F. F.: Metaraminol provocative test: A specific diagnostic test for familial Mediterranean fever. *Lancet* 1:656–657, 1984.

Barnes, A. M., Quan, T. J., Beard, M. L., et al.: Plague in American Indians, 1956–1987. *MMWR* 37:11–16, 1988.

Baron, A. E., Freyer, B. A., and Fixler, D. E.: Longitudinal blood pressures in blacks, whites, and Mexican Americans during adolescence and early adulthood. *Am. J. Epidemiol.* 123:809–817, 1986.

Barrai, I., Schiliro, G., Beretta, M., et al.: Population structure of Sicily: Beta-thalassemia and HbS. *Hum. Genet.* 75:1–3, 1987.

Barrantes, R., Smouse, P. E., Neel, J. V., et al.: Migration and genetic infrastructure of the Central American Guayami and their affinities with other tribal groups. *Am. J. Phys. Anthropol.* 58:201–214, 1982.

Bartholomew, C., Sxinger, W. C., Clark, J. W., et al.: Transmission of HTLV-I and HIV among homosexual men in Trinidad. *JAMA* 257:2604–2608, 1987.

Bassett, M. T., and Krieger, N.: Social class and black–white differences in breast cancer survival. *Am. J. Public Health* 76:1400–1403, 1986.

Basu, A., Namboodiri, K. K., Weitkamp, L. R., et al.: Morphology, serology, dermatoglyphics, and microevolution of some village populations in Haiti, West Indies. *Hum. Biol.* 48:245–269, 1976.

Basu, M. P.: *Anthropological Profile of the Muslims of Calcutta.* Calcutta, Anthropological Survey of India, Department of Culture, 1985.

Bauer, R. L.: Ethnic differences in hip fracture: A reduced incidence in Mexican Americans. *Am. J. Epidemiol.* 127:145–149, 1988.

Bauer, R. L., and Deyo, R. A.: Low risk of vertebral fracture in Mexican American women. *Arch. Intern. Med.* 147:1437–1439, 1987.

Baumgartner, R. N., Roche, A. F., Guo, S., et al.: Adipose tissue distribution: The stability of principal components by sex, ethnicity and maturation stage. *Hum. Biol.* 58:719–735, 1986.

Bayley, A.C.: Aggressive Kaposi's sarcoma in Zambia, 1983. *Lancet* 1:1318–1320, 1984.

Bayoumi, R. A., Bashir, A. H., and Abdulhadi, N. H.: Resistance to falciparum malaria among adults in central Sudan. *Am. J. Trop. Med. Hyg.* 35:45–55, 1986.

Beaglehole, R., Stewart, A. W., and Butler, M.: Comparability of old and new World Health Organization criteria for definite myocardial infarction. *Int. J. Epidemiol.* 16:373–376, 1987.

Beals, R.: Acculturation. In Tax, S. (ed.), *Anthropology Today: Selections.* Chicago, University of Chicago Press, 1962, pp. 372–395.

Beasley, R. P., Hwang, L. Y., Lin, C. C., and Chien, C. S.: Hepatocellular carcinoma and hepatitis B virus. *Lancet* 2:1129–1132, 1981.

Becker, N., Frentzel-Beyme, R., and Wagner, G.: *Atlas of Cancer Mortality in the Federal Republic of Germany*, second edition. Berlin, Springer-Verlag, 1984.

Becker, T., Magder, L., Harrison, H. R., et al.: The epidemiology of infection with the human herpesviruses in Navajo children. *Am. J. Epidemiol.* 127:1071–1078, 1988.

Beckles, G. L. A., Kirkwood, B. R., Carson, D. C., Miller, G. J., et al.: High total and cardiovascular disease mortality in adults of Indian descent in Trinidad, unexplained by coronary risk factors. *Lancet* 2:1198–1201, 1986.

Beckman, L., Beckman, G., and Nylander, P. O.: Gc subtypes in Finns, Swedes, and Swedish Lapps. *Hum. Hered.* 38:18–21, 1988.

Beckstead, J. H., Wood, G. S., and Fletcher, V.: Evidence for the origin of Kaposi's sarcoma from lymphatic endothelium. *Am. J. Pathol.* 119:294–300, 1985.

Benatar, S. R.: Sarcoidosis in South Africa. *S. Afr. Med. J.* 52:602–606, 1977.

Benfante, R. J., Hoffman, P. M., Garruto, R. M., and Gajdusek, D. C.: HL-A antigens in the Chamorros of the Mariana Islands and comparisons with other Pacific populations. *Hum. Biol.* 51:210–212, 1979.

Benkmann, H. G., Hanssen, H. P., Ovenbeck, R., et al.: Distribution of alpha-1-antitrypsin and haptoglobin phenotypes in bladder cancer patients. *Hum. Hered.* 37:290–293, 1987.

Bennet, N. H., and Shea, S.: Hypertensive emergency: Case criteria, sociodemographic profile, and previous care of 100 cases. *Am. J. Public Health* 78:636–640, 1988.

Berenson, G. S., Webber, L. S., Srinivasan, S. R., et al.: Black–white contrasts as determinants of cardiovascular risk in childhood. *Am. Heart J.* 108:672–683, 1984.

Berg, J. W., Ross, R., and Latourette, H. B.: Economic status and survival of cancer patients. *Cancer* 39:467–477, 1977.

Berger, L. R.: Suicides and pesticides in Sri Lanka. *Am. J. Public Health* 78:826–828, 1988.

Berry, R. J., Buehler, J. W., Strauss, L. T., et al.: Birth weight-specific infant mortality due to congenital anomalies, 1960 and 1980. *Public Health Rep.* 102:171–181, 1987.

Bhargava, D. K., and Chopra, P.: Colorectal adenomas in a tropical country. *Dis. Colon Rectum* 31:692–693, 1988.

Bharucha, N. E., Bharucha, E. P., Dastur, H. D., et al.: Pilot survey of the prevalence of neurologic disorders in the Parsi community of Bombay. *Am. J. Prevent. Med.* 3:293–299, 1987.

Bhattacharyya, A. K., Malcom, G. T., Guzman, M. A., et al.: Differences in adipose tissue fatty acid composition between black and white men in New Orleans. *Am. J. Clin. Nutr.* 46:41–46, 1987.

Bhuiya, A., Wojtyniak, B., D'Souza, S., et al.: Measles case fatality among the under-fives: A multivariate analysis of risk factors in a rural area of Bangladesh. *Soc. Sci. Med.* 24:439–443, 1987.

Biggar, R. J.: The AIDS problem in Africa. *Lancet* 1:79–83, 1986.

Birchall, J. D., and Chappell, J. S.: Aluminum, chemical physiology and Alzheimer's disease. *Lancet* 2:1008–1010, 1988.

Birdsell, J. B., Simmons, R. T., and Graydon, J.: Microdifferentiation in blood group frequencies among twenty-eight adjacent aboriginal tribal isolates in western Australia. Occasional Papers in Human Biology, No. 2, Australian Institute of Aboriginal Studies, Canberra, 1979.

Bissada, A., and Al-Ghussain, E.: Kuwait. In Howe, G. (ed.), *Global Geocancerology.* Edinburgh, Churchill Livingstone, 1986, pp. 253–258.

Bittles, A. H., Devi, A. R. R., and Rao, N. A.: Inbreeding and the incidence of recessive disorders in the populations of Karnataka, South India. In Roberts, D. F., and De Stefano, G. P. (eds.), *Genetic Variation and Its Maintenance.* Cambridge, U.K., Cambridge University Press, 1986, pp. 220–227.

Bjerregaard, P., and Dyerberg, J.: Fish oil and ischaemic heart disease in Greenland. *Lancet* 2:514, 1988.

Bjorkholm, E.: Blood groups and ovarian cancer. *Int. J. Epidemiol.* 13:15–17, 1984.

Black, L., David, R. J., Brouillette, R. T., and Hunt, C. E.: Effects of birth weight and ethnicity on incidence of sudden infant death syndrome. *J. Pediatr.* 108:209–214, 1986.

Black, R. H., Brown, K. H., Becker, S., and Yunis, M.: Longitudinal studies of infectious diseases and physical growth of children in rural Bangladesh. I. Patterns of morbidity. *Am. J. Epidemiol.* 115:305–314, 1982a.

Black, R. E., Brown, K. H., Becker, S., Abdul Ahim, A. R. M., and Huq, I.: Longitudinal studies of infectious diseases and physical growth of children in rural Bangladesh. II. Incidence of diarrhea and association with known pathogens. *Am. J. Epidemiol.* 115:315–324, 1982b.

Black, W. C., and Key, C. H.: Epidemiologic pathology of cancer in New Mexico's tri-ethnic population. *Pathol. Annu.* 15(pt. 2):181–194, 1980.

Black, W. C., and Wiggins, C.: Melanoma among southwestern American Indians. *Cancer* 55:2899–2902, 1985.

Blair, D., Habicht, J. P., Sims, E. A. H., et al.: Evidence for an increased risk of hypertension with centrally located body fat and the effect of race and sex on this risk. *Am. J. Epidemiol.* 119:526–540, 1984.

Blake, N. M., Hawkins, B. R., Kirk, R. L., et al.: A population genetic study of the Banks and Torres Islands (Vanuatu) and of the Santa Cruz Islands and Polynesian outliers (Solomon Islands). *Am. J. Phys. Anthropol.* 62:343–361, 1983.

Block, A. B., and Snider, D. E. Jr.: How much tuberculosis in children must we accept? *Am. J. Public Health* 76:14–15, 1986.

Block, G.: A review of validation of dietary assessment methods. *Am. J. Epidemiol.* 115:492–505, 1982.

Bloom, B.: Use of selective preventive care procedures, United States, 1982. Data from the National Health Survey, Series 10, No. 157 (PHS 86-1585). Hyattsville, MD, U.S. Public Health Service, 1986.

Blot, W. J., McLaughlin, J. K., Winn, D. M., et al.: Smoking and drinking in relation to oral and pharyngeal cancer. *Cancer Res.* 48:3282-3287, 1988.

Bodmer, J. G., Kennedy, L. J., Lindsay, J., et al.: Applications of serology and the ethnic distribution of three locus HLA haplotypes. *Br. Med. Bull.* 43:94-121, 1987.

Bogin, B., and Sullivan, T.: Socioeconomic status, sex, age, and ethnicity as determinants of body fat distribution for Guatemalan children. *Am. J. Phys. Anthropol.* 69:527-535, 1986.

Bonham, G. S.: Prevalence of chronic skin and musculoskeletal conditions. Data from the National Health Survey, Series 10, No. 124, publication No. PHS 79-1552. Hyattsville, MD, U.S. Public Health Service, 1978.

Bonnevie, O.: Changing demographics of peptic ulcer disease. *Digest. Dis. Sci.* 30 (Suppl): 8S-14S, 1985.

Boon, M. E., Deng, Z., Baowen, G., and Ryd, W.: Koilocyte frequency in positive cervical smears as indicator of sexual promiscuity. *Lancet* 1:205, 1986.

Bortolini, E. R., and Zatz, M.: Duchenne muscular dystrophy: Comparison among different racial groups. *Am. J. Med. Genet.* 28:925-929, 1987.

Botha, J. F., Ritchie, M. J. J., Dushieko, G. M., et al.: Hepatitis virus carrier state in black children in Ovamboland: Role of perinatal and horizontal infection. *Lancet* 1:1210-1212, 1984.

Botha, J. L., and Bradshaw, D.: African vital statistics—a black hole? *S. Afr. Med. J.* 67:977-981, 1985.

Botha, J. L., Irwig, L. M., and Strebel, P. M.: Excess mortality from stomach cancer, lung cancer, and asbestosis and/or mesothelioma in crocidolite mining districts in South Africa. *Am. J. Epidemiol.* 123:30-40, 1986.

Botha, J. L., Bradshaw, D., Gonin, R., et al.: The distribution of health needs and services in South Africa. *Soc. Sci. Med.* 26:845-851, 1988.

Bowden, D. K., Hill, A. V. S., Higgs, D. R., and Clegg, J. B.: Relative roles of genetic factors, dietary deficiency, and infection in anaemia in Vanuatu, South-West Pacific. *Lancet* 2:1025-1028, 1985.

Bowden, D. K., Hill, A. V. S., Weatherall, D. J., et al.: High frequency of β thalassemia in a small island population in Melanesia. *J. Med. Genet.* 24:357-361, 1987.

Bower, G.: Intrathoracic sarcoidosis: A review of 69 cases. *Chest* 44:457-468, 1963.

Bowles, G. T.: *The People of Asia.* New York, Scribner's, 1977.

Bowry, J. R., Pade, J., Omari, M., and Chemtai, A.: A pilot study of hepatitis B virus seroepidemiology suggests widespread immunosuppression in the nomadic inhabitants of Turkana District of Kenya. *East Afr. Med. J.* 62:501-506, 1985.

Brabin, L., and Brabin, B. J.: Cultural factors and transmission of heptatitis B virus. *Am. J. Epidemiol.* 122:725-730, 1985.

Bracken, M. B., Brinton, L. A., and Hayashi, K.: Epidemiology of hydatidiform mole and choriocarcinoma. *Epidemiol. Rev.* 6:52-75, 1984.

Branda, R. F., and Eaton, J. W.: Skin color and nutrient photolysis: An evolutionary hypothesis. *Science* 201:625-626, 1978.

Bresnitz, E. A., and Strom, B. L.: Epidemiology of sarcoidosis. *Epidemiol. Rev.* 5:124-156, 1983.

Brignone, G., Cusimano, R., Dardanoni, G., et al.: A case-control study on breast cancer risk factors in a southern European population. *Int. J. Epidemiol.* 16:356-361, 1987.

Brinton, L. A., and Fraumeni, J. F. Jr.: Epidemiology of uterine cervical cancer. *J. Chron. Dis.* 39:1051-1065, 1986.

Brissonnette, L. G. G., and Fareed, D. S.: Cardiovascular diseases as a cause of death in the island of Mauritius, 1972–1980. *World Health Stat. Q.* 38:163–170, 1985.

Brittenham, G. M., Schechter, A. N., and Noguchi, T.: Hemoglobin S polymerization: Primary determinant of the hemolytic and clinical severity of the sickling syndromes. *Blood* 65:183–189, 1985.

Brooks, A. M. V., and Gillies, W. E.: Blood groups as genetic markers in glaucoma. *Br. J. Ophthalmol.* 72:270–273, 1988.

Brooks, R., Capell, F., Benn, S., et al.: Smoking prevalence and cessation in selected states, 1981–1983 and 1985—the behavioral risk factor survey. *MMWR* 35:740–741, 1986.

Broun, G. O., Herbig, F. K., and Hamilton, J. R.: Leukopenia in negroes. *N. Engl. J. Med.* 275:1410–1413, 1966.

Brown, L. M., Pottern, L. M., Hoover, R. N., et al.: Testicular cancer in the United States: Trends in incidence and mortality. *Int. J. Epidemiol.* 15:164–170, 1986.

Brown, P. J., and Konner, M.: An anthropological perspective on obesity. *Ann. N. Y. Acad. Sci.* 499:29–46, 1987.

Brues, A. M.: *People and Races.* New York, Macmillan, 1977.

Buckley, J. D., Henderson, B. E., Morrow, C. P., et al.: Case-control study of gestational choriocarcinoma. *Cancer Res.* 48:1004–1010, 1988.

Budowle, B., Dearth, J., Bowman, P., et al.: Genetic predisposition to acute lymphocytic leukemia in American blacks. *Cancer* 55:2880–2882, 1985.

Bulka, R. P.: Smoking: A religious view. *J. Relig. Health* 25:221–226, 1986.

Burbank, F., and Fraumeni, J. F. Jr.: U.S. cancer mortality: Nonwhite predominance. *JNCI* 49:649–659, 1972.

Burke, G. L., Voors, A. W., Shear, C. L., et al.: Blood pressure. *Pediatrics* 80 (Suppl.):784–788, 1987.

Burke, S. W., Macey, T. I., Roberts, J. M., and Johnston, C. III: Congenital dislocation of the hip in the American black. *Clin. Orthop.* 192:120–123, 1985.

Burt, R. W., Bishop, D. T., Cannon, L. A., et al.: Dominant inheritance of adenomatous colonic polyps and colorectal cancer. *N. Engl. J. Med.* 312:1540–1544, 1985.

Burton, R. F.: *Wit and Wisdom from West Africa.* (Originally published in 1865.) New York, Biblo and Tannen, 1969.

Byard, P. J.: Quantitative genetics of human skin color. *Yearbook Phys. Anthropol.* 24:123–137, 1981.

Byers, T., Graham, S., Rzepka, T., et al.: Lactation and breast cancer. *Am. J. Epidemiol.* 121:664–674, 1985.

Caetano, R.: Drinking patterns and alcohol problems among Hispanics in the U.S.: A review. *Drug Alcohol Depend.* 18:1–15, 1983.

Calkins, B. M., and Mendeloff, A. I.: Epidemiology of inflammatory bowel disease. *Epidemiol. Rev.* 8:60–91, 1986.

Camaschella, C., Saglio, G., Serra, A., Cremonesi, L., Travi, M., and Ferrari, M.: Fetal diagnosis of β-thalassemia by DNA analysis in Italy. *Lancet* 1:390, 1986.

Cambien, F., Warnet, J. M., Vernier, V., et al.: An epidemiologic appraisal of the association between the fatty acids esterifying serum cholesterol and some cardiovascular risk factors in middle-aged men. *Am. J. Epidemiol.* 127:75–86, 1988.

Cameron, P.: Kinsey sex surveys. *Science* 240:867, 1988.

Campion, M. J., McCance, D. J., Cuzick, J., et al.: Progressive potential of mild cervical atypia: Prospective cytological, colposcopic, and virological study. *Lancet* 2:237–240, 1986.

Canella, R., Barbujani, G., Cucchi, P., et al.: Biological performance in β-thal heterozygotes and normals: Results of a longitudinal comparison in a former malarial environment. *Ann. Hum. Genet.* 51:337–343.

Cannon, W. B.: 'Voodoo' death. *Am. Anthropol.* 44:169–181, 1942.

Capocaccia, R., and Farchi, G.: Mortality from liver cirrhosis in Italy: Proportion associated with consumption of alcohol. *J. Clin. Epidemiol.* 41:347–357, 1988.

Carestia, C., Pagano, L., Fioretti, G., et al.: β-Thalassemia in Campania: DNA polymorphism analysis in $β^A$ and $β^{thal}$ chromosomes and its usefulness in prenatal diagnosis. *Br. J. Haematol.* 67:231–234, 1987.

Carter, C., McGee, D., and Yano, K.: Morbidity and mortality rates in Okinawan Japanese vs. mainland Japanese: The Honolulu Heart Program. *Hum. Biol.* 56:339–353, 1984.

Carucci, P. M.: Reliability of statistical and medical information reported on birth and death certificates. New York State Department of Health Monograph No. 15, Albany, May 1979.

Cathala, F., Brown, P., LeCanuet, P., et al.: High incidence of Creutzfeldt-Jakob disease in North African immigrants to France. *Neurology* 35:894–895, 1985.

Catovsky, D., Greaves, M. F., Rose, M., Galton, D. A. G., Goolden, R. W. C., McCluskey, D. R., et al.: Adult T-cell lymphoma–leukemia in blacks from the West Indies. *Lancet* 1:639–644, 1982.

Causse, G., and Meheus, A.: La lutte contre les maladies sexuellement transmissibles (MST) et les tréponématoses endemiques. *World Health Stat. Q.* 41:82–101, 1988.

Cavalli-Sforza, L. L. (ed.): *African Pygmies.* Orlando, FL, Academic Press, 1986.

Chakraborty, R.: Relationship between heterozygosity and genetic distance in the three major races of man. *Am. J. Phys. Anthropol.* 65:249–258, 1984.

Chakraborty, R.: Gene admixture in human populations: Models and predictions. *Yearbook Phys. Anthropol.* 29:1–43, 1986.

Chakraborty, R., and Weiss, K. M.: Frequencies of complex diseases in hybrid populations. *Am. J. Phys. Anthropol.* 70:489–503, 1986.

Chakraborty, R., Walter, H., Mukherjee, B. N., et al.: Gene differentiation among ten endogamous groups of West Bengal, India. *Am. J. Phys. Anthropol.* 71:295–309, 1986.

Chalmanov, V. N.: Epidemiological studies of Parkinsonism in Sofia. *Neuroepidemiology* 5:171–177, 1986.

Chalmers, J., and Ho, K. C.: Geographical variations in senile osteoporosis. The association with physical activity. *J. Bone Joint Surg.* 52B:667–675, 1970.

Chan, S. H., Chew, C. T., Prasad, U., et al.: HLA and nasopharyngeal carcinoma in Malays. *Br. J. Cancer* 51:389–392, 1985.

Chan, V., Chan, T. K., Ghosh, A., et al.: Application of DNA polymorphisms for prenatal diagnosis of β thalassemia in Chinese. *Am. J. Hematol.* 25:409–415, 1987a.

Chan, V., Chan, T. K., Chehab, F. F., et al.: Distribution of β-thalassemia mutations in South China and their association with haplotypes. *Am. J. Hum. Genet.* 41:678–685, 1987b.

Chehab, F. F., Honig, G. R., and Kan, Y. W.: Spontaneous mutation in β-thalassemia producing the same nucleotide substitution as that in a common hereditary form. *Lancet* 1:3–5, 1986.

Chehl, S., Job, C. K., and Hastings, R. C.: Transmission of leprosy in nude mice. *Am. J. Trop. Med. Hyg.* 34:1161–1168, 1985.

Chen, C. J., Chuang, Y. C., Lin, T. M., and Wu, H. Y.: Malignant neoplasms among residents of a Blackfoot disease-endemic area in Taiwan: High arsenic artesian well water and cancers. *Cancer Res.* 45:5895–5899, 1985.

Chen, D. S., Hsu, N. H. M., Sung, J. L., et al.: A mass vaccination program in Taiwan against hepatitis B virus infection in infants of hepatitis B surface antigen-carrier mothers. *JAMA* 257:2597–2603, 1987.

Chen, K. H., Cann, H., Van West, B., and Cavalli-Sforza, I.: Genetic markers of an aboriginal Taiwanese population. *Am. J. Phys. Anthropol.* 66:327–337, 1985.

Chen, L. C.: Primary health care in developing countries: Overcoming operational, technical, and social barriers. *Lancet* 2:1260–1265, 1986.

Chin, J., Von Reyn, C. F., Esteves, K., et al.: Update: Acquired immunodeficiency syndrome (AIDS)—worldwide. *MMWR* 37:286–295, 1988.

China Map Press: *Atlas of Cancer Mortality in the People's Republic of China.* Beijing, China Map Press, 1981.

Chirikos, T. N., and Horner, R. D.: Economic status and survivorship in digestive system cancers. *Cancer* 56:210–217, 1985.

Chou, M. Y., and Malison, M. D.: Outbreak of acute hemorrhagic conjunctivitis due to Coxsackie A24 variant—Taiwan. *Am. J. Epidemiol.* 127:795–800, 1988.

Chrisman, N. J., and Maretzki, T. W. (eds.): *Clinically Applied Anthropology.* Boston, D. Reidel, 1982.

Chung, C. S., Bixler, D., Watanabe, T., et al.: Segregation analysis of cleft lip with or without cleft palate: A comparison of Danish and Japanese data. *Am. J. Hum. Genet.* 39:603–611, 1986a.

Chung, C. S., Runck, D. W., Bilben, S. E., and Kau, M. C. W.: Effects of interracial crosses on cephalometric measurements. *Am. J. Phys. Anthropol.* 69:465–472, 1986b.

Clark, A. G.: The use of multiple restriction fragment length polymorphisms in prenatal risk estimation. *Hum. Hered.* 37:41–53, 1987.

Clarke, M., Halil, T., and Salmon, N.: Peptic ulceration in men. *Br. J. Prev. Soc. Med.* 30:115–122, 1976.

Clarke-Finnegan, M., and Fahy, T. J.: Suicide rates in Ireland. *Psychol. Med.* 13:385–391, 1983.

Clemens, J. D., and Stanton, B. F.: An educational intervention for altering water-sanitation behaviors to reduce childhood diarrhea in urban Bangladesh. *Am. J. Epidemiol.* 125:284–291, 1987.

Clemens, J. D., Sack, D. A., Harris, J. R., Chakraborty, J., et al.: Field trial of oral cholera vaccines in Bangladesh. *Lancet* 2:124–127, 1986.

Clifford, P.: Malignant disease of the nasopharynx and paranasal sinuses in Kenya. In C. S. Muir and K. Shanmugaratnam (eds.), *Cancer of the Nasopharynx.* Copenhagen, Munkbgaard, 1967, pp. 82–94.

Clugston, G. A., and Bagchi, K.: Tackling iodine deficiency in South-East Asia. *World Health Forum* 7:33–36, 1986.

Cocchi, S. L., Markowitz, L. E., Joshi, D. D., et al.: Control of epidemic group A meningococcal meningitis in Nepal. *Int. J. Epidemiol.* 16:91–97, 1987.

Cochrane, R., and Bal, S. S.: Ethnic density is unrelated to incidence of schizophrenia. *Br. J. Psychiat.* 153:363–366, 1988.

Cohen, J. B., Wofsy, C., Gill, P., et al.: Antibody to human immunodeficiency virus in female prostitutes. *JAMA* 257:2011–2012, 1987.

Colliver, J., Doernberg, D., Grant, B., et al.: Trends in mortality from cirrhosis and alcoholism—United States, 1945–1983. *MMWR* 35:703–705, 1986.

Colton, T.: *Statistics in Medicine.* Boston, Little Brown, 1974.

Comess, L. J., Bennett, P. H., and Burch, T. A.: Clinical gallbladder disease in Pima Indians. Its high prevalence in contrast to Framingham, Massachusetts. *N. Engl. J. Med.* 277:894–898, 1967.

Comstock, G. W.: Tuberculosis: A bridge to chronic disease epidemiology. *Am. J. Epidemiol.* 124:1–16, 1986.

Connett, J. E., and Stamler, J.: Responses of black and white males to the special intervention program of the multiple risk factor intervention trial. *Am. Heart J.* 108:839–848, 1984.

Constans, J., Hazout, S., Garruto, R. M., et al.: Population distribution of the human vitamin D binding protein: Anthropological considerations. *Am. J. Phys. Anthropol.* 68:107–122, 1985.

Cook, I. F., Cochrane, J. P., and Epstein, M. D.: Race linked differences in serum concentrations of dapsone, monoacetyldapsone and pyrimethamine during malaria prophylaxis. *Trans. R. Soc. Trop. Med. Hyg.* 80:897–901, 1986.

Cook-Mozaffari, P.: East and central Africa. In Howe, G. M. (ed.), *Global Geocancerology.* Edinburgh, Churchill Livingstone, 1986, pp. 331–337.

Cooke, R.: The colorful people of Papua–New Guinea. Some of their habits and some diseases which result from these habits. *Pathol. Annu.* 21 (Pt. 2):311–346, 1986.

Coon, C. S.: *The Living Races of Man.* New York, Knopf, 1965.

Cooper, D. N., and Clayton, J. F.: DNA polymorphism and the study of disease associations. *Hum. Genet.* 78:299–312, 1988.

Cooper, D. N., and Schmidtke, J.: Restriction fragment length polymorphisms in the human genome. In Roberts, D. F., and De Stefano, G. F. (eds.), *Genetic Variation and Its Maintenance.* Cambridge, U.K., Cambridge University Press, 1986, pp. 57–75.

Cooper, E. S.: Cerebrovascular disease in blacks. In Hall, W. D., Saunders, E., and Shulman, N. B., *Hypertension in Blacks: Epidemiology, Pathophysiology and Treatment.* Chicago, Yearbook Medical Publishers, 1985, pp. 83–103.

Coulehan, J. L., Lerner, G., Helzlsouer, K., et al.: Acute myocardial infarction among Navajo Indians, 1976–83. *Am. J. Public Health* 76:412–414, 1986.

Covington, D. L., Carl, J., Daley, J. G., et al.: Effects of the North Carolina prematurity prevention program among public patients delivering at New Hanover Memorial Hospital. *Am. J. Public Health* 78:1493–1495, 1988.

Cox, P.: Epidemiology and research at low cost. *Br. Med. J.* 288:1814–1816, 1984.

Crawford, F. C., and Sofaer, J. A.: Cleft lip with or without cleft palate: Identification of sporadic cases with a high level of genetic predisposition. *J. Med. Genet.* 24:163–169, 1987.

Crawford, M. H.: The anthropological genetics of the black Caribs (Garifuna) of Central America and the Caribbean. *Yearbook Phys. Anthropol.* 26:161–192, 1983.

Cresanta, J. L., Croft, J. B., Webber, L. S., et al.: Racial differences in hemoglobin concentration of young adults. *Prev. Med.* 16:659–669, 1987.

Crews, D. E.: Body weight, blood pressure and the rise of total and cardiovascular mortality in an obese population. *Hum. Biol.* 60:417–433, 1988.

Cristofolini, M., Francheschi, S., Tasin, L., et al.: Risk factors for cutaneous malignant melanoma in a northern Italian population. *Int. J. Cancer* 39:150–154, 1987.

Crombie, K.: Racial differences in melanoma incidence. *Br. J. Cancer* 40:185–193, 1979.

Cummings, K. M.: Changes in the smoking habits of adults in the United States and recent trends in lung cancer mortality. *Cancer Detect. Prev.* 7:125–134, 1984.

Cunningham, L. S., and Kelsey, J. L.: Epidemiology of musculoskeletal impairments and associated disability. *Am. J. Public Health* 74:574–579, 1984.

Curran, J. W., Jaffe, H. W., Hardy, A. M., et al.: Epidemiology of HIV infection and AIDS in the United States. *Science* 239:610–616, 1988.

Curry, C. L., Oliver, J., and Mumtaz, F. B.: Coronary artery disease in blacks: Risk factors. *Am. Heart J.* 108:653–657, 1984.

Dabis, F., Sow, A., Waldman, R. J., et al.: The epidemiology of measles in a partially vaccinated population in an African city: Implications for immunization programs. *Am. J. Epidemiol.* 127:171–178, 1988.

Dales, L. G., Friedman, G. D., Ury, H. K., Grossman, S., and Williams, S. R.: A case-control study of relationships of diet and other traits to colorectal cancer in American blacks. *Am. J. Epidemiol.* 109:132–144, 1978.

Damon, A.: Race, ethnic group, and disease. *Social Biol.* 16:69–80, 1969.

Damon, A.: Race, ethnic group and disease. In Osborne, R. H. (ed.), *The Biological and Social Meaning of Race.* San Francisco, W. H. Freeman, 1971, pp. 57–74.

Damon, A. (ed.): *Physiological Anthropology.* New York, Oxford University Press, 1975.

Damon, A.: *Human Biology and Ecology.* New York, Norton, 1977.

Danker-Hopfe, H.: Menarcheal age in Europe. *Yearbook Phys. Anthropol.* 29:81–112, 1986.

Darabi, K. F., and Ortiz, V.: Childbearing among young Latino women in the United States. *Am. J. Public Health* 77:25–28, 1987.

Darwish, M. J., and Armenian, H. K.: A case-control study of rheumatoid arthritis in Lebanon. *Int. J. Epidemiol.* 16:420–424, 1987.

David, R., and Jenkins, T.: Genetic markers in glaucoma. *Br. J. Ophthalmol.* 64:227–231, 1980.

Davies, D. P.: Cot death in Hong Kong: A rare problem. *Lancet* 2:1346–1347, 1985.

Davies, J. N. P.: Mortality from pneumococcal meningitis. *Lancet* 1:255, 1977.

Davis, D. L., and Whitten, R. G.: The cross-cultural study of human sexuality. *Annu. Rev. Anthropol.* 16:69–98, 1987.

Dawson, D. A., Hendershot, G. E., and Bloom, B.: Trends in routine screening examinations. *Am. J. Public Health* 77:1004–1005, 1987.

Dayal, H., Goldberg-Alberts, R., Kinman, J., et al.: Patterns of mortality from selected causes in an urban population. *J. Chron. Dis.* 39:877–888, 1986.

DeCeulaer, K., McMullen, K. W., Maude, G. H., Keatinge, R., and Serjeant, G. R.: Pneumonia in young children with homozygous sickle cell disease: Risk and clinical features. *Eur. J. Pediatr.* 144:255–258, 1985.

Dembert, M. L., Shaffer, R. A., Baugh, N. L., et al.: Epidemiology of viral hepatitis among U.S. Navy and Marine Corps Personnel, 1984–1985. *Am. J. Public Health* 77:1446–1447, 1987.

Denia, F., Barin, F., Gershy-Damet, G., et al.: Prevalence of human T-lymphotropic retroviruses type III (HIV) and type IV in Ivory Coast. *Lancet* 1:408–411, 1987.

Dennett, G., and Connell, J.: Acculturation and health in the highlands of Papua New Guinea. *Curr. Anthropol.* 29:273–299, 1988.

Denny, F. W., and Loda, F. A.: Acute respiratory infections are the leading cause of death in children in developing countries. *Am. J. Trop. Med. Hyg.* 35:1–2, 1986.

Detheridge, F. M., Guyer, P. B., and Barker, D. J.: European distribution of Paget's disease of bone. *Br. Med. J.* 285:1005–1008, 1982.

Devesa, S. S., and Diamond, E. L.: Association of breast cancer and cervical cancer incidences with income and education among whites and blacks. *JNCI* 65:515–528, 1980.

Devesa, S. S., and Diamond, E. L.: Socioeconomic and racial differences in lung cancer incidence. *Am. J. Epidemiol.* 118:818–831, 1983.

Devi, A. R. R., Rao, N. A., and Bittles, A. H.: Inbreeding and the incidence of childhood genetic disorders in Karnataka, South India. *J. Med. Genet.* 24:362–365, 1987.

DeVita, V. T. Jr.: Cancer prevention awareness program: Testing black Americans. *Public Health Rep.* 100:253–254, 1985.

DeVries, R. R. P., Mehra, N. K., Vaidya, M. C., et al.: HLA-linked control of susceptibility to tuberculoid leprosy and association with HLA-DR types. *Tissue Antigens* 16:294–304, 1980.

De Wals, P., Dolk, H., Weatherall, J. A. C., et al.: Prevalence of neural tube defects in 16 regions of Europe, 1980–1983. *Int. J. Epidemiol.* 16:246–251.

Dewey, J. R., Bartley, M. H. Jr., and Armelagos, G. J.: Rates of femoral cortical bone loss in two Nubian populations. *Clin. Orthop.* 65:61–66, 1969.

Deyo, R. A.: Pitfalls in measuring the health status of Mexican Americans: Comparative validity of the English and Spanish sickness impact profile. *Am. J. Public Health* 74:569–573, 1984.

Digard, J. P.: On the family and change in the Middle East. *Curr. Anthropol.* 27:45, 1986.

Dischinger, P., Tyroler, H. A., McDonough, R. Jr., et al.: Blood fibrinolytic activity, social class and habitual physical activity. I. A study of black and white men in Evans County, Georgia. *J. Chron. Dis.* 33:283–290, 1980.

Dobson, A. J., Gibberd, R. W., and Leeder, S. R.: Death certification and coding for ischemic heart disease in Australia. *Am. J. Epidemiol.* 117:397–405, 1983.

Donahue, R. P., Abbott, R. D., Bloom, E., et al.: Central obesity and coronary heart disease in men. *Lancet* 1:821–824, 1987.

Dorn, H. F.: Methods of analysis in follow-up studies. *Hum. Biol.* 22:238–248, 1950.

Dowdle, W.: The search for an AIDS vaccine. *Public Health Rep.* 101:232–233, 1986.

Downing, R. G., Eglin, R. P., and Bayley, A. C.: African Kaposi's sarcoma and AIDS. *Lancet* 1:478–480, 1984.

Dozy, A. M., Kan, Y. W., Embury, S. H., et al.: Alpha globin gene organization in blacks precludes the severe form of alpha thalassemia. *Nature* 280:605–607, 1979.

Dressler, W. W., and Badger, L. W.: Epidemiology of depression symptoms in black community: A comparative analysis. *J. Nerv. Ment. Dis.* 173:212–220.

Drizd, T., Dannenberg, A. L., and Engel, A.: Blood pressure levels in persons 18–74 years of age in 1976–80, and trends in blood pressure from 1960 to 1980 in the United States. Data from the U.S. National Health Survey, Series 11, No. 234, 1986.

Dubos, R.: *Man Adapting.* New Haven, CT, Yale University Press, 1965.

Dunk, A. A., Spiliadis, H., Sherlock, S., et al.: Hepatocellular carcinoma: Clinical, aetiological and pathological features in British patients. *Int. J. Cancer* 41:17–23, 1988.

Dunnigan, M. G., and Robertson, I.: Residence in Britain as a risk factor for Asian rickets and osteomalacia. *Lancet* 1:770, 1980.

Durrington, P. N., Ishola, M., Hunt, L., et al.: Apolipoprotein (a), AI, and B and parental history in men with early onset ischaemic heart disease. *Lancet* 1:1070–1073, 1988.

Durst, R., and Rosca-Rebaudengo, P.: Koro secondary to a tumor of the corpus callosum. *Br. J. Psychiat.* 153:251–254, 1988.

Dwyer, D. E., Collignon, P. J., MacLeod, C., et al.: Extrapulmonary tuberculosis—a continuing problem in Australia. *Aust. N.Z. J. Med.* 17:507–511, 1987.

Dykes, D. D., Crawford, M. H., and Polesky, H. F.: Population distribution in North and Central America of PGM_1 and Gc subtypes as determined by isoelectric focusing (IEF). *Am. J. Phys. Anthropol.* 62:137–145, 1983.

Eales, L. J., Nye, K. E., Parkin, J. M., et al.: Association of different allelic forms of group specific complement with susceptibility to and clinical manifestation of human immunodeficiency virus infection. *Lancet* 1:999–1002, 1987.

Edmondstone, W. M., and Wilson, A. G.: Sarcoidosis on Caucasians, blacks, and Asians in London. *Br. J. Dis. Chest* 79:27–36, 1985.

Efremov, G. D., Gjorgovski, I., Stojanovski, N., et al.: One haplotype is associated with the Swiss type of hereditary persistence of fetal hemoglobin in the Yugoslavian population. *Hum. Genet.* 77:132–136, 1987.

Ehnholm, C., Huttunen, J. K., Pietinen, P., et al.: Effect of diet on serum lipoproteins in a population with a high risk of coronary heart disease. *N. Engl. J. Med.* 307:850–855, 1982.

Eimas, P. D., and Kavanagh, J. F.: Otitis media, hearing loss, and child development: A NICHD conference summary. *Public Health Rep.* 101:289–293, 1986.

El-Hazmi, M. A. F., and Warsy, A. S.: Beta-globin gene polymorphism in Saudis: 5.6 Hpa I fragment. *Hum. Hered.* 37:237–240, 1987.

El-Islam, M. F., Malasi, T. H., and Abu-Dagga, S. I.: Interparental differences in attitudes and cultural change in Kuwait. *Soc. Psychiat. Psychiatr. Epidemiol.* 23:109–113, 1988.

El-Najjar, M. Y.: Human treponematosis and tuberculosis: Evidence from the New World. *Am. J. Phys. Anthropol.* 51:599–618, 1979.

Elston, R. C.: The estimation of admixture in racial hybrids. *Ann. Hum. Genet.* 35:9–17, 1971.

Embury, S. H., Dozy, A. M., Miller, J., Davis, J. R. Jr., Kleman, K. M., et al.: Concurrent sickle-cell anemia and a-thalassemia. Effect on severity of anemia. *N. Engl. J. Med.* 306: 270–274, 1982.

Engel, A., Johnson, M. L., and Haynes, S. G.: Health effects of sunlight exposure in the United States. *Arch. Dermatol.* 124:72–79, 1988.

Enwonwu, C. O.: The role of dietary aflatoxin in the genesis of hepatocellular cancer in developing countries. *Lancet* 2:956–958, 1984.

Epstein, M. A.: Recent studies on a vaccine to prevent EB–virus-associated cancers. *Br. J. Cancer* 54:1–5, 1986.

Erickson, D., Swenson, I., Ehlinger, E., et al.: Maternal and infant outcomes among Caucasians and Hmong refugees in Minneapolis, Minnesota. *Hum. Biol.* 59:799–808, 1987.

Esry, S. A., and Habicht, J. P.: Epidemiologic evidence for health benefits from improved water and sanitation in developing countries. *Epidemiol. Rev.* 8:117–128, 1986.

Evans, A. S.: Ruminations on infectious disease epidemiology: Retrospective, curspective, and prospective. *Int. J. Epidemiol.* 14:205–212, 1985.

Eveleth, P. B.: Differences between populations in body shape of children and adolescents. *Am. J. Phys. Anthropol.* 49:373–382, 1978.

Excoffier, L., Pellegrini, B., Sanchez-Mazas, A., et al.: Genetics and history of sub-Saharan Africa. *Yearbook Phys. Anthropol.* 30:151–194, 1987.

Farer, L. S., Lowell, A. M., and Meador, M. P.: Extrapulmonary tuberculosis in the United States. *Am. J. Epidemiol.* 109:205–217, 1979.

Farmer, M. E., White, L. R., Brody, J. A., et al.: Race and sex differences in hip fracture incidence. *Am. J. Public Health* 74:1374–1380, 1984.

Farrell, S. W., Kohl, H. W. and Rogers, T.: The independent effect of ethnicity on cardiovascular fitness. *Hum. Biol.* 59:657–666, 1987.

Feret, E., Larouze, B., Diop, B., et al.: Epidemiology of hepatitis B virus infection in the rural community of Tip, Senegal. *Am. J. Epidemiol.* 125:140–149, 1987.

Filice, G. A., Van Etta, L. L., Darby, C. P., and Fraser, D. W.: Bacteremia in Charleston County, South Carolina. *Am. J. Epidemiol.* 123:128–136, 1986.

Finch, M. J., Morris, J. G. Jr., Kavitti, J., et al.: Epidemiology of antimicrobial resistant cholera in Kenya and East Africa. *Am. J. Trop. Med. Hyg.* 39:484–490, 1988.

Fine, P. E. M.: Immunogenetics of susceptibility to leprosy, tuberculosis and leishmaniasis: An epidemiological perspective. *Int. J. Leprosy* 49:437–454, 1981.

Fine, P. E. M.: Leprosy: The epidemiology of a slow bacterium. *Epidemiol. Rev.* 4:161–188, 1982.

Firebaugh, G., and Davis, K. E.: Trends in antiblack prejudice, 1972–1984: Region and cohort effects. *Am. J. Sociol.* 94:251–272, 1988.

Fischer, J.: Negroes and whites and rates of mental illness: Reconsideration of a myth. *Psychiatry* 32:428–446, 1969.

Fix, A. G.: Kin group and trait selection: Population structure and epidemic disease selection. *Am. J. Phys. Anthropol.* 65:201–212, 1984.

Fix, A. G., and Lie-Injo, L. E.: Genetic microdifferentiation in the Semai Senoi of Malaysia. *Am. J. Phys. Anthropol.* 43:47–56, 1975.

Flegal, K. M., Harlan, W. R., and Landis, J. R.: Secular trends in body mass index and skinfold thickness with socioeconomic factors in young adult women. *Am. J. Clin. Nutr.* 48:535–543, 1988.

Fleiss, J.: *Statistical Methods for Rates and Proportions.* New York, Wiley, 1974.

Fleming, A. F.: Maternal anemia in northern Nigeria: Causes and solutions. *World Health Forum* 8:339–343, 1987.

Folstein, S. E., Chase, G. A., Wahl, W. E., et al.: Huntington's disease in Maryland: Clinical aspects and racial variation. *Am. J. Hum. Genet.* 41:168–179, 1987.

Ford, E., Nelson, K. E., and Warren, D.: Epidemiology of epidemic keratoconjunctivitis. *Epidemiol. Rev.* 9:244–261, 1987.

Ford, E., Cooper, R., Simmons, B., et al.: Sex differences in high density lipoprotein cholesterol in urban blacks. *Am. J. Epidemiol.* 127:753–761, 1988a.

Ford, E., Cooper, R. S., Castaner, A., et al.: Differential utilization of coronary arteriography and coronary artery bypass surgery among whites and blacks. *Am. J. Epidemiol.* 128:922, 1988b.

Foster, A., Kavishe, F., Sommer, A., and Taylor, H. R.: A simple surveillance system for xerophthalmia and childhood corneal ulceration. *Bull. WHO* 64:725–728, 1986.

Fox, E., Khalig, A. A., and Strickland, G. T.: Chloroquine-resistant *Plasmodium falciparum*: Now in Pakistani Punjab. *Lancet* 1:1432–1435, 1985.

Fox, M. H., Webber, L. S., Thurmon, T. F., and Berenson, G. S.: ABO blood group associations with cardiovascular risk factor variables. II. Blood pressure, obesity and their anthropometric covariables. The Bogalusa Heart Study. *Hum. Biol.* 58:549–584, 1986.

Franco, L. J., Stern, M. P., Rosenthal, M., et al.: Prevalence, detection, and control of hypertension in a biethnic community. The San Antonio heart study. *Am. J. Epidemiol.* 121:684–696, 1985.

Franco, M. H., Weiner, T. A., and Salzano, F. M.: Blood polymorphisms and racial admixture in two Brazilian populations. *Am. J. Phys. Anthropol.* 58:127–132, 1982.

Frank, E., Weiss, S. H., Compas, J. C., Bienstock, J., et al.: AIDS in Haitian-Americans: A reassessment. *Cancer Res.* (Suppl.) 45:4619s–4620s, 1985.

Franklin, R. R., Jacobs, C. F., and Betrand, W. E.: Illness in black Africans. In Rothschild, H. (ed.), *Biocultural Factors in Disease.* New York, Academic Press, 1981, pp. 484–530.

Fraser, G. E.: *Preventive Cardiology.* New York, Oxford University Press, 1986.

Fraser, G. E., Dysinger, W., Best, C., et al.: Ischemic heart disease risk factors in middle-aged Seventh-Day Adventists and their neighbors. *Am. J. Epidemiol.* 126:638–646, 1987.

Fratiglioni, L., Massey, E. W., Schoenberg, D. G., et al.: Mortality from cerebrovascular disease: International comparisons and temporal trends. *Neuroepidemiology* 2:101–116, 1983.

Freedman, D. S., Srinivasan, S. R., Shear, C. L., et al.: Cigarette smoking initiation and longitudinal changes in serum lipids and lipoproteins in early adulthood: The Bogalusa heart study. *Am. J. Epidemiol.* 124:207–219, 1986.

Frerichs, R. R., Chapman, J. M., and Maes, E. F.: Mortality due to all causes and to cardiovascular diseases among seven race-ethnic populations in Los Angeles county, 1980. *Int. J. Epidemiol.* 13:291–298, 1984.

Fried, L. P., and Pearson, T. A.: The association of risk factors with arteriographically defined coronary artery disease: What is the appropriate control group? *Am. J. Epidemiol.* 125:844–853, 1987.

Friedlaender, J. S., Howells, W. W., and Rhoads, J. G.: *The Solomon Islands Project.* New York, Oxford University Press, 1987.

Friedlander, Y., and Kark, J. D.: Complex segregation analysis of plasma lipid and lipoprotein variables in a Jerusalem sample of nuclear families. *Hum. Hered.* 37:7-19, 1987.

Friedlander, Y., Kark, J. D., and Stein, Y.: Religious observance and plasma lipids and lipoproteins among 17-year-old Jewish residents of Jerusalem. *Prev. Med.* 16:70-79, 1987.

Friedman, E. G., Koch, R., and Azen, C.: Maternal phenylketonuria collaborative study (MPKUCS): USA and Canada. *Am. J. Hum. Genet.* 41:A60, 1987.

Friedman, M. J., and Trager, W.: The biochemistry of resistance to malaria. *Sci. Am.* 244:154-164, 1981.

Friedman-Kien, A., Laubenstein, L., Marmor, M., et al.: Kaposi's sarcoma and *Pneumocystis* pneumonia among homosexual men—New York City and California. *MMWR* 30:305-308, 1981.

Friedman-Kien, A. E., Laubenstein, L. J., Rubenstein, P., et al.: Disseminated Kaposi's sarcoma in homosexual men. *Ann. Intern. Med.* 96:693-700, 1982.

Frisancho, A. R., Leonard, W. R., and Bolletino, L. A.: Blood pressure in blacks and whites and its relationship to dietary sodium and potassium intake. *J. Chron. Dis.* 37:515-519, 1984.

Fruchter, R. G., Remy, J. C., Burnett, W. S., and Boyce, J. G.: Cervical cancer in immigrant women. *Am. J. Public Health* 76:797-799, 1986.

Fujimoto, W. Y., Leonetti, D. L., Kinyoun, J. L., et al.: Prevalence of diabetes mellitus and impaired glucose tolerance among second-generation Japanese-American men. *Diabetes* 36:721-729, 1987.

Fujishima, S., Tochikubo, O, and Kaneko, Y.: Environmental and physiological characteristics in adolescents genetically predisposed to hypertension. *Jpn. Circ. J.* 47:267-286, 1983.

Fulwood, R., Johnson, C. L., Bryner, J. D., et al.: *Hematological and Nutritional Biochemistry Reference Data for Persons 6 Months-74 Years of Age: United States, 1976-80.* Data from the National Health Survey, Series 11, No. 232 (PHS 83-1682). Hyattsville, MD, U.S. Public Health Service, 1983.

Fulwood, R., Kalsbeek, W., Rifkind, B., et al.: *Total Serum Cholesterol Levels of Adults 20-74 Years of Age, United States, 1976-1980.* Data from the National Health Survey, Series 11, No. 236, PHS 86-1686. Hyattsville, MD, U.S. Public Health Service, 1986.

Furstenberg, A. L., and Mezey, M. D.: Differences in outcome between black and white elderly hip fracture patients. *J. Chron. Dis.* 40:931-938, 1987.

Gad-el-Mawla, N., El-Deeb, B. B., Abu-Gabal, A., et al.: Pediatric Hodgkin's disease in Egypt. *Cancer* 52:1129-1131, 1983.

Gallagher, J. C., Melton, L. J., Riggs, B. L., et al.: Epidemiology of fractures of the proximal femur in Rochester, Minnesota. *Clin. Orthoped.* 150:163-171, 1980.

Gao, Y. T., Tu, J. T., Jin, F., and Gao, R. N.: Cancer mortality in Shanghai during the period 1963-1977. *Br. J. Cancer* 43:183-195, 1981.

Gao, Y. T., Blot, W. J., Zheng, W., et al.: Lung cancer among Chinese women. *Int. J. Cancer* 40:604-609, 1981.

Garcia-Palmieri, M. R., Sorlie, P. D., Havlik, R. J., et al.: Urban–rural differences in 12 year coronary heart disease mortality: The Puerto Rico heart health program. *J. Clin. Epidemiol.* 41:285-292, 1988.

Gardner, J. W., and Lyon, J. L.: Cancer in Utah Mormon men by lay priesthood level. *Am. J. Epidemiol.* 116:243-257, 1982a.

Gardner, J. W., and Lyon, J. L.: Cancer in Utah Mormon women by church activity level. *Am. J. Epidemiol.* 116:258-265, 1982b.

Gardner, L. T., Stern, M. P., Haffner, S. M., et al.: Prevalence of diabetes in Mexican Americans. *Diabetes* 33:86–92, 1984.

Garn, S. M.: *Human Races.* Springfield, IL: C. C Thomas, 1971.

Garn, S. M., Rohman, C. G., and Wagner, B.: Bone loss as a general phenomenon in man. *Fed. Proc.* 26:1729–1736, 1967.

Garn, S. M., Rohmann, C. G., Wagner, B., Davila, G. H., and Ascoli, W.: Population similarities in the onset and rate of adult endosteal bone loss. *Clin. Orthop.* 65:51–60, 1969.

Garruto, R. M., Gadjusek, D. C., and Chen, K. M.: Amyotrophic lateral sclerosis and Parkinsonism-dementia among Filipino migrants to Guam. *Ann. Neurol.* 10:341–350, 1981.

Gartside, P. S., Khoury, P. K., and Glueck, C. J.: Determinants of high-density lipoprotein cholesterol in blacks and whites: The second National Health and Nutrition Examination Survey. *Am. Heart J.* 108:641–653, 1984.

Gazzolo, L., Robert-Guroff, H., Jennings, A., Duc-Dodon, M., Najberg, G., Mangi Peti, M., and De-The, G.: Type-I and Type-III HTLV antibodies in hospitalized and out-patient Zairians. *Int. J. Cancer* 36:373–378, 1985.

Gerber, L. M.: Diabetes mortality among Chinese immigrants to New York City. *Hum. Biol.* 56:449–458, 1984.

Gerber, L. M., and Madhavan, S.: Epidemiology of coronary heart disease in migrant Chinese populations. *Med. Anthropol.* 4:307–320, 1980.

Gergen, P. J., and Turkeltaub, P. C.: *Percutaneous Immediate Hypersensitivity to Eight Allergens, United States, 1976–80.* Data from the National Health Survey, Series 11, No. 235. Hyattsville, MD, U.S. Public Health Service, 1986.

Ghadirian, P., Vobecky, J., and Vobecky, J. S.: Factors associated with cancer of the esophagus: An overview. *Cancer Detect. Prev.* 11:225–234, 1988.

Giachello, A. L., Bell, R., Aday, L. A., et al.: Uses of the 1980 Census for Hispanic health services research. *Am. J. Public Health* 73:266–274, 1983.

Gifford, R. W. Jr.: Epidemiology and clinical manifestations of renovascular hypertension. In Stanley, J. C., Ernst, C. B., and Fry, W. J. (eds.), *Renovascular Hypertension.* Philadelphia, W. B. Saunders, 1984, pp. 77–99.

Gillum, R. F.: Ischemic heart disease mortality in American Indians, United States, 1969–71 and 1979–81. *Am. Heart J.* 115:1141–1144, 1988.

Gillum, R. F., and Liu, K. C.: Coronary heart disease mortality in United States blacks, 1940–1978: Trends and unanswered questions. *Am. Heart J.* 108:728–732, 1984.

Gittelsohn, A., and Senning, J.: Studies on the reliability of vital and health records. I. Comparison of cause of death and hospital record diagnoses. *Am. J. Public Health* 69:680–689, 1979.

Glass, B.: On the unlikelihood of significant admixture of genes from the North American Indians in the present composition of the Negroes of the United States. *Am. J. Hum. Genet.* 7:368–385,1955.

Glass, R. I., Holmgren, J., Haley, C. E., et al.: Predisposition for cholera of individuals with O blood group. *Am. J. Epidemiol.* 121:791–796, 1985.

Gleuck, C. J., Gartside, P., Laskarzewski, P. M., et al.: High-density lipoprotein cholesterol in blacks and whites: Potential ramifications for coronary heart disease. *Am. Heart J.* 108:815–826, 1984.

Glickman, L. T., Magnaval, J. F., and Domanski, L. M.: Visceral larva migrans in French adults: A new disease syndrome? *Am. J. Epidemiol.* 125:1019–1034, 1987.

Glynn, R. J., Campion, E. W., Bouchard, G. R., et al.: The development of benign prostatic hyperplasia among volunteers in the normative aging study. *Am. J. Epidemiol.* 121:78–80, 1985.

Goede, H. W., Benkmann, H. G., Kriese, L., et al.: Population genetic studies in three Chinese minorities. *Am. J. Phys. Anthropol.* 64:277–284, 1984.

Goedert, J. J., Weiss, S. H., Biggar, R. J., Landesman, S. H., et al.: Lesser AIDS and tuberculosis. *Lancet* 2:52, 1985.

Goel, K. M., Sweet, E. M., Campbell, S., Attenburrow, A., et al.: Reduced prevalence of rickets in Asian children in Glasgow. *Lancet* 2:405–407, 1981.

Goh, K. T., Ding, J. L., Monteiro, E. H., et al.: Hepatitis B in households of acute cases. *J. Epidemiol. Community Health* 41:123–126, 1987.

Goldson, A., Henschke, U., Leffall, L. D., and Schneider, R. L.: Is there a genetic basis for the differences in cancer incidence between Afro-Americans and Euro-Americans? *J. Natl. Med. Assoc.* 73:701–706, 1981.

Goodman, A. H., Allen, L. H., Hernandez, G. P., et al.: Prevalence and age at development of enamel hyperplasias in Mexican children. *Am. J. Phys. Anthropol.* 72:7–19, 1987.

Goodman, R. M.: *Genetic Disorders Among the Jewish People.* Baltimore: Johns Hopkins University Press, 1979.

Goodman, R. M., and Motulsky, A. G. (eds.): *Genetic Diseases Among Ashkenazi Jews.* New York, Raven, 1979.

Goodwin, M. H., Shaw, J. R., and Feldman, C. M.: Distribution of otitis media among four Indian populations. *Public Health Rep.* 95:589–594, 1980.

Gottlieb, K.: Genetic demography of Denver, Colorado: Spanish surname as a marker of Mexican ancestry. *Hum. Biol.* 55:227–234, 1983.

Grady, G. F.: The here and now of hepatitis B immunization. *N. Engl. J. Med.* 315:350–352, 1986.

Graham, D. Y., Klein, P. D., Evans, D. J. Jr., et al.: *Campylobacter pylori* detected noninvasively by the ^{13}C-urea breath test. *Lancet* 1:1174–1177, 1987.

Gratten, M., Naraqi, S., and Hansman, D.: High prevalence of penicillin-insensitive pneumococci in Port Moresby, Papua New Guinea. *Lancet* 2:192–195, 1980.

Gray, G. E., Henderson, B. E., and Pike, M. C.: Changing ratio of breast cancer incidence rates with age of black females compared with white females in the United States. *JNCI* 64:461–463, 1980.

Greenberg, J. H., Turner, C. G., and Zagura, S. L.: The settlement of the Americas: A comparison of the linguistic, dental, and genetic evidence. *Curr. Anthropol.* 27:477–497, 1986.

Greenberg, M. A., Wiggins, C. L., Kutvirt, D. K., et al.: Cigarette use among Hispanic and non-Hispanic white school children. Albuquerque, New Mexico. *Am. J. Public Health* 77:621–622, 1987.

Greenwald, P.: Prostate. In Schottenfeld, D., and Fraumeni, J. F. Jr. (eds.), *Cancer Epidemiology and Prevention.* Philadelphia, W. B. Saunders, 1982, pp. 938–946.

Greenwald, P., Korns, R. F., Nasca, P. C., et al.: Cancer in United States Jews. *Cancer Res.* 35:3507–3512, 1975.

Greenwood, B. M., Blakebrough, I. S., Bradley, A. K., Wali, S., and Whittle, H. C.: Meningococcal disease and season in sub-Saharan Africa. *Lancet* 1:1339–1342, 1984.

Greenwood, B. M., Greenwood, A. M., Bradley, A. K., et al.: Comparison of two strategies for control of malaria within a primary health care programme in the Gambia. *Lancet* 1:1121–1127, 1988.

Gregg, I.: Epidemiological research in asthma: The need for a broad perspective. *Clin. Allergy* 16:17–23, 1986.

Greiner, J., Spengler, D. H., Kruger, J., et al.: The secretor locus as a marker for prenatal prediction of myotonic dystrophy (DM). *Hum. Genet.* 78:330–332, 1988.

Griesel, R. D., and Richter, L. M.: Psycho-social studies of malnutrition in southern Africa. *World Rev. Nutr. Diet.* 54:71–104, 1987.

Grossman, R. A., Benenson, M. W., Scott, R. M., et al.: An epidemiologic study of hepatitis B virus in Bangkok, Thailand. *Am. J. Epidemiol.* 101:144–159, 1975.

Grover, R., Newman, S., Wethers, D., Anyane-Yeboa, K., and Pass, K.: Newborn screening for the hemoglobinopathies: The benefit beyond the target. *Am. J. Public Health* 76:1236–1237, 1986.

Grubb, G. S.: Human papillomavirus and cervical neoplasia: Epidemiological considerations. *Int. J. Epidemiol.* 15:1–7, 1986.

Grufferman, S., and Delzell, E.: Epidemiology of Hodgkin's disease. *Epidemiol. Rev.* 6:76–106, 1984.

Gu, Y. C., Nakatsuji, T., and Huisman, T. H. J.: Detection of a new hybrid a2 globin gene among American blacks. *Hum. Genet.* 79:68–72, 1988.

Guileyardo, J. M., Johnson, W. D., Welsh, R. A., Akazaki, K., and Correa, P.: Prevalence of latent prostate carcinoma in two U.S. populations. *JNCI* 65:311–316, 1980.

Guilleminault, C., Heldt, G., Powell, N., and Riley, R.: Small upper airway in near-miss sudden death syndrome infants and their families. *Lancet* 1:402–407, 1986.

Gulaid, J. A., Onwuachi-Saunders, E. C., Sacks, J. J., et al.: Differences in death rates due to injury among blacks and whites, 1984. *MMWR* 37(SS3) 25–31, 1988.

Gupta, P. C., Mehta, F. S., Pindborg, J. J., et al.: Intervention study for primary prevention of oral cancer among 36000 Indian tobacco users. *Lancet* 1:1235–1239, 1986.

Gurnack, A. M.: Determinants of health provider selection in a West Dallas, Mexican-American community. *Am. J. Prev. Med.* 1:34–40, 1985.

Guttridge, B., Ferrer, H. P., Thompson, E., et al.: Distribution of meningococcal meningitis in England and Wales, 1982–86. *Lancet* 2:567–568, 1986.

Guyer, F. B., and Chamberlain, A. T.: Paget's disease of bone in two American cities. *Br. Med. J.* 1:985, 1980.

Haaga, J. G.: Evidence of a reversal of the breastfeeding decline in Peninsular Malaysia. *Am. J. Public Health* 76:245–251, 1986.

Haddy, T. B.: Cancer in black children. *Am. J. Pediatr. Hematol. Oncol.* 4:285–292, 1982.

Haenszel, W.: Cancer mortality among the foreign-born in the United States. *JNCI* 26:37–132, 1961.

Haenszel, W.: Migrant studies. In Schottenfeld, D. S. (ed.), *Cancer Epidemiology.* Philadelphia, W. B. Saunders, 1982, pp. 194–207.

Haenszel, W., Loveland, D. B., and Sirken, M. G.: Lung cancer mortality as related to residence and smoking histories. I. White males. Appendix C. *JNCI* 28:1000–1001, 1962.

Haenszel, W., and Kurihara, M.: Studies of Japanese migrants. I. Mortality from cancer and other diseases among Japanese in the United States. *JNCI* 40:43–68, 1968.

Haenszel, W., Kurihara, M., Segi, M., and Lee, R. K. C.: Stomach cancer among Japanese in Hawaii. *JNCI* 49:969–988, 1972.

Haffner, S. M., Stern, M. P., Hazuda, H. P., et al.: Hyperinsulinemia in a population at high risk for non-insulin-dependent diabetes mellitus. *N. Engl. J. Med.* 315:220–224, 1986a.

Haffner, S. M., Stern, M. P., Hazuda, H. P., et al.: Role of obesity and fat distribution in non-insulin-dependent diabetes mellitus in Mexican Americans and non-Hispanic whites. *Diabetes Care* 9:153–161, 1986b.

Haffner, S. M., Stern, M. J., Hazuda, H. P., et al.: The role of behavioral variables and fat patterning in explaining ethnic differences in serum lipids and lipoproteins. *Am. J. Epidemiol.* 123:830–839, 1986c.

Haffner, S. M., Stern, M. P., Hazuda, H. P., et al.: Increased insulin concentration in nondiabetic offspring of diabetic parents. *N. Engl. J. Med.* 319:1297–1301, 1988.

Haile, R. W., Hodge, S., and Iselius, L.: Genetic susceptibility to multiple sclerosis: A review. *Int. J. Epidemiol.* 12:8–16, 1983.

Hakulinen, T., Hansluwka, H., Lopez, A. D., and Nakada, T.: Global and regional mortality patterns by cause of death in 1980. *Int. J. Epidemiol.* 15:227–233, 1986.

Halberstein, R. A., and Davies, J. E.: Biosocial aspects of high blood pressure in people of the Bahamas. *Hum. Biol.* 56:317–328, 1984.

Halfon, S. T., Green, M. S., and Heiss, G.: Smoking status and lipid and lipid levels in adults of different ethnic origins: The Jerusalem lipid research clinic program. *Int. J. Epidemiol.* 13:177–183, 1984.

Hall, R. L., and Dexter, D.: Smokeless tobacco use and attitudes toward smokeless tobacco among Native Americans and other adolescents in the Northwest. *Am. J. Public Health* 78:1586–1588, 1988.

Hall, W. D.: Secondary causes of hypertension in blacks. In Hall, W. D., Saunders, E., and Shulman, N. B. (eds.), *Hypertension in Blacks.* Chicago, Year Book, 1985, pp. 144–152.

Hall, W. D., Saunders, E., and Shulman, N. B.: *Hypertension in Blacks: Epidemiology, Pathophysiology and Treatment.* Chicago, Year Book, 1985.

Halle, L., Castellano, F., Kaplan, C., et al.: HLA haplotype and HIV infection. *Lancet* 2:342, 1988.

Halperin, D. C., Belgrade, M. E., and Mohar, A.: Stomach cancer cluster in Mexico. *Lancet* 1:1055, 1988.

Hamill, P. V., Johnston, F. E., and Lemeshow, S.: Body weight, stature, and sitting height: White and Negro youths 12–17 years. Data from the U.S. National Health Survey, Series 1, No. 126. Hyattsville, MD, U.S. Public Health Service, 1973.

Hamilton, P. J. S., and Persaud, V.: Cancer among blacks in the West Indies. In Mettlin, C., and Murphy, G. P. (eds.), *Cancer Among Black Populations.* New York, Alan R. Liss, 1981, pp. 1–15.

Hanis, C. L., Ferrell, R. E., Barton, S. A., et al.: Diabetes among Mexican-Americans in Starr County, Texas. *Am. J. Epidemiol.* 118:659–672, 1983.

Hanis, C. L., Ferrell, R. E., Tulloch, B. R., and Schull, W. J.: Gallbladder disease epidemiology in Mexican Americans in Starr County, Texas. *Am. J. Epidemiol.* 122:820–829, 1985.

Hanna, J. M., and Baker, P. T.: Biocultural correlates to the blood pressure of Samoan migrants in Hawaii. *Hum. Biol.* 51:481–497, 1979.

Harburg, E., Gleibermann, L., and Harburg, J.: Blood pressure and skin color: Maupiti, French Polynesia. *Hum. Biol.* 54:283–298, 1982.

Hardy, A. M., Allen, J. R., Morgan, W. M., and Curran, J. W.: The incidence rate of acquired immunodeficiency syndrome in selected populations. *JAMA* 253:215–220, 1985.

Harinasuta, T., Bunnag, D., Lasserre, R., Leimer, R., and Vinijanont, S.: Trials of mefloquine in vivax and of mefloquine plus 'fansidar' in falciparum malaria. *Lancet* 1:885–888, 1983.

Harlan, W. R., Hull, A. L., Schmouder, R. L., et al.: Blood pressure and nutrition in adults. The National Health and Nutrition Examination Survey. *Am. J. Epidemiol.* 120:17–28, 1984.

Harpending, H. C., and Chasko, W. Jr.: Heterozygosity and population structure in southern Africa. In Giles, E., and Friedlaender, J. S. (eds.), *The Measures of Man.* Cambridge, MA, Peabody Museum Press, 1976.

Harpending, H. C., and Jenkins, T.: Genetic distance among southern African populations. In Crawford, M. H., and Workman, P. L. (eds.), *Method and Theory in Anthropological Genetics.* Albuquerque, University of New Mexico Press, 1973, pp. 177–199.

Harper, A. B., Laughlin, W. S., and Mazess, R. B.: Bone mineral content in St. Lawrence Island Eskimos. *Hum. Biol.* 56:63–77, 1984.

Harries, A. D., Fryatt, R., Walker, J., et al.: Schistosomiasis in expatriates to Britain from the tropics: A controlled study. *Lancet* 1:86–88, 1986.

Harris, A., Quinlan, C., and Bobrow, M.: Cystic fibrosis typing with DNA probes: Experience of a screening laboratory. *Hum. Genet.* 79:76–79, 1988.

Harris, M.: Epidemiologic characteristics of impaired glucose tolerance in the United States population. In Baba, S., Gould, M. K., and Zimmet, P. (eds.), *Diabetes Mellitus.* New York, Academic Press, 1984, pp. 105–109.

Hart, K. A., Hodgson, S., Walker, A., et al.: DNA deletions in mild and severe Becker muscular dystrophy. *Hum. Genet.* 75:281–285, 1987.

Hartz, A., Houts, P., Arnold, S., et al.: A method to quantify confounding in regression analyses applied to data on diet and CHD incidence. *J. Clin. Epidemiol.* 41:331–337, 1988.

Harwood, A.: *Ethnicity and Medical Care.* Cambridge, MA, Harvard University Press, 1981.

Hatton, C. S. R., Peto, T. E. A., Bunch, C., et al.: Frequency of severe neutropenia associated with amodiaquine prophylaxis against malaria. *Lancet* 1:411–414, 1986.

Hattori, H., Asai, C., and Segi, R. (eds.): *Age-Adjusted Death Rates for Cancer for Selected Sites (A-classification) in 43 Countries in 1977.* Nagoya, Japan, Segi Institute of Cancer Epidemiology, 1982.

Hawkins, B. R., Lam, K. S. L., Ma, J. T. C., et al.: Strong association of HLA-Dr3/Drw9 heterozygosity with early-onset insulin-dependent diabetes mellitus in Chinese. *Diabetes* 36:1297–1300, 1987.

Haynes, R.: Cancer and urbanization in China. *Int. J. Epidemiol.* 15:268–271, 1986a.

Haynes, R.: Chile. In Howe, G. M. (ed.), *Global Geocancerology.* Edinburgh, Churchill Livingstone, 1986b, pp. 106–117.

Hayward, R. A., Shapiro, M. F., Freeman, H. E., et al.: Inequities in health services among insured Americans: Do working-class adults have less access to medical care than the elderly? *N. Engl. J. Med.* 318:1507–1512, 1988.

Hazell, S. L., and Lee, A.: *Campylobacter pyloridis,* urease, hydrogen ion back diffusion, and gastric ulcers. *Lancet* 2:15–17, 1986.

Hazuda, H. P., and Stern, M. P.: A comparison of three indicators for identifying Mexican Americans in epidemiological research. *Am. J. Epidemiol.* 123:96–112, 1986.

Hazuda, H. P., Stern, M. P., Gaskill, S. P., et al.: Ethnic differences in health knowledge and behaviors related to the prevention and treatment of coronary heart disease. *Am. J. Epidemiol.* 117:717–728, 1983.

Heath, D. B.: Anthropology and alcohol studies. *Annu. Rev. Anthropol.* 16:99–120, 1987.

Hediger, M. L., and Katz, S. H.: Fat patterning, overweight, and adrenal androgen interactions in black adolescent females. *Hum. Biol.* 58:585–600, 1986.

Heer, D. M.: Intermarriage and racial amalgamation in the United States. *Eugen. Q.* 14:112–120, 1967.

Hegele, R. A., Huang, L. S., Herbert, P. N., et al.: Apolipoprotein B-gene DNA polymorphisms associated with myocardial infarction. *N. Engl. J. Med.* 315:1509–1515, 1986.

Heinonen, O. P., Slone, D., and Shapiro, S.: *Birth Defects and Drugs in Pregnancy.* Littleton, MA: Publishing Sciences Group, 1977.

Heiss, G., Schonfeld, G., Johnson, J. L., et al.: Black–white differences in plasma levels of apolipoproteins: The Evans County heart study. *Am. Heart J.* 108:807–814, 1984.

Held, P. J., Pauly, M. V., Bovbjberg, R. R., et al.: Access to a kidney transplantation. *Arch. Intern. Med.* 148:2594–2600, 1988.

Helmick, C. G., Wrigley, M., Zack, M. M., et al.: Cluster of cases in Key West, Fla. *Neuroepidemiology* 7:48, 1988.

Hendershot, G. E.: Coitus-related cervical cancer risk factors: Trends and differentials in racial and religious groups. *Am. J. Public Health* 73:299–301, 1983.

Henderson, E. E.: Physiochemical–viral synergism during Epstein-Barr virus infection: A review. *JNCI* 80:476–483, 1988.

Henneberger, P. K., Galaid, E. I., and Marr, J. S.: The descriptive epidemiology of pneumococcal meningitis in New York City. *Am. J. Epidemiol.* 117:484–491, 1983.

Hennekens, C. H.: Vitamin A analogues in cancer chemoprevention. In DeVita, V. T. Jr., and Rosenberg, S. A. (eds.), *Oncology 1986.* Philadelphia, W. B. Saunders, 1986, pp. 23–35.

Henry, J. P.: Stress, salt and hypertension. *Soc. Sci. Med.* 26:293–302, 1988.

Heshmat, M. Y.: Nutrition and prostate cancer: A case-control study. *Prostate* 6:7–17, 1985.

Hetzel, B. S.: Bridging the knowledge application gap—the international council of iodine deficiency disorders. *Int. J. Epidemiol.* 15:153–154, 1986.

Heyman, A., Karp, H. R., Bartel, A., et al.: Cerebrovascular disease in the bi-racial population of Evans County, Georgia. *Stroke* 2:509–518, 1971.

Heymann, D. L., Murphy, K., Brigaud, M., et al.: Oral poliovirus vaccine in tropical Africa: Greater impact on incidence of paralytic disease than expected from coverage surveys and seroconversion rates. *Bull. WHO* 65:495–501, 1987.

Heymsfield, S., Kraus, J., Lee, E. S., et al.: Race, education and prevalence of hypertension. *Am. J. Epidemiol.* 106:351–361, 1977.

Hiatt, H. H.: *America's Health in the Balance: Choice or Chance?* New York, Harper and Row, 1987.

Hiernaux, J.: *The Peoples of Africa.* New York, Scribner's, 1975.

Higgs, D. R., Aldridge, B. E., Lamb, J., Clegg, J. B., et al.: The interaction of alpha-thalassemia and homozygous sickle-cell disease. *N. Engl. J. Med.* 306:1441–1446, 1982.

Hill, A. B.: *Principles of Medical Statistics,* 9th Ed. New York, Oxford University Press, 1971.

Hill, P., Wynder, E. L., Garbaczewski, L., et al.: Diet and menarche in different ethnic groups. *Eur. J. Cancer* 16:519–525, 1980.

Hiller, R., Sperduto, R. D., and Ederer, F.: Epidemiologic associations with nuclear, cortical, and posterior subcapsular cataracts. *Am. J. Epidemiol.* 124:916–925, 1986.

Himmelstein, D. U., and Woolhandler, S.: Pitfalls of private medicine: Health care in the USA. *Lancet* 2:391–394, 1984.

Hirayama, T.: Japan. In Howe, G. M. (ed.), *Global Geocancerology.* Edinburgh, Churchill Livingstone, 1986, pp. 284–293.

Hirayama, T.: Actions suggested by the Japanese retrospective and prospective studies. *Cancer Lett.* 39 (Suppl.):S20, 1988.

Hisamichi, S., Suguwara, N., and Fukao, A.: Effectiveness of gastric mass screening in Japan. *Cancer Detect. Prevent.* 11:323–329, 1988.

Hitzeroth, H. W.: On the genetic interrelationships of South African Negroes. *Am. J. Phys. Anthropol.* 69:389–401, 1986.

Hjalmarsson, K.: Distribution of alpha-1-antitrypsin phenotypes in Sweden. *Hum. Hered.* 38:37–40, 1988.

Hoff, C., Wertlecki, W., Dutt, J., et al.: Sickle cell trait, maternal age and pregnancy outcome in primiparous women. *Hum. Biol.* 55:763–770, 1983.

Hoffman-Goetz, L.: Malnutrition and immunological function with special reference to cell-mediated immunity. *Yearbook Phys. Anthropol.* 29:139–159, 1986.

Hofman, K., Valle, D., Kazazian, H., et al.: Haplotype analysis of the phenylalanine hydroxylase (PH) gene in US blacks with phenyltketonuria (PKU). *Am. J. Hum. Genet.* 41:A256, 1987.

Holdiness, M. R.: Adverse cutaneous reactions to antituberculosis drugs. *Int. J. Dermatol.* 24:280–285, 1985.

Holme, I., Helgeland, A., Hjermann, I., et al.: Correlates of blood pressure change in middle-aged male mild hypertensives: Results from the untreated control group in the Oslo hypertension trial. *Am. J. Epidemiol.* 127:742–752, 1988.

Holt, M., Hogan, P. F., and Nurse, G. T.: The ovalocytosis polymorphism on the western border of Papua New Guinea. *Hum. Biol.* 53:23–34, 1981.

Honigfeld, L. S., and Kaplan, D. W.: Native American postneonatal mortality. *Pediatrics* 80:575–578, 1987.

Hook, E. B.: Down's syndrome: Its frequency in human populations and some factors pertinent to variation in rates. In De la Cruz, F. F., and Gerald, P. S. (eds.), *Trisomy 21 (Down's Syndrome): Research Perspectives.* Baltimore, University Park Press, 1981, pp. 8–67.

Hook, E. B., and Cross, P. K.: Maternal cigarette smoking, Down syndrome in live births, and infant race. *Am. J. Hum. Genet.* 42:482–489, 1988.

Hopkins, D. R.: Dracunculiasis eradication: The tide has turned. *Lancet* 2:148–150, 1988.

Hoppe, S. K., and Martin, H. W.: Patterns of suicide among Mexican Americans and Anglos, 1960–1980. *Soc. Psychiatry* 21:83–88, 1986.

Horowitz, I., and Enterline, P. E.: Lung cancer among the Jews. *Am. J. Public Health* 60:275–282, 1970.

Hovi, T., Cantell, K., Huovilainen, A., et al.: Outbreak of paralytic poliomyelitis in Finland: Widespread circulation of antigenically altered poliovirus type 3 in a vaccinated population. *Lancet* 1:1427–1432, 1986.

Howe, G. M. (ed.): *Global Geocancerology.* Edinburgh, Churchill Livingstone, 1986.

Howe, G. R., Harrison, L., and Jain, M.: A short diet history for assessing dietary exposure to N-nitrosamines in epidemiologic studies. *Am. J. Epidemiol.* 124:595–602, 1986.

Howells, W. W.: The meaning of race. In Osborne, R. H. (ed.), *The Biological and Social Meaning of Race.* San Francisco, W. H. Freeman, 1971, pp. 3–10.

Howells, W. W.: Requiem for a lost people. *Harvard Mag.* Jan.–Feb.:48–55, 1977.

Howson, C. P., Hiyama, T., and Wynder, E. L.: The decline of gastric cancer: Epidemiology of an unplanned triumph. *Epidemiol. Rev.* 8:1–27, 1986.

Hu, D. N.: Prevalence and mode of inheritance of major genetic eye diseases in China. *J. Med. Genet.* 24:584–588, 1987.

Huang, H. J., Stoming, T. A., Haris, H. F., et al.: The Greek $^A\gamma\beta^+$-HPFH observed in a large black family. *Am. J. Hematol.* 25:401–408, 1987.

Huang, Y. Y.: Prevalence and unawareness of hypertension in the petrochemical industrial population in China. *Prev. Med.* 15:643–651, 1986.

Hudson, H. M., and Rockett, I. R. H.: An environmental and demographic analysis of otitis media in rural Australian aborigines. *Int. J. Epidemiol.* 13:73–82, 1984.

Huff, W. G.: Patterns of economic development of Singapore. *J. Dev. Areas* 21:305–326, 1987.

Hughes, K.: Trends in mortality from ischaemic heart disease in Singapore, 1959 to 1983. *Int. J. Epidemiol.* 15:44–50, 1986.

Hughes, T., Benn, S., Conn, R., et al.: Sex-, age-, and region-specific prevalence of sedentary lifestyle in selected states in 1985—the behavioral risk factor surveillance system. *MMWR* 36:195–204, 1987.

Hulse, F. S.: Race as an evolutionary episode. *Am. Anthropol.* 64:929–945, 1962.

Hulse, F. S.: Habits, habitats, and heredity: A brief history of studies in human plasticity. *Am. J. Phys. Anthropol.* 56:495–501, 1981.

Humphries, S. E., Cook, M., Dubowitz, M., et al.: Role of genetic variation at the fibrinogen locus in determination of plasma fibrinogen concentration. *Lancet* 1:1452–1455, 1987.

Hutchinson, J.: Association between stress and blood pressure variation in a Caribbean population. *Am. J. Phys. Anthropol.* 71:69–79 1986.

Hutchinson, J., and Crawford, M. H.: Genetic determinants of blood pressure among the black Caribs of St. Vincent. *Hum. Biol.* 53:453–466, 1981.

Huvos, A. G., Butler, A., and Bretsky, S. S.: Osteogenic sarcoma in the American black. *Cancer* 52:1959–1965, 1983.

Huxley, A.: *Brave New World*, 2d Ed. New York, Bantam Books, 1946.

Hyman, L., Leske, M. C., and Polednak, A. P.: Epidemiology of ocular melanoma. In Nathanson, L. (ed.), *Melanoma*. Boston, Martinus Nijhoff, 1987.

Ibarra, B., Vaca, G., De la Mora, E., et al.: Genetic heterogeneity of thalassemias in Mexican mestizo patients with hemolytic anemia. *Hum. Hered.* 38:95–100, 1988.

Idahosa, P. E.: Blood pressure and salt supplies in West Africa. *Lancet* 2:43–44, 1986.

Idahosa, P. E.: Hypertension: An ongoing health hazard in Nigerian workers. *Am. J. Epidemiol.* 125:85–91, 1987.

Ikeda, M., Kasahara, M., Koizum, A., and Watanabe, T.: Correlation of cerebrovascular disease standardized mortality ratio and the sodium/potassium ratio among the Japanese population. *Prev. Med.* 15:46–59, 1986.

Imaizumi, Y.: A recent survey of consanguineous marriages in Japan: Religion and socioeconomic class effects. *Ann. Hum. Biol.* 13:317–330, 1986.

Ingram, V. M.: *Hemoglobins in Genetics and Evolution*. New York, Columbia University Press, 1963.

Isaacson, C.: *Pathology of a Black African Population*. Berlin, Springer-Verlag, 1982.

Isaacson, C., Bothwell, T. H., MacPhail, A. P., and Simon, M.: The iron status of urban black subjects with carcinoma of the oesophagus. *S. Afr. Med. J.* 67:591–593, 1985.

Ishii, T., Guzman, M. A., Newman, W. P. III, et al.: Atherosclerosis in Japan and the USA. *Lancet* 1:339, 1984.

Iskrant, A. P., and Joliet, P. V.: *Accidents and Homicides*. Cambridge, MA, Harvard University Press, 1968.

Issitt, P. D., Wren, M. R., Rueda, E., et al.: Red cell antigens in Hispanic blood donors. *Transfusion* 27:117, 1987.

Jackson, J. J.: Urban black Americans. In Harwood, A. (ed.), *Ethnicity and Medical Care*. Cambridge, MA, Harvard University Press, 1981, pp. 37–129.

Jackson, L., Taylor, R., Faaiuso, S., Ainuu, S. P., et al.: Hyperuricemia and gout in Western Samoans. *J. Chron. Dis.* 34:65–75, 1981.

Jackson, R., and Beaglehole, R.: Trends in dietary fat and cigarette smoking and the decline in coronary heart disease in New Zealand. *Int. J. Epidemiol.* 16:377–382, 1987.

Jackson, R. T., and Jackson, L. C.: Biological and behavioral contributors to anemia during pregnancy in Liberia, West Africa. *Hum. Biol.* 59:585–597, 1987.

Jacobson, M., and Liebman, B. F.: Dietary sodium and the risk of hypertension. *N. Engl. J. Med.* 303:817–818, 1980.

James, G. D., Baker, P. T., Jenner, D. A., et al.: Variation in lifestyle characteristics and catecholamine excretion rates among young Western Samoan men. *Soc. Sci. Med.* 25:981–986, 1987.

James, S. A., Strogatz, D. S., Wing, S. B., et al.: Socioeconomic status, John Henryism, and hypertension in blacks and whites. *Am. J. Epidemiol.* 126:664–673, 1987.

James, W. P. T., Ralph, A., and Sanchez-Castillo, C. P.: The dominance of salt in manufactured food in the sodium intake of affluent societies. *Lancet* 1:426–429, 1987.

Janerich, D. T., Kelly, J. H., Ziegler, F. D., et al.: Age trends in the prevalence of the sickle cell trait. *Health Services Rep.* 88:804–807, 1973.

Jarvis, G. K., and Northcott, H. C.: Religion and differences in morbidity and mortality. *Soc. Sci. Med.* 25:813–824, 1987.

Jayant, K.: Cancers of the cervix uteri and breast: Changes in incidence rates in Bombay over the last two decades. *Bull. WHO* 64:431–435, 1986.

Jayant, K.: Additive effect of two risk factors in the aetiology of cancer of the cervix uteri. *Br. J. Cancer* 56:685–686, 1987.

Jenner, D. A., Harrison, G. A., Prior, A. M., et al.: Interpopulation comparisons of catecholamine excretion. *Ann. Hum. Biol.* 14:1–9, 1987.

Jenesi, R., Makumbe, K., Munemo, A., Munemo, J., et al.: Endemic goitre in Chinamora, Zimbabwe. *Lancet* 1:1198–1200, 1986.

Jezek, Z., Khodakevich, L. N., and Wickett, J. F.: Smallpox and its post-eradication surveillance. *Bull. WHO* 65:425–434, 1987.

Jin, O. C.: Liver cancer in Singapore. *Singapore Med. J.* 28:410–414, 1987.

Joachim, G., Hadler, J. L., Goldberg, M., et al.: Relationship of syphilis to drug use and prostitution—Connecticut and Philadelphia, Pennsylvania. *MMWR* 37:755–758, 1988.

Joesoef, M. R., Annest, J. L., and Utomo, B.: A recent increase in breastfeeding duration in Jakarta, Indonesia. *Am. J. Public Health* 79:36–38, 1989.

Johnson, J. L., Heineman, E. F., Heiss, G., et al.: Cardiovascular disease risk factors and mortality among black and white women aged 40–64 years. *Am. J. Epidemiol.* 123:209–220, 1986.

Johnson, R. C., Bowman, K. S., Schwitters, S. Y., et al.: Ethnic, familial, and environmental influences on lactose tolerance. *Hum. Biol.* 56:307–316, 1984.

Johnson, S., Echeverria, P., Taylor, D. N., et al.: Enteritis necroticans among Khmer children at an evacuation site in Thailand. *Lancet* 2:496–500, 1987.

Johnston, P. E., Hamill, P. V. V., and Lemeshow, S.: *Skinfold Thickness in Children 6–11 Years.* U.S. National Health Survey, Series 11, No. 120. Rockville, MD, U.S. Department of Health, Education and Welfare, 1972.

Johnston, P. E., Hamill, P. V. V., and Lemeshow, S.: *Skinfold Thickness in Children 12–17 Years.* U.S. National Health Survey, Series 11, No. 132. U.S. Department of Health, Education, and Welfare, 1974.

Jorde, L. B.: The genetic structure of the Utah Mormons: Migration analysis. *Hum. Biol.* 54:583–597, 1982.

Jorde, L. B.: Human genetic distance studies: Present status and future prospects. *Annu. Rev. Anthropol.* 14:343–373, 1985.

Jorde, L. B. and Durbize, P.: Opportunity for natural selection in the Utah Mormons. *Hum. Biol.* 58:97–114, 1986.

Joseph, J. G., Prior, I. A. M., Salmond, C. E., et al.: Elevation of systolic and diastolic blood pressure associated with migration: The Tokelau Island migrant study. *J. Chron. Dis.* 36:507–516, 1983.

Jussawalla, D. J., Yeole, B., and Natekar, M. V.: Cancer in Indian Moslems. *Cancer* 55:1149–1158, 1985.

Juttijudata, P., Chiemchaisri, C., Palavatana, C., et al.: A high incidence of cholangiocarcinoma in patients with biliary obstructive (malignant) disease in Thailand. *JNCI* 71:229, 1983.

Juttijudata, P., Prichanond, S., Churnratanakul, S., et al.: Hilar intrahepatic cholangiocarcinoma and its etiology. *J. Clin. Gastroenterol.* 6:503–504, 1984.

Kaer, T., Roin, J., Djurhuus, J., et al.: Epidemiological aspects of peptic ulcer on the Faroe Islands: An interim report. *Scand. J. Gastroenterol.* 20:1157–1162, 1985.

Kagan, A., Harris, B. R., Winkelstein, W., et al.: Epidemiologic studies of coronary heart disease and stroke in Japanese men living in Japan, Hawaii and California: Demographic, physical, dietary, and biochemical characteristics. *J. Chron. Dis.* 27:345–363, 1974.

Kahn, C. R.: Insulin resistance: A common feature of diabetes mellitus. *N. Engl. J. Med.* 315:252–254, 1986.

Kahn, H. A.: The Dorn study of smoking and mortality among U.S. veterans: Report of eight and one-half years of observation. In Haenszel, W. (ed.), *Epidemiological Approaches to the Study of Cancer and Other Diseases.* Washington, DC, U.S. Government Printing Office, National Cancer Institute Monograph No. 19, 1966.

Kalafatova, O.: Geographic and climatic factors and multiple sclerosis in some districts of Bulgaria. *Neuroepidemiology* 6:116–119, 1987.

Kalow, W., Goedde, H. W., and Agarwal, D. P.: *Ethnic Differences in Reactions to Drugs and Xenobiotics.* New York, Alan R. Liss, 1986.

Kamboh, M. I., and Ferrell, R. E.: Human transferrin polymorphism. *Hum. Hered.* 37:65–81, 1987.

Kan, Y. W., and Dozy, A. M.: Evolution of hemoglobin S and C genes in world populations. *Science* 209:388–391, 1980.

Katsanis, E., Hsu, E., Luke, K. H., et al.: Systemic lupus erythematosus and sickle hemoglobinopathies: A report of two cases and review of the literature. *Am. J. Hematol.* 25:211–214, 1987.

Kar, B. C., Satapathy, B. F., Kulozik, M., Sirr, S., et al.: Sickle cell disease in Orissa state, India. *Lancet* 2:1198–1201, 1986.

Kark, J. D., and Friedlander, Y.: ABO and RH blood groups and blood pressure in Jerusalem 17 year olds. *Hum. Biol.* 56:759–769, 1984.

Kashiwagi, S., Hayashi, J., Ikematsu, H., et al.: Transmission of hepatitis B among siblings. *Am. J. Epidemiol.* 120:617–625, 1984.

Kashiwagi, S., Hayashi, J., Nomura, H., et al.: Changing pattern of intrafamilial transmission of heptatitis B virus in Okinawa, Japan. *Am. J. Epidemiol.* 127:783–787, 1988.

Kasprisin, D. O., Crow, M., McClintock, C., et al.: Blood types of the native Americans of Oklahoma. *Am. J. Phys. Anthropol.* 73:1–7, 1987.

Kattamis, C., Tzotzos, S., Kahavakis, E., et al.: Correlation of clinical phenotype to genotype in haemoglobin H disease. *Lancet* 1:442–444, 1988.

Keil, J. E., Loadholt, C. B., Weinrich, M. C., et al.: Incidence of coronary heart disease in blacks in Charleston, South Carolina. *Am. Heart J.* 108:779–786, 1984.

Kelsey, J. L.: *Epidemiology of Musculoskeletal Disorders.* New York, Oxford University Press, 1982.

Kelson, M., and Farebrother, M.: The effect of inaccuracies in death certification and coding practices in the European Economic Community (EEC) on international cancer mortality statistics. *Int. J. Epidemiol.* 16:411–414, 1987.

Kennedy, D. H.: Tuberculous meningitis. *Lancet* 2:261, 1981.

Kessler, I. I.: Epidemiologic studies of Parkinson's disease. II. A hospital-based survey. *Am. J. Epidemiol.* 95:308–318, 1972.

Kessler, R. C., and Neighbors, H. W.: A new perspective on the relationship among social class, and psychological distress. *J. Health Soc. Behav.* 27:107–115, 1986.

Keys, A.: Diet and blood cholesterol in population survey—Lessons from analysis of the data from a major survey in Israel. *Am. J. Clin. Nutr.* 48:1161–1165, 1988.

Keys, A., et al.: *Seven Countries. A Multivariate Analysis of Death and Coronary Heart Disease.* Cambridge, MA, Harvard University Press, 1980.

Keys, A., Arvannis, C., Blackburn, H., et al.: Serum cholesterol and cancer mortality in the Seven Countries Study. *Am. J. Epidemiol.* 121:870–883, 1985.

Keys, A., Menotti, A., Karvonen, M. J., et al.: The diet and 15-year death rate in the Seven Countries Study. *Am. J. Epidemiol.* 124:903–915, 1986.

Khaw, K. T., and Barrett-Connor, E.: Dietary fiber and reduced IHD mortality rates in men and women: A 12-year prospective study. *Am. J. Epidemiol.* 126:1093–1102, 1987.

Khaw, K. T., and Barrett-Connor, E.: The association between blood pressure, age, and dietary sodium and potassium: A population study. *Circulation* 77:53–61, 1988.

Khlat, M.: Social correlates of consanguineous marriages in Beirut. *Hum. Biol.* 60:541–548, 1988.

Khoury, M. J., Beaty, T. H., Newill, C. A., et al.: Genetic-environmental interactions in chronic airways obstruction. *Int. J. Epidemiol.* 15:64–71, 1986.

Khoury, M. J., Cohen, B. H., Diamond, E. L., et al.: Inbreeding and prereproductive mortality in the Old Order Amish. I. Genealogic epidemiology of inbreeding. *Am. J. Epidemiol.* 125:453–461, 1987.

Khoury, P., Morrison, J. A., Mellies, M. J., and Glueck, C. J.: Weight change since age 18 years in 30- to 55-year-old whites and blacks. *JAMA* 250:3179–3187, 1983.

Kiely, M.: The prevalence of mental retardation. *Epidemiol. Rev.* 9:194–218, 1987.

Kim, Y. S.: Cancer mortality of the Korean population in Japan, 1968–1977. *Int. J. Epidemiol.* 13:11–14, 1984.

Kim, Y. S.: Seasonal variation in carbon monoxide poisoning in urban Korea. *J. Epidemiol. Community Health* 39:79–81, 1985.

Kim-Farley, R. J., Rutherford, G., Lichfield, P., et al.: Outbreak of paralytic poliomyelitis, Taiwan. *Lancet* 2:1322–1324, 1984.

Kimura, K.: Studies of growth and development in Japan. *Yearbook Phys. Anthropol.* 27:179–214, 1984.

King, H., Balkau, B., Zimmet, P., et al.: Diabetic retinopathy in Nauruans. *Am. J. Epidemiol.* 117:659–667, 1983.

King, H., Zimmet, P., Raper, L. R., and Balkau, R.: Risk factors for diabetes in three Pacific populations. *Am. J. Epidemiol.* 119:396–409, 1984.

King, H., Collins, A., King, L. F., et al.: Blood pressure in Papua, New Guinea: A survey of two highland villages in the Asaro Valley. *J. Epidemiol. Community Health* 39:215–219, 1985a.

King, H., Li, J. Y., Locke, F. B., et al.: Patterns of site-specific displacement in cancer mortality among migrants: The Chinese in the United States. *Am. J. Public Health* 75:237–242, 1985b.

Kingston, M. E., Harder, E. J., Al-Jaberim, M. M., et al.: Acquired immune deficiency syndrome in the Middle East from imported blood. *Transfusion* 25:317–318, 1985.

Kirk, R., and Szathmary, E. (eds.): *Out of Asia: Peopling of the Americas and the Pacific.* Canberra, Australia (*Journal of Pacific History*) (Distributed by Canadian Association for Physical Anthropology, McMaster University, 1985.)

Kirk, R. L., Serjeantson, S. W., King, H., and Zimmet, P.: The genetic epidemiology of diabetes mellitus. In Chakraborty, R., and Szathmary, E. J. E. (eds.), *Diseases of Complex Etiology in Small Populations.* New York, Alan R. Liss, 1985, pp. 119–145.

Klain, M., Coulehan, J. L., Arena, V. C., et al.: More frequent diagnosis of acute myocardial infarction among Navajo Indians. *Am. J. Public Health* 78:1351–1352, 1988.

Kleinbaum, D. G., Kupper, L. L., and Morgenstern, H.: *Epidemiologic Research. Principles and Quantitative Methods.* Belmont, CA, Lifetime Learning Publications, 1982.

Kleinman, A. (ed.): *Studies in the Anthropology and Cross-Cultural Psychiatry of Affective Disorder.* Berkeley, University of California Press, 1985.

Kleinman, A.: *Social Origins of Distress and Disease: Depression, Neurasthenia, and Pain in Modern China.* New Haven, CT, Yale University Presss, 1986.

Kliewer, E. V., and Ward, R. H.: Convergence of immigrant suicide rates to those in the destination country. *Am. J. Epidemiol.* 127:640–653, 1988.

Knowler, W. C., Williams, R. C., Pettitt, D. J., et al.: Gm[3;5,13,14] and type 2 diabetes mellitus: An association in American Indians with genetic admixture. *Am. J. Hum. Genet.* 43:520–526, 1988.

Kobliansky, E., and Livshits, G.: A morphological approach to the problem of the biological similarity of Jewish and non-Jewish populations. *Ann. Hum. Biol.* 12:203–212, 1985.

Koh, S. J. G., and Johnson, W. W.: Cancer of the large bowel in children. *South. Med. J.* 79:931–935, 1986.

Kohonen-Corish, M. R. J., and Serjeantson, S. W.: RFLP analysis of HLA-DR and -DQ genes and their linkage relationships in the Pacific. *Am. J. Hum. Genet.* 39:751–762, 1986.

Kondo, K., Takasu, T., and Ahmed, A.: Neurological diseases in Karachi, Pakistan— elevated occurrence of subacute sclerosing panencephalitis. *Neuroepidemiology* 7:66–80, 1988.

Kono, S., Isa, A. R., Ogimoto, I., et al.: Cause-specific mortality among Koreans, Chinese and Americans in Japan, 1973–1982. *Int. J. Epidemiol.* 16:415–419, 1987.

Koo, L. C., Ho, J. H. C., Saw, D., et al.: Measurement of passive smoking and estimates of lung cancer risk among non-smoking Chinese females. *Int. J. Cancer* 39:162–169, 1987.

Korey, K. A.: Skin colorimetry and admixture measurement: Some further considerations. *Am. J. Phys. Anthropol.* 53:123–128, 1980.

Kovar, M. G., Harris, M. T., and Hadden, W. C.: The scope of diabetes in the United States population. *Am. J. Public Health* 77:1549–1550, 1987.

Koyama, H., Moji, K., Suzuki, S.: Blood pressure, urinary sodium/potassium, and body mass index in rural and urban populations of West Java. *Hum. Biol.* 60:263–272, 1988.

Krambovitis, E., McIllmurray, M. B., Lock, P. E., et al.: Rapid diagnosis of tuberculous meningitis by latex particle agglutination. *Lancet* 2:1229–1231, 1984.

Kramer, S., Meadows, A. T., Jarrett, P., and Evans, A. E.: Incidence of childhood cancer: Experience of a decade in a population-based registry. *JNCI* 70:49–55, 1983.

Kraus, J. F., Borhani, N. O., and Franti, C. E.: Socioeconomic status, ethnicity, and risk of coronary heart disease. *Am. J. Epidemiol.* 111:407–414, 1980.

Kreiss, J. K., Koech, D., Plummer, F. A., et al.: AIDS virus infection in Nairobi prostitutes: Spread of the epidemic to East Africa. *N. Engl. J. Med.* 314:414–418, 1985.

Kristein, M.: Japanese lung cancer mortality rates, 1947–1980 and per capita cigarette consumption in Japan. *Int. J. Epidemiol.* 15:140–141, 1986.

Kromhout, D., Bosschieter, E. B., and Couhander, C. D. L.: The inverse relation between fish consumption and 20-year mortality from coronary heart disease. *N. Engl. J. Med.* 312:1205–1209, 1985.

Kuller, L. H., Perper, J. A., Dai, W. S., et al.: Sudden death and the decline in coronary heart disease mortality. *J. Chron. Dis.* 39:1001–1019, 1986.

Kumanyika, S.: Obesity in black women. *Epidemiol. Rev.* 9:31–50, 1987.

Kune, S., Kune, G. A., and Watson, L.: The Melbourne colorectal cancer study: Incidence findings by age, sex, site, migrants and religion. *Int. J. Epidemiol.* 15:483–493, 1986.

Kuo, W. H., and Tsai, Y. M.: Social networking, hardiness and immigrant's mental health. *J. Health Soc. Behav.* 27:133–149, 1986.

Kuratsune, M., Honda, T., Englyst, H. N., et al.: Dietary fiber in the Japanese diet as investigated in connection with colon cancer risk. *Jpn. J. Cancer Res.* 77:736–738, 1986.

Kurihara, M., Aoki, K., and Tominaga, S. (eds.): *Cancer Mortality Statistics in the World.* Nagoya, Japan, University of Nagoya Press, 1984.

Kurland, L. T.: Epidemiological investigations of amyotropic lateral sclerosis. III. A genetic interpretation of incidence and geographic distribution. *Mayo Clin. Proc.* 32:449–462, 1957.

Kusin, J. A., Van Rens, M. M., Lakhani, S., and Jansen, A. A. J.: Vitamin A status of pregnant and lactating women as assessed by serum levels in Machakos area, Kenya. *East Afr. Med. J.* 62:476–479, 1985.

Laborde, J. M., Dando, W. A., and Teetzen, M. L.: Climate, diffused solar radiation and multiple sclerosis. *Soc. Sci. Med.* 27:231–238, 1988.

Lachant, N. A.: Hemoglobin E: An emerging hemoglobinopathy in the United States. *Am. J. Hematol.* 25:449–462, 1987.

Laga, M., Plummer, F. A., Nzanze, H., et al.: Epidemiology of ophthalmia neonatorum in Kenya. *Lancet* 2:1145–1149, 1986.

Laguerre, M. S.: Haitian Americans. In Harwood, A. (ed.), *Ethnicity and Medical Care.* Cambridge, MA, Harvard University Press, 1981, pp. 172–210.

Lamm, G., Csukas, M., Gyarfas, J., et al.: Risk factors for coronary heart disease in rural Hungary. *Int. J. Epidemiol.* 14:327–329, 1985.

Langendorfer, A., Davenport, W., London, W. T., et al.: Sex-related differences in transmission of hepatitis B infection in a Melanesian population. *Am. J. Phys. Anthropol.* 64:243–254, 1984.

Lanier, A. P., Kilkenny, S. J., and Wilson, J. F.: Esophageal cancer in Alaskan natives. *Int. J. Epidemiol.* 14:79–85, 1985.

LaPorte, R. E., Tajima, N., Dorman, J. S., et al.: Differences between blacks and whites in epidemiology of insulin-dependent diabetes mellitus in Allegheny County, Pennsylvania. *Am. J. Epidemiol.* 123:592–603, 1986.

Lasker, G. W.: Migration and physical differentiation. A comparison of immigrant with American-born Chinese. *Am. J. Phys. Anthropol.* 4:273–300, 1946.

Lasker, G. W.: *Surnames and Genetic Structure.* Cambridge, U.K., Cambridge University Press, 1985.

Lasker, G. W., and Tyzzer, R. N.: *Physical Anthropology*, 3d Ed. New York, Holt, Rinehart and Winston, 1982.

La Vecchia, C., and DeCarli, A.: Trends in ischemic heart disease mortality in Italy, 1968–78. *Am. J. Public Health* 76:454–456, 1986.

La Vecchia, C., DeCarli, A., Mezzanotte, C., et al.: Mortality from alcohol related disease in Italy. *J. Epidemiol. Community Health* 40:257–261, 1986.

La Vecchia, C., DeCarli, A., Parazzini, F., et al.: General epidemiology of breast cancer in northern Italy. *Int. J. Epidemiol.* 16:347–355, 1987.

Leck, I.: The geographical distribution of neural tube defects and oral clefts. *Br. Med. Bull.* 40:390–395, 1984.

Lee, H. P., Duffy, S. W., Day, N. E., et al.: Recent trends in cancer incidence among Singapore Chinese. *Int. J. Cancer* 42:159–166, 1988.

Lee, J.: An insight on the use of multiple logistic regression analysis to estimate association between risk factor and disease occurrence. *Int. J. Epidemiol.* 15:22–29, 1986.

Lee, T. D., Zhao, T. M., Mickey, R., et al.: The polymorphism of HLA antigens in the Chinese. *Tissue Antigens* 32:188–208, 1988.

Lehmann, H., and Carrell, R. W.: Nomenclature of the α-thalassemias. *Lancet* 1:552–553, 1984.

LeMarchand, L., Kolonel, L. N., and Nomura, A. M. Y.: Breast cancer survival among Hawaii Japanese and Caucasian women. *Am. J. Epidemiol.* 122:571–578, 1985.

Lenoir, G. M., O'Conor, G. T., and Olweny, C. L. M. (eds.): *Burkitt's Lymphoma: A Human Cancer Model.* International Agency for Research on Cancer (IARC) Public. No. 60. Lyon, France, IARC, 1985.

Leonard, B., Leonard, C., and Wilson, R.: Zuni diabetes project. *Public Health Rep.* 101:282–288, 1986.

Leonard, B. E., Wilson, R. H., Gohdes, D., et al.: Community-based exercise intervention—the Zuni diabetes project. *MMWR* 36:661–663, 1987.

Lepers, J. P., Deloron, P., Fontenille, D., et al.: Reappearance of falciparum malaria in central highland plateaux of Madagascar. *Lancet* 1:586, 1988.

Leske, M. C.: The epidemiology of open-angle glaucoma: A review. *Am. J. Epidemiol.* 118:166–191, 1983.

Leske, M. C.: Results of pilot study of glaucoma in Barbados. Personal communication, 1987.

Levell, M. J., Rowe, E., Glashas, R. W., et al.: Free testosterone in carcinoma of the prostate. *Prostate* 7:363–367, 1985.

Levine, P. H., McKay, F. W., and Connelly, R. R.: Patterns of nasopharyngeal cancer mortality in the United States. *Int. J. Cancer* 39:133–137, 1987.

Levy, J. E., and Kunitz, S. J.: A suicide prevention program for Hopi youth. *Soc. Sci. Med.* 25:931–940, 1987.

Lewis, B., Turner, P. R., Revill, J., et al.: Metabolic epidemiology of plasma cholesterol. Mechanisms of variation of plasma cholesterol within populations and between populations. *Lancet* 2:991–996, 1986.

Li, F. P.: Cancer mortality in China, 1972–2000: Implications for cancer control. *Cancer Detect. Prev.* 3:499–506, 1980.

Li, J.-Y.: Investigation of geographic patterns of cancer mortality in China. *Natl. Cancer Inst. Monogr.* 62:17–42, 1982.

Li, S. C., Schoenberg, B. S., Wang, C. C., et al.: Cerebrovascular disease in the People's Republic of China: Epidemiological and clinical features. *Neurology* 35:1708–1713, 1985.

Li, V. C., Hua, H. J., Manlan, Z., et al.: Behavioral aspects of cigarette smoking among industrial college men of Shanghai, China. *Am. J. Public Health* 78:1550–1553, 1988.

Lichter, D. T.: Racial differences in underemployment in American cities. *Am. J. Sociol.* 93:771–792, 1988.

Lie, R. T., Irgens, L. M., Skjaerven, R., et al.: Secular changes in early neonatal mortality in Norway, 1967–1981. *Am. J. Epidemiol.* 125:1011–1078, 1987.

Liegeois, J. P.: *Gypsies: An Illustrated History.* London, Al Saqi Books, 1986.

Lilienfeld, A. M.: *Cancer Epidemiology.* Baltimore, Johns Hopkins University Press, 1967.

Lilienfeld, A. M. (ed.): *Times, Places, and Persons.* Baltimore, Johns Hopkins University Press, 1980.

Lilienfeld, A. M., and Lilienfeld, D. E.: *Foundations of Epidemiology*, 2d Ed. New York, Oxford University Press, 1980.

Lilienfeld, A. M., Levin, M. L., and Kessler, I. I.: *Cancer in the United States.* Cambridge, MA, Harvard University Press, 1972.

Lindlof, M., Sistonen, P., and De la Chapelle, A.: Linked polymorphic DNA markers in the prediction of X-linked muscular dystrophy. *Ann. Hum. Genet.* 51:317–328, 1987.

Linet, M. S., and Stewart, W. F.: Migraine headache: Epidemiologic perspectives. *Epidemiol. Rev.* 6:114–139, 1984.

Lingmei, Z., and Hui, D.: Analysis of two causes of maternal death in China. *Bull. WHO* 66:387–390, 1988.

Linke, U.: AIDS in Africa. *Science* 231:203, 1986.

Lisker, R., Perez-Briceno, R., Granados, J., et al.: Gene frequencies and admixture estimates in a Mexico City population. *Am. J. Phys. Anthropol.* 71:203–207, 1986.

Liu, L. S., and Lai, S. H.: Relationship between salt excretion and blood pressure in various regions of China: Part 2. *Bull. WHO* 64:729–733, 1986.

Livingstone, F. B.: Natural selection and the origin and maintenance of standard genetic marker systems. *Yearbook Phys. Anthropol.* 23:25–42, 1980.

Livingstone, F. B.: The Duffy blood groups, vivax malaria, and malaria selection: A review. *Hum. Biol.* 56:413–425, 1984.

Livingstone, F. B.: *Frequencies of Hemoglobin Variants, Thalassemia, the Glucose-6-Phosphate Dehydrogenase Deficiency, G6PD Variants and Ovalocytosis in Human Populations.* New York, Oxford University Press, 1985.

Logan, W. P. D.: Cancer Mortality by Occupational and Social Class, 1851–1971. IARC Scientific Publication No. 36. London, Her Majesty's Stationery Office, 1982.

London, W. T., and Blumberg, B. S.: Comments on the role of epidemiology in the investigation of hepatitis B virus. *Epidemiol. Rev.* 7:59–78, 1985.

Love, D. C., Rapkin, J., Lesser, G. R., et al.: Temporal arteritis in blacks. *Ann. Intern. Med.* 105:387–389, 1986.

Lowenfels, A. B.: Gallstones and glaciers: The stone that came in from the cold. *Lancet* 1:1385–1386, 1988.

Lowenfels, A. B., Linstrom, C. G., Conway, M. J., and Hastings, P. R.: Gallstones and risk of gallbladder cancer. *JNCI* 75:77–80, 1985.

Lu, J. B., and Qin, Y. M.: Correlation between high salt intake and mortality rates for oesophageal and gastric cancers in Henan Province, China. *Int. J. Epidemiol.* 16:171–176, 1987.

Luft, F. C., Grim, C. E., Higgins, J. J. Jr.: Differences in response to sodium administration in normal white and black subjects. *J. Lab. Clin. Med.* 90:555–559, 1977.

Lugosi, L.: Trends in childhood tuberculosis in Hungary 1953–1983: Quantitative methods for evaluation of BCG policy. *Int. J. Epidemiol.* 14:304–312, 1985.

Lukacs, J. R. (ed.): *The People of South Asia.* New York, Plenum Press, 1985.

Lule, G. N., Otieno, L. S., and Kinuthia, D. M. W.: Hypertension over a 4-year period at Kenyatta National Hospital (KNH). *East Afr. Med. J.* 62:365–371, 1985.

Lutalo, S. K. K., and Mabonga, N.: Some clinical and epidemiological aspects of diabetes mellitus on an endemic disease register in Zimbabwe. *East Afr. Med. J.* 62:435–445, 1985.

Lyon, J. L., Wetzler, H. P., Gardner, J. W., et al.: Cardiovascular mortality in Mormons and non-Mormons in Utah, 1969–1971. *Am. J. Epidemiol.* 108:357–366, 1978.

MacDonald, M. J., Famyiwa, O. O., Nwabuelo, I. A., et al.: HLA-DR associations in black type 1 diabetes in Nigeria. *Diabetes* 35:583–589, 1986.

Mackenbach, J. P., Van Duyne, W. J., and Kelson, M. C.: Certification and coding of two underlying causes of death in the Netherlands and other countries of the European community. *J. Epidemiol. Community Health* 41:156–160, 1987.

MacLean, C. J., Adams, M. S., Leyshan, W. C., et al.: Genetic studies on hybrid populations. III. Blood pressure in an American black community. *Am. J. Hum. Genet.* 26:614–626, 1974.

MacMahon, B., and Pugh, T. F.: *Epidemiology. Principles and Methods.* Boston, Little, Brown, 1970.

MacMahon, B., Trichopoulos, D., Brown, J., et al.: Age at menarche, probability of ovulation and breast cancer risk. *Int. J. Cancer* 29:13–16, 1982.

MacMahon, S. W., and Leeder, S. R.: Blood pressure levels and mortality from cerebrovascular disease in Australia and the United States. *Am. J. Epidemiol.* 120:865–875, 1984.

Majeed, H. A., Yousof, A. M., Khuffash, F. A., et al.: The natural history of acute rheumatic fever in Kuwait: A prospective six year follow-up report. *J. Chron. Dis.* 39:361–369, 1986.

Malina, R. M., Martorell, R., and Mendoza, F.: Growth status of Mexican American children and youths: Historical trends and contemporary issues. *Yearbook Phys. Anthropol.* 29:45–79, 1986.

Malina, R. M., Brown, K. H., and Zavaleta, A. N.: Relative lower extremity length in Mexican American and in American black and white youth. *Am. J. Phys. Anthropol.* 72:89–94, 1987.

Malmgren, R., Warlow, C., Bamford, J., et al.: Geographical and secular trends in stroke incidence. *Lancet* 2:1196–1200, 1987.

Manciaux, M., and Romer, C. J.: Accidents in children, adolescents and young adults: A major public health problem. *World Health Statist. Q.* 39:227–231, 1986.

Maniam, T.: Suicide and parasuicide in a hill resort in Malaysia. *Br. J. Psychiat.* 153:222–225, 1988.

Mann, J. M.: The global AIDS situation. *World Health Stat. Q.* 40:185–192, 1987.

Mann, J. M., Francis, H., Davachi, F., et al.: Risk factors for human immunodeficiency virus seropositivity among children 1–24 months old in Kinshasa, Zaire. *Lancet* 2:654–657, 1986.

Mann, J., Quinn, T. C., Pitot, P., et al.: Condom use and HIV infection among prostitutes in Zaire. *N. Engl. J. Med.* 316:345, 1987.

Marcus, A. C., and Crane, L. A.: Smoking behavior among U.S. Latinos. *Am. J. Public Health* 75:169–172, 1985.

Marinig, C., Fiorini, G., Boneschi, V., et al.: Immunologic and immunogenetic features of primary Kaposi's sarcoma. *Cancer* 55:1899–1901, 1985.

Markides, K. S., and Coreil, J.: The health of Hispanics in the southwestern United States: An epidemiologic paradox. *Public Health Rep.* 101:253–265, 1986.

Marquez, C., Taintor, Z., and Schwartz, M. A.: Diagnosis of manic depressive illness in blacks. *Compr. Psychiatry* 26:337–341, 1985.

Marsella, A. J.: Depressive experience and disorder across cultures. In Triandis, H. C., and Draguns, J. G. (eds.), *Handbook of Cross-Cultural Psychology*, Vol. 6: *Psychopathology*. Boston, Allyn and Bacon, pp. 237–252, 1980.

Martin, A. O., Dunn, J. K., Simpson, J. L., et al.: Cancer mortality in a human isolate. *JNCI* 65:1109–1113, 1980.

Martin, C. N., Garner, R. C., Tursi, F., et al.: An ELISA procedure for assaying aflatoxin-B. In Berlin, A., Draper, M., Hemminki, K., et al. (eds.), *Monitoring Human Exposure to Carcinogenic and Mutagenic Agents*. Lyon, France, International Agency for Research on Cancer, 1985.

Martin, J., and Suarez, L.: Cancer mortality among Mexican Americans and other whites in Texas, 1969–80. *Am. J. Public Health* 77:851–853, 1987.

Martin, M. J., Hullet, S. B., Browner, W. S., et al.: Serum cholesterol, blood pressure, and mortality: Implications from a cohort of 361 662 men. *Lancet* 2:933–936, 1986.

Martorell, R.: Interrelationships between diet, infectious disease, and nutritional status. In Greene, L. S., and Johnston, F. E. (eds.), *Social and Biological Predictors of Nutritional Status, Physical Growth and Neurological Development*. New York, Academic Press, 1980, pp. 81–106.

Martyn, C. N., Barker, D. J. P., and Osmond, C.: Motoneuron disease and past poliomyelitis in England and Wales. *Lancet* 1:1319–1322, 1988.

Mascie-Taylor, C. G. N., and Boldsen, J. L.: Recalled age of menarche in Europe. *Ann. Hum. Biol.* 13:253–257, 1986.

Mason, T. J., McKay, F. W., Hoover, R., et al.: *Atlas of Cancer Mortality Among U.S.*

Nonwhites: 1950–1969. DHEW Pub. No. NIH 76-1204. Washington, U.S. Public Health Service, 1976.

Mason, T. J., Fraumeni, J. F. Jr., Hoover, R., et al.: *An Atlas of Mortality from Selected Diseases.* NIH Publication No. 81-2397. Washington, U.S. Government Printing Office, 1981.

Massey, D. S., and Denton, N. A.: Trends in the residential segregation of blacks, Hispanics, and Asians: 1970–1980. *Am. Sociol. Rev.* 52:802–825, 1987.

Matkovic, V., Kostial, K., Simonovic, I., et al.: Bone status and fracture rates in two regions of Yugoslavia. *Am. J. Clin. Nutr.* 32:540–549, 1979.

Matsumoto, H., Miyazaki, T., Xu, X., et al.: Distribution of Gm and Km allotypes among five populations in China. *Am. J. Phys. Anthropol.* 70:161–165, 1986.

Matutes, E., Dalgleish, A. G., Weiss, R. A., et al.: Studies in healthy human T-cell-leukemia lymphoma virus (HTLV-I) carriers from the Caribbean. *Br. J. Cancer* 38:41–45, 1986.

Mavrou, A., Syrrou, M., Tsenghi, C., et al.: Martin–Bell syndrome in Greece, with report of another 47,XXY fragile X patient. *Am. J. Med. Genet.* 31:735–739, 1988.

Mayo, J. A.: The significance of sociocultural variables in the psychiatric treatment of black outpatients. *Compr. Psychiatry* 15:471–482, 1974.

McClellan, W., Hall, W. D., Brogan, D., et al.: Isolated systolic hypertension: Declining prevalence in the elderly. *Prev. Med.* 16:686–695, 1987.

McElroy, A., and Townsend, P. K.: *Medical Anthropology in Ecological Perspective.* Boulder, Westview Press, 1985 (reprint of 1979 edition).

McGarvey, S. T., and Baker, P. T.: The effects of modernization and migration on Samoan blood pressures. *Hum. Biol.* 51:461–479, 1979.

McGarvey, S. T., and Schendel, D. E.: Blood pressure of Samoans. In Baker, P. T., Hanna, J. M., and Baker, T. S. (eds), *The Changing Samoans.* New York, Oxford University Press, 1986, pp. 350–393.

McGeer, P. L., Itagaki, S., and McGeer, E. G.: Expression of the histocompatibility glycoprotein HLA-DR in neurological disease. *Acta Neuropathol.* 76:550–557, 1988.

McGill, N. W., and Gow, P. J.: Juvenile rheumatoid arthritis in Auckland: A long-term follow-up study with particular reference to uveitis. *Aust. N.Z. J. Med.* 17:305–308, 1987.

McGlashan, N. D., and Harrington, J. S.: Lung cancer 1978–1981 in the black peoples of South Africa. *Br. J. Cancer* 52:339–346, 1985.

McGlynn, K. A., Lustbader, E. D., and London, W. T.: Immune responses to hepatitis B virus and tuberculosis infections in Southeast Asian refugees. *Am. J. Epidemiol.* 122:1032–1036, 1985.

McKenna, J. J.: An anthropological perspective on the sudden infant death syndrome (SIDS). *Med. Anthropol.* 10:9–53, 1986.

McKusick, V. A.: The ethnic distribution of disease in the United States. *J. Chron. Dis.* 20:115–118, 1967.

McKusick, V. A.: *Mendelian Inheritance in Man.* Baltimore, Johns Hopkins University, 1983.

McKusick, V. A.: The morbid anatomy of the human genome (four parts). *Medicine* 66, 67, 1986–88.

McMichael, A. J., and Giles, G. G.: Cancer in migrants to Australia: Extending the descriptive epidemiological data. *Cancer Res.* 48:751–756, 1988.

McNeill, W. H.: *Plagues and Peoples.* New York, Doubleday (Anchor), 1976.

McWhorter, W. P., and Mayer, W. J.: Black/white differences in type of initial breast cancer treatment and implications for survival. *Am. J. Public Health* 77:1515–1517, 1987.

Meade, T. W., Mellows, S., Brozovic, M., et al.: Haemostatic function and ischaemic heart disease: Principal results of the Northwick Park heart study. *Lancet* 2:533–537, 1986.

Meade, T. W., Imeson, J., and Stirling, Y.: Effects of changes in smoking and other characteristics on clotting factors and the risk of ischaemic heart disease. *Lancet* 2:986–988, 1987.

Mehta, F. S., Gupta, P. C., Bhonsle, R. S., et al.: Detection of oral cancer using basic health workers in an area of high oral cancer incidence in India. *Cancer Detect. Prev.* 9:219–225, 1986.

Meikle, A. W., Smith, J. A., and Stringham, J. D.: Production, clearance and metabolism of testosterone in men with prostatic cancer. *Prostate* 10:25–31, 1987.

Meindl, R. S.: Hypothesis: A selective advantage for cystic fibrosis heterozygotes. *Am. J. Phys. Anthropol.* 74:39–45, 1987.

Melbye, M., Kestens, L., and Biggar, R. J.: HLA studies of endemic African Kaposi's sarcoma patients and matched controls: No association with HLA-DR5. *Int. J. Cancer* 39:182–184, 1987.

Melia, R. J. W., and Swan, A. V.: International trends in mortality rates for bronchitis, emphysema and asthma during the period 1971–1980. *World Health Statist. Q.* 39:206–216, 1986.

Mellemgaard, A., and Gaarslev, K.: Risk of hepatobiliary cancer in carriers of *Salmonella typhi. JNCI* 80:288, 1988.

Menakanit, W., Muir, C. S., and Jain, D. K.: Cancer in Chiang Mai, North Thailand. A relative frequency study. *Br. J. Cancer* 25:226–236, 1971.

Menck, H. R., Henderson, B. E., Pike, M. C., Mack, T., et al.: Cancer incidence in the Mexican-American. *JNCI* 55:531–536, 1975.

Mendeloff, A. I., and Dunn, J. P.: *Digestive Diseases.* Cambridge, MA, Harvard University Press, 1971.

Mendes de Leon, C. F., and Markides, K. S.: Depressive symptoms among Mexican Americans: A three-generation study. *Am. J. Epidemiol.* 127:150–160, 1988.

Merbs, C. F., and Miller, R. J. (eds.): *Health and Disease in the Prehistoric Southwest.* Tempe, Arizona State University Press, 1985.

Messer, E.: Some like it sweet: Estimating sweetness preferences and sucrose intake from ethnographic and experimental data. *Am. Anthropol.* 88:637–647, 1986.

Mickelson, K. N. P., Dixon, M. W., Hill, P. J., et al.: Influence of α thalassemia on haematological parameters in Polynesian patients. *N.Z. Med. J.* 98:1036–1038, 1985.

Micozzi, M. S.: Nutrition, body size and breast cancer. *Yearbook Phys. Anthropol.* 28:175–206, 1985.

Milan, F. A.: *The Human Biology of Circumpolar Populations.* International Biological Programme, No. 21. Cambridge, U.K., Cambridge University Press, 1980.

Millar, W. J., and Stephens, T.: The prevalence of overweight and obesity in Britain, Canada and the United States. *Am. J. Public Health* 77:38–41, 1987.

Miller, L. H., Howard, R. J., Carter, R., et al.: Research toward malaria vaccines. *Science* 234:1349–1356, 1986.

Miller, R. W.: Cancer epidemics in the People's Republic of China. *JNCI* 60:1195–1203, 1978.

Millikan, L. E., Krotoski, W. A., Mroczkowski, T. F., Douglas, J. T., and Courrege, M. L.: Preliminary study of a *Mycobacterium leprae* bacterin vaccine in a human volunteer population in a nonendemic area. *Int. J. Dermatol.* 25:245–248, 1985.

Milne, A., Allwood, G. K., Moyes, C. D., et al.: A seroepidemiological study of the prevalence of heptatitis B infections in a hyperendemic New Zealand community. *Int. J. Epidemiol.* 16:84–90, 1987.

Mitacek, E. J., St. Vallieres, D., and Polednak, A. P.: Cancer in Haiti 1979–84: Distribution of various forms of cancer according to geographical area and sex. *Int. J. Cancer* 38:9–16, 1986.

Mitchell, B. D., and Lepkowski, J. M.: The epidemiology of cataract in Nepal. *Hum. Biol.* 58:975–990, 1986.

Modan, M., Halkin, H., Karasik, A., and Lusky, A.: Effectiveness of glycolysated hemoglobin, fasting plasma glucose, and a single post load plasma glucose level in population screening for glucose intolerance. *Am. J. Epidemiol.* 119:431–444, 1984.

Modell, B., Ward, R. H. T., Rodeck, C., White, J. M., et al.: Effect of fetal diagnostic testing on birth-rate of thalassemia major in Britain. *Lancet* 2:1383–1386, 1984.

Mohs, E.: Acute respiratory infections in children: Possible control measures. *Bull. Pan Am. Health Org.* 19:82–87, 1985.

Montagu, A. M. F.: *Manual of Physical Anthropology.* Springfield, IL, C. C Thomas, 1960.

Montes, J. H.: *Annotated Bibliography of the Literature on Cancer in Hispanics for the Hispanic Cancer Control Program.* Bethesda, MD, Division of Cancer Prevention and Control, National Cancer Institute, 1986.

Monzon, C. M., Fairbanks, V. F., Burgert, E. O., et al.: Hereditary red cell disorders in Southeast Asian refugees and the effect on the prevalence of thalassemia disorders in the United States. *Am. J. Med. Sci.* 291:147–151, 1986.

Moore, J. W., Key, T. J. A., Bulbrook, R. D., et al.: Sex hormone binding globulin and risk factors for breast cancer in a population of normal women who had never used exogenous sex hormones. *Br. J. Cancer* 56:661–666, 1987.

Moosa, A.: The health of children in South Africa: Some food for thought. *Lancet* 1:779–782, 1984.

Morgan, J. W., Fraser, G. E., Phillips, R. L., et al.: Dietary factors and colon cancer incidence among Seventh Day Adventists. *Am. J. Epidemiol.* 128:918, 1988.

Morgan, K., Holmes, T. M., Grace, M., et al.: Patterns of cancer in geographic and endogamous subdivisions of the Hutterite brethren of Canada. *Am. J. Phys. Anthropol.* 62:3–10, 1983.

Morin, M. M., Pickle, L. W., and Mason, T. J.: Geographic patterns of ethnic groups in the United States. *Am. J. Public Health* 74:133–139, 1984.

Moriyama, I. M., Krueger, D. E., and Stamler, J.: *Cardiovascular Diseases in the United States.* Cambridge, MA, Harvard University Press, 1971.

Morrison, A. S., Ahlbom, A., Verhoek, W. G., et al.: Occupation and bladder cancer in Boston, USA, Manchester, UK, and Nagoya, Japan. *J. Epidemiol. Community Health* 39:294–300, 1985.

Morton, N. E.: Genetic markers in atherosclerosis: A review. *J. Med. Genet.* 13:81–90, 1976.

Mourant, A. E., Kopec, A., and Domaniewska-Sobczak, K.: *The Distribution of the Human Blood Groups and Other Polymorphisms*, 2d Ed. London, Oxford University Press, 1976.

Mourant, A. E., Kopec, A. C., and Domaniewska-Sobczak, K.: *The Genetics of the Jews.* Oxford, U.K., Clarendon Press, 1978.

Moyes, C. D., Milne, A., Dimitrakakis, M., et al.: Very-low-dose hepatitis B vaccine in newborn infants: An economic option for control in endemic areas. *Lancet* 1:29–31, 1987.

Mu, L., Derun, L., Chengyi, Q., et al.: Endemic goitre in central China caused by excessive iodine intake. *Lancet* 2:257–259, 1987.

Mugambi, M.: Epidemiological report from East Africa. In Gross, F., and Strasser, T. (eds.), *Mild Hypertension: Recent Advances.* New York, Raven, 1983, pp. 55–60.

Muir, C. S., and Nectoux, J.: International patterns of cancer. In Schottenfeld, D., and

Fraumeni, J. F. Jr. (eds.), *Cancer Epidemiology and Prevention*. Philadelphia, W. B. Saunders, 1982.

Muir, C. S., Waterhouse, J., Mack, T., et al.: *Cancer Incidence in Five Continents*, Vol. V. International Association for Research on Cancer. Lyon, France, 1987.

Munoz, L. M., Lonnerdal, B., Keen, C. L., et al.: Coffee consumption as a factor in iron deficiency anemia among pregnant women and their infants in Costa Rica. *Am. J. Clin. Nutr.* 48:645–651, 1988.

Murdock, G. P.: *Atlas of World Cultures*. Pittsburgh, University of Pittsburgh Press, 1981.

Murphy, H. B. M., and Raman, A. C.: The chronicity of schizophrenia in indigenous tropical peoples. *Br. J. Psychiatry* 118:489–497, 1971.

Murphy, J. M.: Psychiatric labeling in cross-cultural perspective. *Science* 191:1019–1028, 1976.

Murphy, S., Hayward, A., Troup, G., Devor, E. J., and Coons, T.: Gene enrichment in an American Indian population: An excess of severe combined immunodeficiency disease. *Lancet* 2:502–505, 1980.

Mustaffa, B. E.: Diabetes in the ASEAN region. In Baba, S., Gould, M. K., and Zimmet, P. (eds.), *Diabetes Mellitus*. New York, Academic Press, 1984, pp. 95–103.

Myerowitz, R., and Hogikyan, N. D.: Different mutations in Ashkenazi Jewish and non-Jewish French Canadians with Tay-Sachs disease. *Science* 232:1646–1648, 1986.

Myrianthopoulos, N. C.: *Malformations in Children from One to Seven Years*. New York, Alan R. Liss, 1985.

Nadim, A., and Nasseri, K.: Iran. In Howe, G. (ed.), *Global Geocancerology*. Edinburgh, Churchill Livingstone, 1986, pp. 241–252.

Naggan, L., and MacMahon, B.: Ethnic differences in the prevalence of anencephaly and spina bifida in Boston, Massachusetts. *N. Engl. J. Med.* 277:1119–1123, 1967.

Najean, Y., Mugnier, P., Dresch, C., et al.: Polycythemia vera in young people: An analysis of 58 cases diagnosed before 40 years. *Br. J. Haematol.* 67:285–291, 1987.

Nanji, A. A., and French, S. W.: Relationship between pork consumption and cirrhosis. *Lancet* 1:681–683, 1985.

Neel, J.: Diabetes mellitus: A "thrifty" genotype rendered detrimental by 'progress'? *Am. J. Hum. Genet.* 14:353–362, 1962.

Nei, M., and Roychoudhury, A. K.: Gene differences between Caucasian, Negro and Japanese populations. *Science* 177:434–436, 1972.

Nei, M., and Roychoudhury, A. K.: Genetic variation within and between the major races of man, Caucasoids, Negroids, and Mongoloids. *Am. J. Hum. Genet.* 26:421–443, 1974.

Nei, M., and Roychoudhury, A. K.: Genetic relationship and evolution of human races. *Evol. Biol.* 14:1–59, 1982.

Neighbors, H. W.: Socioeconomic status and psychologic distress in adult blacks. *Am. J. Epidemiol.* 124:779–793, 1986.

Nelson, J. K., and Nelson, K. R.: Skinfold profiles of black and white boys and girls ages 11–13. *Hum. Biol.* 58:379–390, 1986.

Nelson, L. M., Hamman, R. F., Thompson, D. S., et al.: Higher than expected prevalence of multiple sclerosis in northern Colorado: Dependence on methodologic issues. *Neuroepidemiology* 5:17–28, 1986.

Nepom, G. T., Seyfried, C. E., Holbeck, S. L., et al.: Identification of HLA-Dw14 genes in Dr4$^+$ rheumatoid arthritis. *Lancet* 2:1002–1004, 1986.

Nervi, F., Duarte, I., Gomez, G., et al.: Frequency of gallbladder cancer in Chile, a high-risk area. *Int. J. Cancer* 41:657–660, 1988.

Neser, W. B., Thomas, J., Semenya, K., et al.: Obesity and hypertension in a longitudinal study of black physicians: The Meharry cohort study. *J. Chron. Dis.* 39:105–113, 1986.

Newill, V. A.: Distribution of cancer among ethnic subgroups of the white population of New York City, 1953–58. *JNCI* 26:405–417, 1961.

Newsome, F., and Choudhuri, S. B. G.: Sarcoid in a Nigerian: Geographical variation of the frequency of sarcoid among blacks considered. *Trans. R. Soc. Trop. Med. Hyg.* 78:663–664, 1984.

Ng, T. P.: A case-referent study of cancer of the nasal cavity and sinuses in Hong Kong. *Int. J. Epidemiol.* 15:171–175, 1986.

Ngugi, E. N., Plummer, F. A., Simonsen, J. N., et al.: Prevention of transmission of human immunodeficiency virus in Africa: Effectiveness of condom promotion and health education among prostitutes. *Lancet* 2:887–890, 1988.

Nicklas, T. A., Farris, R. P., Major, C., et al.: Dietary intakes. *Pediatrics* 80 (Suppl.):797–806, 1987a.

Nicklas, T. A., Frank, G. C., Webber, L. S., et al.: Racial contrasts in hemoglobin levels and dietary patterns related to hematopoiesis in children: The Bogalusa Heart Study. *Am. J. Public Health* 77:1320–1323, 1987b.

Nixon, R. B., and Phelps, C. D.: Glaucoma. In Renie, W. A., and Goldberg, M. F. (eds.), *Goldberg's Genetic and Metabolic Eye Disease*, 2d Ed. Boston, Little, Brown, 1986, pp. 275–296.

Noah, N. D.: Vaccination against pneumococcal infection. *Br. Med. J.* 297:1351–1352, 1988.

Noguchi, C. T., Rodgers, G. P., Serjeant, G., et al.: Levels of fetal hemoglobin necessary for treatment of sickle cell disease. *N. Engl. J. Med.* 318:96–99, 1988.

Nolan, R. J. Jr.: Childhood tuberculosis in North Carolina: A study of the opportunity for intervention in the transmission of tuberculosis to children. *Am. J. Public Health* 76:26–30, 1986.

Nomomura, A., Hayashi, M., Watanabe, K., et al.: Studies on the pathogenesis of hepatocellular carcinoma in HBV-negative alcoholic cirrhotics. *Acta Pathol. Jpn.* 36:1297–1305, 1986.

Nomura, A., Yamakawa, H., Ishidate, T., Kamiyama, S., et al.: Intestinal metaplasis in Japan: Association with diet. *JNCI* 68:401–405, 1982.

Nomura, A. M. Y., Lee, J., Kolonel, L. N., and Hirohata, T.: Breast cancer in two populations with different risk factors for the disease. *Am. J. Epidemiol.* 119:496–502, 1984.

Noordeen, S. K., and Bravo, L. L.: The world leprosy situation. *World Health Stat. Q.* 39:122–128, 1986.

Norgan, N. G.: Fat patterning in Papua New Guineans: Effects of age, sex and acculturation. *Am. J. Phys. Anthropol.* 74:385–392, 1987.

Norio, R.: Diseases of Finland and Scandinavia. In Rothschild, H. (ed.), *Biocultural Aspects of Disease*. New York, Academic Press, 1981, pp. 359–403.

Norman, J. E. Jr., Kurtzke, J. F., and Beebe, G. W.: Epidemiology of multiple sclerosis in U.S. veterans: 2. Latitude, climate and risk of multiple sclerosis. *J. Chron. Dis.* 36:551–559, 1983.

Nunn, A. J., Darbyshire, J. M., Fox, W., et al.: Changes in annual tuberculosis notification rates between 1978/79 and 1983 for the population of Indian subcontinent ethnic origin resident in England. *J. Epidemiol. Community Health* 40:357–363, 1986.

Nurse, G. T., Weiner, J. S., and Jenkins, T.: *The Peoples of Southern Africa and Their Affinities*. New York, Oxford University Press, 1985.

Nute, P. E., and Stamatoyannopoulos, G.: Estimating mutation rates using abnormal human hemoglobins. *Yearbook Phys. Anthropol.* 27:135–151, 1984.

O'Brien, E., Jorde, L. B., Ronnlof, B., et al.: Founder effect and genetic diseases in Sottunga, Finland. *Am. J. Phys. Anthropol.* 77:335–346, 1988.

Ober, C., Bombard, A., Dhaliwal, R., et al.: Studies of cystic fibrosis in Hutterite females using linked DNA probes. *Am. J. Hum. Genet.* 41:1145–1151, 1987.

Oen, K., Chalmers, I. M., Ling, N., et al.: Rheumatic diseases in an Inuit population. *Arthritis Rheum.* 29:65–74, 1986.

Oettlé, A. G.: Geographical and racial differences in the frequency of Kaposi's sarcoma as evidence of environmental or genetic causes. *Acta Un. Int. Cancer* 18:330–363, 1962.

Oganov, R. G., Glasunov, I. S., Britov, A. N., et al.: Intensifying the fight against high blood pressure. *World Health Forum* 9:88–91, 1988.

Ogawa, S. K., Smith, M. A., Brennessel, D. J., et al.: Tuberculous meningitis in an urban medical center. *Medicine* 66:317–326, 1987.

Ogunnowo, P. O., Odesanmi, W. O., and Andy, J. J.: Coronary artery pathology in 111 consecutive Nigerians. *Trans. R. Soc. Trop. Med. Hyg.* 80:923–926, 1986.

Okoye, R. C., Williams, E., Alonso, A., Doyle, P., et al.: HLA polymorphisms in Nigerians. *Tissue Antigens* 25:142–155, 1985.

Olshansky, S. J., and Ault, A. B.: The fourth stage of the epidemiologic transition: The age of delayed degenerative diseases. *Milbank Mem. Fund Q.* 64:355–391, 1986.

Omar, M. A. K., Hammond, M. G., Seedat, M. A., and Asmal, A. C.: HLA antigens and non-insulin-dependent diabetes mellitus in young South African Indians. *S. Afr. Med. J.* 67:130–132, 1985.

Omene, J. A., and Onwuejeogwu, M. A.: Blood pressure and salt supplies in West Africa. *Lancet* 2:44–45, 1986.

Omenn, G. S.: Genetic investigations of alcohol metabolism and alcoholism. *Am. J. Hum. Genet.* 43:579–581, 1988.

Opler, M. K. (ed.): *Culture and Mental Health.* New York, Macmillan, 1959.

Oppenheimer, S. J., Higgs, D. R., Weatherall, D. J., Barker, J., and Spark, R. A.: α Thalassemia in Papua New Guinea. *Lancet* 1:424–426, 1984.

Oppenheimer, S. J., Gibson, F. D., MacFarlane, S. B., et al.: Iron supplementation increases prevalence and effects of malaria: Report on clinical studies in Papua New Guinea. *Trans. R. Soc. Med. Hyg.* 80:603–612, 1986a.

Oppenheimer, S. J., MacFarlane, S. B., Moody, J. B., et al.: Effect of iron prophylaxis on morbidity due to infectious disease: Report of clinical studies in Papua New Guinea. *Trans. R. Soc. Trop. Med. Hyg.* 80:596–602, 1986b.

Orchard, T. J., Dorman, J. S., LaPorte, R. E., et al.: Host and environmental interactions in diabetes mellitus. *J. Chron. Dis.* 39:979–999, 1986.

O'Rourke, D. H., Suarez, B. K., and Crouse, J. D.: Genetic variation in North Amerindian populations: Covariance with climate. *Am. J. Phys. Anthropol.* 67:241–250, 1985.

Orren, A., Taljaard, D., and Du Toit, E.: HLA-A, B, C and DR antigen associations in insulin dependent diabetes mellitus (IDDM) in South African Negro (black) and Cape Coloured people. *Tissue Antigens* 26:332–339, 1985.

Osborne, R. H. (ed.): *The Biological and Social Meaning of Race.* San Francisco, W. H. Freeman, 1971.

Ottenhoff, T. H. M., Torres, P., De las Aguas, J. T., et al.: Evidence for an HLA-DR4-associated immune-response gene for *Mycobacterium tuberculosis. Lancet* 2:310–313, 1986.

Ottolenghi, S., Camaschella, C., Comi, P., et al.: A frequent $^{A}\partial$-hereditary persistence of fetal hemoglobin in northern Sardinia: Its molecular basis and hematologic phenotype in heterozygotes and compound heterozygotes with B-thalassemia. *Hum. Hered.* 79:13–17, 1988.

Ovuga, E. B. L.: The different faces of depression. *East Afr. Med. J.* 63:109–114, 1985.

Owen, G. M., and Yanochik-Owen, A.: Should there be a different definition of anemia in black and white children? *Am. J. Public Health* 67:865–868, 1977.

Oyejide, O. C., et al.: Sickle-cell patients: No difference between Ibadan, Nigeria and Oakland, California patients in morbidity. *Int. J. Epidemiol.* 13:107–111, 1984.

Pabinger, I., Lechner, K., Kyrle, P. A., et al.: HLA haplotype and HIV infection. *Lancet* 2:342–343, 1988.

Padian, N., and Pickering, J.: Female-to-male transmission of AIDS: A reexamination of the African sex ratio of cases. *JAMA* 256:590, 1986.

Page, L. B., Damon, A., and Moellering, R. C. Jr.: Antecedents of cardiovascular disease in six Solomon Islands societies. *Circulation* 49:1132–1146, 1974.

Pandey, V. S., Ouhelli, H., and Moumen, A.: Epidemiology of hydatidosis/echinococcosis in Ouarzazate, the pre-Saharan region of Morocco. *Ann. Trop. Med. Parasitol.* 82:461–470, 1988.

Papiha, S. S.: Some implications of improved electrophoresis techniques for population genetics. In Roberts, D. F., and De Stefano, G. F. (eds.), *Genetic Variation and Its Maintenance.* Cambridge, U.K., Cambridge University Press, 1986, pp. 11–27.

Papiha, S. S., Mukherjee, B. N., Chahal, S. M. S., et al.: Genetic heterogeneity and population structure in north-west India. *Ann. Hum. Biol.* 9:235–251, 1982.

Papiha, S. S., Wentzel, J., Roberts, D. F., et al.: HLA antigen frequency in the Koya tribe of Andhra Pradesh, India. *Am. J. Phys. Anthropol.* 62:147–150, 1983.

Papiha, S. S., White, I., Singh, B. N., et al.: Group-specific component (Gc) subtypes in the Indian subcontinent. *Hum. Hered.* 37:250–254, 1987.

Parker, R.: Acquired immunodeficiency syndrome in urban Brazil. *Med. Anthropol. Q.* 1:155–175, 1987.

Parkin, D. M.: *Cancer in the Developing Countries.* IARC Publication. New York, Oxford University Press, 1986.

Parkin, D. M., Stjernsward, J., and Muir, C. S.: Estimates of the worldwide frequency of twelve major cancers. *Bull. WHO* 62:163–182, 1984.

Parry, E. H. O. (ed.): *Principles of Medicine in Africa*, 2d Ed. Oxford, U.K., Oxford University Press, 1984.

Pascali, V. L., Ranalletta, D., and Spedini, G.: Antitrypsin and Gc polymorphisms in some populations of Congo: An unusual, highly frequent mutant, Pi^{S*}, in Bateke and Babenga. *Ann. Hum. Biol.* 13:267–271, 1986.

Patterson, T. L., Kaplan, R. M., Sallis, J. F., et al.: Aggregation of blood pressure in Anglo-American and Mexican-American families. *Prev. Med.* 16:616–625, 1987.

Pawson, I. G., and Janes, C.: Massive obesity in a migrant Samoan population. *Am. J. Public Health* 71:508–513, 1981.

Payani, G. S.: Rheumatoid arthritis and tuberculosis. *Lancet* 2:816, 1986.

Pearce, N., Newell, K. W., Carter, H.: Incidence of hepatocellular carcinoma in New Zealand, 1974–78: Ethnic, sex and geographical differences. *N.Z. Med. J.* 98:1033–1036, 1985.

Pearce, R. B.: Heterosexual transmission of AIDS. *JAMA* 256:590–591, 1986.

Peers, F., Bosch, X., Kaldor, J., et al.: Aflatoxin exposure, heptatitis B virus infection and liver cancer in Swaziland. *Int. J. Cancer* 39:545–553, 1987.

Perlin, E., and White, J. E.: Increased cancer risk in blacks—Is it true? *J. Natl. Med. Assoc.* 77:177–178, 1985.

Perrine, R. P., Pembrey, M. E., John, P., Perrine, S., and Shoup, F.: Natural history of sickle-cell anemia in Saudi Arabs: A study of 270 subjects. *Ann. Intern. Med.* 88:1–6, 1978.

Persky, V., Pan, W. H., Stamler, J., Dyer, A., and Levy, P.: Time trends in the US racial difference in hypertension. *Am. J. Epidemiol.* 124:724–737, 1986.

Peters, R. K., Thomas, D., Hagan, D. G., et al.: Risk factors for invasive cervical cancer among Latinas and non-Latinas in Los Angeles County. *JNCI* 77:1063–1077, 1986.

Petrakis, N. L.: Some preliminary observations on the influence of genetic admixture on cancer incidence in American Negroes. *Int. J. Cancer* 7:256–258, 1971.

Petrelli, G., Maggini, M., Taggi, F., et al.: Malignant melanoma in Rome, Italy, 1970–9. *Int. J. Epidemiol. Community Health* 39:67–71, 1985.

Petitti, D. B., and Sidney, S.: Obesity and cholecystectomy among women: Implications for prevention. *Am. J. Prev. Med.* 4:327–330, 1988.

Pfeffer, R. I., Afifi, A. A., and Chance, J. M.: Prevalence of Alzheimer's disease in a retirement community. *Am. J. Epidemiol.* 125:420–436, 1987.

Pfeiffer, S.: Paleopathology in an Iroquoian ossuary, with special reference to tuberculosis. *Am. J. Phys. Anthropol.* 65:181–189, 1984.

Phillips, J. H., and Burch, G. E.: A review of cardiovascular diseases in the white and Negro races. *Medicine* 39:241–288, 1960.

Phillipson, B. E., Rothrock, D. W., Connor, W. E., et al.: Reduction of plasma lipids, lipoproteins, and apoproteins by dietary fish oils in patients with hypertriglyceridemia. *N. Engl. J. Med.* 312:1210–1216, 1985.

Phoon, W. O., Fong, N. P., and Leong, H. K.: A study of the prevalence of hepatitis B surface antigen among Chinese adult males in Singapore. *Int. J. Epidemiol.* 16:74–78, 1987.

Picheral, H.: France. In Howe, G. M. (ed.), *Global Geocancerology*. Edinburgh, Churchill Livingstone, 1986, pp. 144–153.

Pickle, L. W., Greene, M. H., Ziegler, R. G., et al.: Colorectal cancer in rural Nebraska. *Cancer Res.* 44:363–369, 1984.

Pickle, L. W., Mason, T. J., Howard, N., et al.: *Atlas of U.S. Cancer Mortality Among Whites: 1950–1980*. U.S. Dept. of Health and Human Services Publication No. 87-2900. Washington, U.S. Government Printing Office, 1987.

Piot, P., and Carael, M.: Epidemiological and sociological aspects of HIV-infection in developing countries. AIDS and HIV infection: The wider perspective. *Br. Med. Bull.* 44:68–88, 1988.

Piot, P., Plummer, F. A., Mhalu, F. S., et al.: AIDS: An international perspective. *Science* 239:573–579, 1988.

Pitchenik, A. E., Fischl, M. A., Dickinson, G. M., et al.: Opportunistic infections and Kaposi's sarcoma among Haitians: Evidence of new acquired immunodeficiency state. *Ann. Intern. Med.* 98:277–284, 1983.

Plapp, F. V., Rachel, J. M., and Sinor, L. T.: Dipsticks for determining ABO blood groups. *Lancet* 1:1465–1466, 1986.

Plaut, G. S.: Multiple sclerosis on islands. *Lancet* 2:277, 1987.

Pocock, S. J., Shaper, A. G., Cook, D. G., et al.: Social class differences in ischaemic heart disease in British men. *Lancet* 2:197–201, 1987.

Polednak, A. P.: Connective tissue responses in Negroes in relation to disease. *Am. J. Phys. Anthropol.* 41:49–58, 1974.

Polednak, A. P.: Primary bone cancer incidence in black and white residents of New York State. *Cancer* 2883–2888, 1985.

Polednak, A. P.: Breast cancer in black and white women in New York State: Case distribution and incidence rates by clinical stage at diagnosis. *Cancer* 58:807–815, 1986a.

Polednak, A. P.: Incidence of soft-tissue cancers in blacks and whites in New York State. *Int. J. Cancer* 38:21–26, 1986b.

Polednak, A. P.: Birth defects in blacks and whites in relation to prenatal development: A review and hypothesis. *Hum. Biol.* 58:317–335, 1986c.

Polednak, A. P.: Connective tissue responses in blacks in relation to diseases: Further observations. *Am. J. Phys. Anthropol.* 74:357–371, 1987a.

Polednak, A. P.: Rates of Paget's disease of bone among hospital discharges, by age and sex. *J. Am. Geriatr. Soc.* 35:550–553, 1987b.

Polednak, A. P.: *Host Factors in Disease. Age, Sex, Racial and Ethnic Group, and Body Build.* Springfield, IL, Charles C. Thomas, 1987c.

Polednak, A. P.: A comparison of survival of black and white female breast cancer cases in Upstate New York. *Cancer Detect. Prev.* 11:245–249, 1988a.

Polednak, A. P.: Mortality among blacks in a high-income area: Suffolk County, New York 1979–85. Submitted for publication, 1988b.

Polednak, A. P.: Mortality from chronic diseases among Hispanics in a high-income area. Submitted for publication, 1988c.

Polednak, A. P., and Janerich, D. T.: Hematocrit among blacks with sickle cell trait. *Hum. Biol.* 47:493–504, 1975.

Polednak, A. P., and Janerich, D. T.: Birth characteristics of blacks with sickle cell trait. *Hum. Biol.* 52:15–21, 1980.

Polednak, A. P., and Janerich, D. T.: Uses of available record systems in epidemiologic studies of reproductive toxicology. *Am. J. Ind. Med.* 4:329–348, 1983.

Pollack, E. S., Nomura, A. M. Y., Heilbrun, L. K., et al.: Prospective study of alcohol consumption and cancer. *N. Engl. J. Med.* 310:617–621, 1984.

Pollitzer, W. S.: The Negroes of Charleston (S.C.); a study of hemoglobin types, serology, and morphology. *Am. J. Phys. Anthropol.* 16:241–264, 1958.

Poolman, J. T., Lind, I., Jonsdottir, K., et al.: Meningococcal serotypes and serogroup B disease in north-west Europe. *Lancet* 2:555–558, 1986.

Popkin, B. M., Akin, J. S., Flieger, W., et al.: Breastfeeding trends in the Philippines, 1973 and 1983. *Am. J. Public Health* 79:32–35, 1989.

Popovich, B. W., Rosenblatt, D. S., Kendall, A. G., et al.: Molecular characterization of an atypical β-thalassemia caused by a large deletion in the 5 β-globin gene region. *Am. J. Hum. Genet.* 39:797–810, 1986.

Porapakkham, Y., and Prasartkul, P.: Cause of death: Trends and differentials in Thailand. In Lopez, A., Porapakkham, Y., and Promote, P. (eds.), *New Developments in Mortality Studies.* Bangkok, Thailand, Mahidol University Press, 1985, pp. 207–237.

Porter, I. H.: Genetic services within a state health department. In Porter, I. H., and Hook, E. B. (eds.), *Service and Education in Medical Genetics.* New York, Academic Press, 1979, pp. 253–269.

Poser, C. M.: Multiple sclerosis on islands. *Lancet* 1:1426, 1987.

Poser, C. M., and Hibberd, P.: Epidemiologic studies on multiple sclerosis. *Arch. Neurol.* 44:351–352, 1987.

Poskanzer, D. C.: Neurological disorders. In Clark, D. W., and MacMahon, B. (eds.), *Prevention and Community Medicine*, 2d Ed. Boston, Little, Brown, 1981, pp. 265–291.

Potter, J. D., and McMichael, A. J.: Diet and cancer of the colon and rectum: A case-control study. *JNCI* 76:557–569, 1986.

Pratt, J. A., Velez, R., Brender, J. D., et al.: Racial differences in acute lymphocytic leukemia mortality and incidence trends. *J. Clin. Epidemiol.* 41:367–371, 1988.

Prener, A., Nielsen, N. H., Hansen, J. P. H., et al.: Cancer pattern among Greenlandic Inuit migrants in Denmark, 1968–1982. *Br. J. Cancer* 56:670–684, 1987.

Preston-Martin, S., Henderson, B. E., and Pike, M. C.: Descriptive epidemiology of cancers of the upper respiratory tract in Los Angeles. *Cancer* 49:2201–2207, 1982.

Preston-Martin, S., Bartsch, H., Pignatelli, B., et al.: Re: 'N-Nitroso compounds and human cancer: A molecular epidemiologic approach.' *Am. J. Epidemiol.* 124:155–156, 1986.

Prineas, R. J., and Gillum, R.: U.S. epidemiology of hypertension in blacks. In Hall, D. W., Saunders, E., and Shulman, N. B. (eds.), *Hypertension in Blacks*. Chicago, Yearbook, 1985, pp. 17–36.

Prior, I.: Epidemiology of rheumatic disorders in the Pacific with particular emphasis on hyperuricemia and gout. *Semin. Arthritis Rheum.* 11:213–229, 1981.

Prior, I. A. M., Stanhope, J. M., Evans, J. G., and Salmond, C. E.: The Tokelau Island migrant study. *Int. J. Epidemiol.* 3:225–232, 1974.

Propert, D. N., and Balkan, B. J.: Selective forces and the maintenance of immunoglobulin polymorphisms. *Hum. Biol.* 58:79–84, 1986.

Pugh, J. A., Stern, M. P., Haffner, S. M., et al.: Excess incidence of treatment of end-stage renal disease in Mexican Americans. *Am. J. Epidemiol.* 127:135–144, 1988.

Pukkala, E., Gustavsson, N., and Teppo, L.: *Suomen Syopakartasto. Atlas of Cancer Incidence in Finland*. Helsinki, Suomen Syoparekisteri, Finnish Cancer Registry, 1987.

Qizilbash, N., and Bates, D.: Incidence of motor neurone disease in the northern region. *J. Epidemiol. Community Health* 41:18–20, 1987.

Quinn, T. C., Piot, P., McCormick, J. B., et al.: Serologic and immunologic studies in patients with AIDS in North America and Africa. *JAMA* 257:2617–2621, 1987.

Rabbani, S., Galvin, M., Louv, W. C., et al.: Risk factor surveys of the adult populations of the state of Alabama and Jefferson County. *Ala. J. Med. Sci.* 24:143–149, 1987.

Radhakrishnan, K., and Mousa, M. E.: Creutzfeldt-Jakob disease in Benghazi, Libya. *Neuroepidemiology* 7:42–43, 1988.

Radhakrishnan, K., Ashok, P. P., Sridharan, R., et al.: Descriptive epidemiology of motor neuron disease in Benghazi, Libya. *Neuroepidemiology* 5:47–54, 1986.

Rahman, M., Wojtyniak, B., Rahaman, M. M., and Aziz, K. M. S.: Impact of environmental sanitation and crowding on infant mortality in rural Bangladesh. *Lancet* 2:28–31, 1985.

Rajanikumari, J., and Srikumari, C. R.: Gene differentiation at the ABO locus in twenty castes and twenty-two tribes of Andhra Pradesh, India. *Am. J. Phys. Anthropol.* 72:95–99, 1987.

Ramsay, M., and Jenkins, T.: α-Thalassemia in Africa: The oldest malaria protective trait? *Lancet* 2:410, 1984.

Ramsay, M., and Jenkins, T.: Globin-gene-associated restriction-fragment-length polymorphisms in southern African peoples. *Am. J. Hum. Genet.* 41:1132–1144, 1987.

Ranford, P., Serjeantson, S. W., Hay, J., et al.: A high frequency of inherited deficiency of complement component C4 in Darwin aborigines. *Aust. N.Z. J. Med.* 17:420–423, 1987.

Rao, P. S. S.: Inbreeding in India. In Lukacs, J. R. (ed.), *The People of South Asia*. New York, Plenum Press, 1984, pp. 260–281.

Rapoport, B.: Approaching an understanding of the genetic basis for autoimmune thyroid disease. *Arch. Intern. Med.* 147:213, 1987.

Raseroka, B. H., and Ormerod, W. E.: Protection of the sleeping sickness trypanosome from chemotherapy by different parts of the brain. *East Afr. Med. J.* 62:452–458, 1985.

Rate, R. G., Morse, H. G., Bonnell, M. D., et al.: 'Navajo arthritis' reconsidered. Relationship to HLA-B27. *Arthritis Rheum.* 23:1299–1302, 1980.

Ratnam, K. V.: Awareness of AIDS among transsexual prostitutes in Singapore. *Singapore Med. J.* 27:519–521, 1986.

Rawls, W. E., Lavery, C., Marrett, L. D., et al.: Comparison of risk factors for cervical cancer in different populations. *Int. J. Cancer* 37:537–546, 1986.

Raymond, C. A.: Worldwide assault on poliomyelitis gathering support, garnering results. *JAMA* 255:1541–1546, 1986.

Reddy, A. P., Mukherjee, B. N., Vijayakumar, M., and Malhotra, K. C.: PGM_1 subtype polymorphism in 14 endogamous Dravidian-speaking populations of South India. *Am. J. Phys. Anthropol.* 71:89–94, 1986.

Redfield, R.: Memorandum on the study of acculturation. *Am. Anthropol.* 38:149–152, 1936.

Reed, D., Labarthe, D., Chen, K. M., and Stallones, R.: A cohort study of amyotrophic lateral sclerosis and parkinsonism-dementia on Guam and Rota. *Am. J. Epidemiol.* 125:92–100, 1987.

Reed, T. E.: Caucasian genes in American negroes. *Science* 165:762–768, 1969.

Reeves, W. C., Brenes, M. M., De Britton, R. C., Valdes, P. F., and Joplin, C. F. B.: Cervical cancer in the Republic of Panama. *Am. J. Epidemiol.* 119:714–724, 1984.

Reeves, W. C., Cuevas, M., Arosemena, J. R., et al.: Human immunodeficiency virus infection in the Republic of Panama. *Am. J. Trop. Med. Hyg.* 39:398–405, 1988.

Regier, D. A., Boyd, J. H., Burke, J. D. Jr., et al.: One month prevalence of mental disorders in the United States. *Arch. Gen. Psychiat.* 45:977–986, 1988.

Reintgen, D. S., McCarthy, K. M. Jr., Cox, E., et al.: Malignant melanoma in black and white American populations. *JAMA* 248:1856–1859, 1983.

Reitnauer, P. J., Roseman, J. M., Barger, B. O., et al.: HLA associations with insulin-dependent diabetes mellitus in a sample of American black population. *Tissue Antigens* 17:286–293, 1981.

Relethford, J. H., and Lees, F. C.: Admixture and skin color in the transplanted Tlaxcalte-can population of Saltillo, Mexico. *Am. J. Phys. Anthropol.* 56:259–267, 1981.

Relman, A. S.: Race and end-stage renal disease. *N. Engl. J. Med.* 306:1290–1291, 1982.

Rezza, G., Titti, F., Rossi, G. B., et al.: Sex as a risk factor for HTLV-I spread among intravenous drug abusers. *Lancet* 1:713, 1988.

Rhoades, R. R., Mason, R. D., Eddy, P., et al.: The Indian Health Services approach to alcoholism among American Indians and Alaskan natives. *Public Health Rep.* 103:621–627, 1988.

Riccardi, G., Vaccaro, O., Rivellese, A., Pignalosa, S., et al.: Reproducibility of the new diagnostic criteria for impaired glucose tolerance. *Am. J. Epidemiol.* 121:422–429, 1985.

Richardson, J. L., Marks, G., Solis, J. M., et al.: Frequency and adequacy of breast cancer screening among elderly Hispanic women. *Prev. Med.* 16:761–774, 1987.

Richardson, S., Stucker, I., and Hemon, D.: Comparison of relative risks obtained in ecological and individual studies: Some methodological considerations. *Int. J. Epidemiol.* 16:111–120, 1987.

Richman, J. A., Gavira, M., Flaherty, J. A., et al.: The process of acculturation: Theoretical perspectives and an empirical investigation in Peru. *Soc. Sci. Med.* 25:839–847, 1987.

Rickwood, A. M. K.: Untreated myelomeningocele. *Lancet* 2:1421, 1985.

Ries, P.: Health care coverage by sociodemographic and health characteristics, United States, 1984. Data from the National Health Survey, Series 10 No. 162. Hyattsville, MD, U.S. Public Health Service, 1987a.

Ries, P.: Physician contacts by sociodemographic and health characteristics, United States, 1982–83. Data from the National Health Survey, Series 10 No. 161. Hyattsville, MD, U.S. Public Health Service, 1987b.

Riggs, B. L., and Melton, L. J. III: Involutional osteoporosis. *N. Engl. J. Med.* 314:1676–1686, 1986.

Rishpon, S., et al.: *Campylobacter jejuni* in Haifa, Israel. *Int. J. Epidemiol.* 13:216–220, 1984.

Roberts, D. F.: The dynamics of racial intermixture in the American Negro—some anthropological considerations. *Am. J. Hum. Genet.* 7:361–367, 1955.

Roberts, D. F.: Applications of polymorphisms in anthropogenetic studies. *Hum. Biol.* 54:175–192, 1982.

Roberts, D. F., Roberts, M. J., and Poskanzer, D. C.: Genetic analysis of multiple sclerosis in Orkney. *J. Epidemiol. Community Health* 33:229–235, 1979.

Roberts, D. F., and De Stefano, G. F. (eds.): *Genetic Variation and Its Maintenance.* Cambridge, U.K., Cambridge University Press, 1986.

Roberts, L.: Diet and health in China. *Science* 240:27, 1988.

Roberts, M., Young, R., Howell, J., et al.: Acquired immunodeficiency syndrome (AIDS) in western Palm Beach county, Florida. *MMWR* 35:609–612, 1986.

Robertson, T. L., Kato, H., Gordon, T., et al.: Epidemiologic studies of coronary heart disease and stroke in Japanese men living in Japan, Hawaii, and California: Coronary heart disease risk factors in Japan and Hawaii. *Am. J. Cardiol.* 39:244–249, 1977.

Robinson, D., and Day, J.: Low plasma triglyceride levels in lake dwelling East African tribesmen—a fishy story? *Int. J. Epidemiol.* 15:183–187, 1986.

Robinson, J. C.: Racial inequality and the probability of occupation-related injury or illness. *Milbank Mem. Fund Q.* 62:567–590, 1984.

Rode, A., and Shephard, R. J.: Growth, development and acculturation—a ten year comparison of Canadian Inuit children. *Hum. Biol.* 56:217–230, 1984.

Rogan, W. J., Gladen, B. C., Hung, K. L., et al.: Congenital poisoning by polychlorinated biphenyls and their contaminants in Taiwan. *Science* 241:334–336, 1988.

Rogers, M. S.: Racial variation in the incidence of trisomy 21. *Br. J. Obstet. Gynaecol.* 93:597–599, 1986.

Roman, G. C., and Sheremata, W. A.: High prevalence of multiple sclerosis in Key West, Fla.: Report of 12 cases in native-born inhabitants. *Neuroepidemiology* 7:48, 1988.

Rosatelli, C., Leoni, G. B., Tuveri, T., et al.: β thalassemia mutations in Sardinians: Implications for prenatal diagnosis. *J. Med. Genet.* 24:97–100, 1987.

Rose, D. P., et al.: Serum and breast duct prolactin and estrogen levels in healthy Finnish and American women and patients with fibrocystic disease. *Cancer* 57:1550–1554, 1986.

Rose, J. C. (ed.): *Gone to a Better Land. A Biohistory of a Rural Black Cemetery in the Post-Reconstruction South.* Fayetteville, Arkansas Archeological Survey Research Series No. 25, 1985.

Rosen, M., Nystrom, L., and Wall, S.: Diet and cancer mortality in the counties of Sweden. *Am. J. Epidemiol.* 127:42–49, 1988.

Rosenwaike, I.: Cancer mortality among Puerto Rican-born residents in New York City. *Am. J. Epidemiol.* 119:177–185, 1984.

Rosenwaike, I.: Mortality differentials among persons born in Cuba, Mexico, and Puerto Rico residing in the United States, 1979–81. *Am. J. Public Health* 77:603–606, 1987.

Rosenwaike, I., and Shai, D.: Trends in cancer mortality among Puerto Rican-born migrants to New York City. *Int. J. Epidemiol.* 15:30–35, 1986.

Roth, E. Jr., Friedman, M., Ueda, Y., Tellez, I., et al.: Sickling rates of human AS red cells infected in vitro with *Plasmodium falciparum* malaria. *Science* 202:650–652, 1978.

Rothhammer, F., Allison, M. J., Nunez, L., Standen, V., and Arriaza, B.: Chagas' disease in pre-Columbian South America. *Am. J. Phys. Anthropol.* 68:495–498, 1985.

Rothschild, H. (ed.): *Biocultural Aspects of Disease.* New York, Academic Press, 1981.

Rotkin, I. D., and Taylor, W. E.: Ethnic comparability of the relation between early coital trends and cervical cancer. *Cancer* 23:458–460, 1969.

Rouse, I.: *Migrations in Prehistory.* New Haven, CT, Yale University Press, 1986.

Roychoudhury, A. K.: Genetic distance and gene diversity among linguistically different tribes of Mexican Americans. *Am. J. Phys. Anthropol.* 42:449–454, 1975.

Royston, E., and Lopez, A.: On the assessment of maternal mortality. *World Health Statist. Q.* 40:214–224, 1987.

Rozen, P., Lynch, H. T., Figer, A., et al.: Familial colon cancer in the Tel-Aviv area and the influence of ethnic origin. *Cancer* 60:2355–2359, 1987.

Sachs, B. P., Brown, D. A. J., Driscoll, S. G., et al.: Hemorrhage, infection, toxemia, and cardiac disease, 1954–85: Causes for their declining role in maternal mortality. *Am. J. Public Health* 78:671–675, 1988.

Saha, N.: A genetic study of blacks from Trinidad. *Hum. Hered.* 37:365–370, 1987.

Saha, N.: Blood genetic markers in Sri Lankan populations—reappraisal of the legend of Prince Vijaya. *Am. J. Phys. Anthropol.* 76:217–225, 1988.

Saiki, R., Chang, C. A., Levenson, C. H., et al.: Diagnosis of sickle cell anemia and β-thalassemia with enzymatically amplified DNA and nonradioactive allele-specific oligonucleotide probes. *N. Engl. J. Med.* 319:537–541, 1988.

Salmond, C. E., Joseph, J. G., Prior, I. A. M., et al.: Longitudinal analysis of the relationship between blood pressure and migration: The Tokelau Island migrant study. *Am. J. Epidemiol.* 122:291–301, 1985.

Salzano, F. M.: Changing patterns of disease among South American Indians. In Chakraborty, R., and Szathmary, E. J. E. (eds.), *Diseases of Complex Etiology in Small Populations.* New York, Alan R. Liss, 1985, pp. 301–323.

Samet, J. M., Kutvirt, D. M., Waxweiler, R. J., et al.: Uranium mining and lung cancer in Navajo men. *N. Engl. J. Med.* 310:1481–1484, 1984.

Samet, J. M., Coultras, D. B., Howard, C. A., et al.: Diabetes, gallbladder disease, obesity, and hypertension among Hispanics in New Mexico. *Am. J. Epidemiol.* 128:1302–1311, 1988.

Sappenfield, W. M., Buehler, J. W., Binkin, N. J., et al.: Differences in neonatal and postneonatal mortality by race, birth weight, and gestational age. *Public Health Rep.* 102:182–192, 1987.

Sartorius, N., Jablensky, A., Cooper, J. E., et al.: Psychiatric classification in an international perspective. *Br. J. Psychiat.* 152 (Suppl.):1–52, 1988.

Satariano, W. A.: Race, socioeconomic status, and health: A study of age differences in a depressed area. *Am. J. Prev. Med.* 2:1–5, 1986.

Satariano, W. A., Belle, S. H., and Swanson, G. M.: The severity of breast cancer at diagnosis: A comparison of age and extent of disease in black and white women. *Am. J. Public Health* 76:779–782, 1986.

Savage, D., Lindenbaum, J., Van Ryzin, J., et al.: Race, poverty and survival in multiple myeloma. *Int. J. Health Serv.* 15:321–338, 1985.

Savitz, D. A.: Changes in Spanish-surname cancer rates, relative to other whites, Denver area, 1969–71 to 1979–81. *Am. J. Public Health* 76:1210–1215, 1986.

Sawchuk, L. A., and Herring, D. A.: Respiratory tuberculosis mortality among the Sephardic Jews of Gibraltar. *Hum. Biol.* 56:291–306, 1984.

Sayetta, R. B.: Rates of senile dementia-Alzheimer's type in the Baltimore longitudinal study. *J. Chron. Dis.* 39:271–286, 1986.

Schaap, G. J. P., Bijkerk, H., Coutinho, R. A., et al.: The spread of wild poliovirus in the well-vaccinated Netherlands in connection with the 1978 epidemic. *Prog. Med. Virol.* 29:124–140, 1984.

Schachter, J., Kuller, L. H., and Perfetti, C.: Blood pressure during the first five years of life: Relation to ethnic group (black or white) and to parental hypertension. *Am. J. Epidemiol.* 119:541–553, 1984.

Schatzkin, A., Palmer, J. R., Rosenberg, L., et al.: Risk factors for breast cancer in black women. *JNCI* 78:213–217, 1987.

Schauf, V., Ryan, S., Scollard, D., et al.: Leprosy associated with HLA-DR2 and DQw1 in the population of northern Thailand. *Tissue Antigens* 26:243–247, 1985.

Schechter, A. N., and Bunn, H. F.: What determines severity of sickle-cell disease? *N. Engl. J. Med.* 306:295–297, 1982.

Schiffers, E., Jamart, J., and Renard, V.: Tobacco and occupation as risk factors in bladder cancer: A case-control study in southern Belgium. *Int. J. Cancer* 39:287–292, 1987.

Schiffman, M. H.: Epidemiology of fecal mutagenicity. *Epidemiol. Rev.* 8:92–105, 1986.

Schooneveldt, M., Songer, T., Zimmet, P., et al.: Changing mortality patterns in Nauruans: An example of epidemiological transition. *J. Epidemiol. Community Health* 42:89–95, 1988.

Schoub, B. D., Johnson, S., and McAnerney, J. M.: A comprehensive investigation of immunity to poliomyelitis in a developing country. *Am. J. Epidemiol.* 123:316–324, 1986.

Schurmann, M., Warnecke, R., and Schwinger, E.: Four DNA polymorphisms on the short arm of the X chromosome: Allele frequencies in a German and in a Turkish population. *Hum. Hered.* 37:329–333, 1987.

Schutte, J. E., Townsend, E. J., Hugg, J., et al.: Density of lean body mass is greater in blacks than in whites. *J. Appl. Physiol.* 56:1647–1649, 1984.

Schwabe, A. D., and Monroe, J. B.: Meningitis in familial Mediterranean fever. *Am. J. Med.* 85:715–717, 1988.

Schwartz, A.: Ethnic identity among left-wing American Jews. *Ethnic Groups* 6:65–84, 1984.

Scorza Smeraldi, R., Fabio, G., Lazzarin, A., et al.: HLA-associated susceptibility to acquired deficiency syndrome in Italian patients with immunodeficiency-virus infection. *Lancet* 2:1187–1189, 1986.

Scozzari, R., Torroni, A., Semino, O., et al.: Genetic studies on the Senegal population. I. Mitochondrial DNA polymorphisms. *Am. J. Hum. Genet.* 43:534–544, 1988.

Scrimgeour, E. M., Matz, L. R., and Aaskov, J. G.: A study of arthritis in Papua New Guinea. *Aust. N.Z. J. Med.* 17:51–54, 1987.

Seedat, Y. K., and Hackland, D. B. T.: The prevalence of hypertension in 4,993 rural Zulus. *Trans. R. Soc. Trop. Med. Hyg.* 78:785–789, 1984.

Segall, A. J.: Distribution of cancer mortality among ethnic subgroups of Montreal, 1959–63. Presented at the 57th meeting of the Canadian Public Health Association, Quebec City, June 2, 1966.

Segall, A. J.: Alimentary disorders. In Clark, D. W., and MacMahon, B. (eds.), *Preventive and Community Medicine*, 2d Ed. Boston, Little, Brown, 1981, pp. 247–264.

Segi, M.: Graphic presentation of cancer incidence by site and by area and population. Compiled from data published in *Cancer Incidence in Five Continents*, Vol. III. Nagoya, Japan, Segi Institute of Cancer Epidemiology, 1977.

Seligsohn, U., Zivelin, A., and Zwang, E.: Combined factor V and factor VIII deficiency among non-Ashkenazi Jews. *N. Engl. Med. J.* 307:1191–1195, 1982.

Selik, R. M., Castro, K. M., and Pappaioanou, M.: Racial/ethnic differences in the risk of AIDS in the United States. *Am. J. Public Health* 78:1539–1545, 1988.

Sempos, C., Cooper, R., Kovar, M. G., et al.: Divergence of the recent trends in coronary mortality for the four major race-sex groups in the United States. *Am. J. Public Health* 78:1422–1427, 1988.

Senanayake, N., and Jeyaratnam, J.: Toxic polyneuropathy due to gingili oil contaminated with tri-cresyl phosphate affecting adolescent girls in Sri Lanka. *Lancet* 1:88–89, 1981.

Senba, M., Nakamura, T., Toda, T., et al.: Decreasing frequency, with time, of hepatitis B surface antigen positive liver biopsy in hepatitis, cirrhosis, and liver hepatocellular carcinoma. *Lancet* 1:588–589, 1988.

Serjeant, G. R.: *Sickle Cell Disease.* New York, Oxford University Press, 1986.

Serjeantson, S., and Zimmet, P.: Diabetes in the Pacific: Evidence for a major gene. In Baba, S., Gould, M. K., and Zimmet, P. (eds.), *Diabetes Mellitus.* New York, Academic Press, 1984, pp. 23–30.

Sewardsen, M., and Jialal, I.: CHD in Indians overseas. *Lancet* 2:159, 1986.

Shanmugaratnam, K.: Nasopharynx. In Schottenfeld, D., and Fraumeni, J. F. Jr. (eds.), *Cancer Epidemiology and Prevention.* Philadelphia, W. B. Saunders, 1982, pp. 536–553.

Shanmugaratnam, K., Lee, H. P., and Day, N. E.: *Cancer Incidence in Singapore 1968–1977.* IARC Publication No. 47. Lyon, France, International Agency for Research on Cancer, 1983.

Shann, F., Germer, S., Hazlett, D., Gratten, M., et al.: Aetiology of pneumonia in children in Goroka Hospital, Papua New Guinea. *Lancet* 2:537–541, 1984.

Shaper, A. G.: National trends in mortality from ischaemic heart disease: Implications for prevention. *Lancet* 1:795, 1986.

Shepard, C. C.: Leprosy today. *N. Engl. J. Med.* 307:1640–1641, 1982.

Shimizu, H., Mack, T. M., Ross, R. K., et al.: Cancer of the gastrointestinal tract among Japanese and white immigrants in Los Angeles County. *JNCI* 78:223–228, 1987.

Shu, X. O., Gao, Y. T., Linet, M. S., et al.: Chloramphenicol use and childhood leukaemia in Shanghai. *Lancet* 2:934–937, 1987.

Shulman, S. T. (ed.): *Kawasaki Disease.* New York, Alan R. Liss, 1987.

Shulman, S. T., and Rowley, A. H.: Does Kawasaki disease have a retroviral aetiology? *Lancet* 2:545–546, 1986.

Siegel, S.: *Nonparametric Statistics for the Behavioral Sciences.* New York, McGraw-Hill, 1956.

Sievers, M. L., and Fisher, J. R.: Diseases of North American Indians. In Rothschild, H. (ed.), *Biocultural Aspects of Disease.* New York, Academic Press, 1981, pp. 191–245.

Sievers, M. L., and Fisher, J. R.: Cancer in North American Indians: Environment versus heredity. *Am. J. Public Health* 73:485–486, 1983.

Silman, A., Loysen, E., De Graaf, W., and Sramek, M.: High dietary fat intake and cigarette smoking as risk factors for ischaemic heart disease in Bangladeshi male immigrants in East London. *J. Epidemiol. Community Health* 39:301–303, 1985.

Silman, A. J., Evans, S. J. W., and Loysen, E.: Blood pressure and migration: A study of Bengali immigrants in East London. *J. Epidemiol. Community Health* 41:152–155, 1987.

Simons, R. G. (ed.): *The Culture-Bound Syndromes: Folk Illnesses of Psychiatric and Anthropological Interest.* Hingham, MA, Kluwer, 1985.

Singal, D. P., D'Souza, M., Reid, B., et al.: HLA-DQ beta-chain polymorphism in HLA-DR4 haplotypes associated with rheumatoid arthritis. *Lancet* 2:1118–1120, 1987.

Sinnett, P. F., and Whyte, H. M.: Epidemiologic studies in a total highland population, Tukisenta, New Guinea. Cardiovascular disease and relevant clinical electrocardiographic, radiological and biochemical findings. *J. Chron. Dis.* 26:265–290, 1973.

Siperstein, G. N., Wolraich, M. L., Reed, D., et al.: Medical decisions and prognostications of pediatricians for infants with meningomyelocele. *J. Pediatr.* 113:835–840, 1988.

Sistonen, P., Abdulle, O. A., and Sahid, M.: Evidence for a 'new' Rh gene complex producing the rare C^X (Rh9) antigen in the Somali population of East Africa. *Transfusion* 27:66–68, 1987a.

Sistonen, P., Koistinen, J., and Abdulle, O. A.: Distribution of blood groups in the East African Somali population. *Hum. Hered.* 37:300–313, 1987b.

Sitthi-Amorn, C., Tussaniyom, S., Soontrapa, S., et al.: Mail follow-up of chronic diseases in northeast Thailand. *Int. J. Epidemiol.* 15:263–267, 1986.

Slattery, M. L., Sorenson, W., and Ford, M. H.: Dietary calcium as a mitigating factor in colon cancer. *Am. J. Epidemiol.* 128:504–514, 1988a.

Slattery, M. L., Schumacher, M. C., Smith, K. R., et al.: Physical activity, diet, and risk of colon cancer in Utah. *Am. J. Epidemiol.* 128:989–999, 1988b.

Smith, A. H., Pearce, N. E., and Joseph, J. G.: Major colorectal cancer aetiological hypotheses do not explain mortality trends among Maori and non-Maori New Zealanders. *Int. J. Epidemiol.* 14:79–85, 1985a.

Smith, A. H., Pool, D. I., Pearce, N. E., et al.: Mortality among New Zealand Maori and non-Maori Mormons. *Int. J. Epidemiol.* 14:265–271, 1985b.

Smith, E. A., and Udry, J. R.: Coital and non-coital sexual behaviors of white and black adolescents. *Am. J. Public Health* 75:1200–1203, 1985.

Smith, G. L., and Smith, K. F.: Lack of HIV infection and condom use in licensed prostitutes. *Lancet* 2:1392, 1986.

Smith, G. L., Greenup, R., and Takafuji, E. T.: Circumcision as a risk factor for urethritis in racial groups. *Am. J. Public Health* 77:452–454, 1987.

Smith, J. C.: The vitamin A–zinc connection: A review. *Ann. N.Y. Acad. Sci.* 355:62–75, 1980.

Smith, J. C., Mercy, J. A., and Rosenberg, M. L.: Suicide and homicide among Hispanics in the Southwest. *Public Health Rep.* 101:265–270, 1986.

Smith, M.: Genetics of human alcohol and aldehyde dehydrogenases. In Harris, H., and Hirschhorn, K. (eds.), *Advances in Human Genetics*, Vol. 15. New York, Plenum Press, 1986, pp. 249–290.

Snedecor, G. W., and Cochran, W. G.: *Statistical Methods*, 6th Ed. Ames, Iowa State University Press, 1967.

Sofaer, J. A., Smith, P., and Kaye, E.: Affinities between contemporary and skeletal Jewish and non-Jewish groups based on tooth morphology. *Am. J. Phys. Anthropol.* 70:265–275, 1986.

Solem, E., Pirzer, C., Siege, M., et al.: Mass screening for glucose-6-phosphate dehydrogenase deficiency: Improved fluorescent spot test. *Clin. Chim. Acta* 31:135–142, 1985.

Solomon, L.: Bone density and aging Caucasian and African populations. *Lancet* 2:1326–1330, 1979.

Somboomcharoen, S.: *Cancer Statistics, 1981 [Thailand]*. Bangkok, Department of Medical Services, Ministry of Public Health, 1986.

Sommer, A., Hussaini, G., Tarwotjo, I., Susanto, D., and Soegiharto, T.: Incidence, prevalence, and scale of blinding malnutrition. *Lancet* 1:1407–1408, 1981.

Song, H. Z., and Wu, P. C.: Incidence of hydatidiform mole in China. *Int. J. Epidemiol.* 15:429–430, 1986.

Spedini, G., Walter, H., Capucci, E., et al.: An anthropobiological study in Basse Kotto (Central Africa). I. Erythrocyte and sero-genetic markers: An analysis of the genetic differentiation. *Am. J. Phys. Anthropol.* 60:39–47, 1983.

Spencer, P. S., Nunn, P. B., Hugon, J., et al.: Guam amyotrophic lateral sclerosis–Parkinsonism–dementia linked to a plant excitant neurotoxin. *Science* 237:517–522, 1987a.

Spencer, P. S., Palmer, V. S., Herman, A., et al.: Cycad use and motor neurone disease in Irian Jaya. *Lancet* 2:1273–1274, 1987b.

Spielman, R. S., and Nathanson, N.: The genetics of susceptibility to multiple sclerosis. *Epidemiol. Rev.* 4:45–65, 1982.

Spitz, M. R., Newell, G. R., Sider, J. G., et al.: Ethnic patterns of bone cancer incidence in the United States, 1973–1981. *Cancer J.* 1:344–348, 1987.

Sridama, V., Hara, Y., Fauchet, R., and DeGroot, L. J.: HLA immunogenetic heterogeneity in black American patients with Graves' disease. *Arch. Intern. Med.* 147:229–231, 1987.

Srinivasa, D. K., and D'Souza, V.: Economic aspects of an epidemic of haemorrhagic conjunctivitis in a rural community. *J. Epidemiol. Community Health* 41:79–81, 1987.

Stamatoyannopoulos, G., Nienhuis, A., Leder, P., et al. (eds.): *The Molecular Basis of Blood Diseases.* Philadelphia, Saunders, 1987.

Stamler, J.: Disease of the cardiovascular system. In Clark, D. W., and MacMahon, B. (eds.), *Preventive Medicine and Community Health.* Boston, Little, Brown, 1981, pp. 193–217.

Stanford, J. L., Szklo, M., and Boring, C. C.: A case-control study of breast cancer stratified by estrogen receptor status. *Am. J. Epidemiol.* 125:184–194, 1987.

Stanley, K. E.: Lung cancer and tobacco—a global problem. *Cancer Detect. Prev.* 9:83–89, 1986.

Staszewski, J., and Haenszel, W.: Cancer mortality among the Polish-born in the United States. *JNCI* 35:291–297, 1965.

Stavig, G. R., Igra, A., and Leonard, A. R.: Hypertension among Asians and Pacific Islanders in California. *Am. J. Epidemiol.* 119:677–691, 1984.

Steel, C. M., Ludlam, C. A., Beatson, D., et al.: HLA haplotype A1 B8 DR3 as a risk factor for HIV-related disease. *Lancet* 1:1185–1188, 1988.

Stehr-Green, J. K., and Schantz, P. M.: Trichinosis in Southeast Asian refugees in the United States. *Am. J. Public Health* 76:1238–1239, 1986.

Stein, Z., and Maine, D.: The health of women. *Int. J. Epidemiol.* 15:303–305, 1986.

Steinberg, A. G., and Cook, C. E.: *The Distribution of Human Immunoglobulin Allotypes.* Oxford, U.K., Oxford University Press, 1981.

Steiner, I., Thomas, J. D., and Hutt, M. S. R.: Aortopathies in Ugandan Africans. *J. Pathol.* 109:295–305, 1973.

Steinhorn, S. C., Myers, M. H., Hankey, B. F., and Pelham, V. F.: Factors associated with survival differences between black women and white women with cancer of the uterine corpus. *Am. J. Epidemiol.* 124:85–93, 1986.

Stern, E., Blau, J., Rusecki, Y., et al.: Prevalence of diabetes in Israel. *Diabetes* 37:297–302, 1988.

Stern, M. P.: Hypertension in Mexican Americans. *Int. J. Epidemiol.* 14:644–645, 1985.

Stern, M. P., Rosenthal, M., Haffner, S. M., et al.: Sex difference in the effects of sociocultural status on diabetes and cardiovascular risk factors in Mexican Americans. *Am. J. Epidemiol.* 120:834–851, 1984.

Stevens, C. E., Taylor, P. E., Tong, M. J., et al.: Yeast-recombinant hepatitis B vaccine. Efficacy with hepatitis B immune globulin in prevention of perinatal hepatitis B virus transmission. *JAMA* 257:2612–2616, 1987.

Stevenson, J. C., and Duquesnoy, R. J.: Distribution of HLA antigens in Polish and German populations in Milwaukee, Wisconsin. *Am. J. Phys. Anthropol.* 50:19–22, 1979.

Stevenson, J. C., Brown, R. J., and Schanfield, M. S.: Surname analysis as a sampling method for recovery of genetic information. *Hum. Biol.* 55:219–225, 1983.

Stevenson, J. C., Schanfield, M. S., and Sandler, S. G.: Immunoglobulin allotypes in Jewish populations living in Israel and the United States. *Am. J. Phys. Anthropol.* 67:195–207, 1985.

Stewart, J. S. W., Matutes, E., Lampert, I. A., Goolden, A. W. G., and Catovsky, D.: HTLV-I-positive T-cell lymphoma–leukemia in an African resident in UK. *Lancet* 2:984–985, 1984.

Strogatz, D. S., and James, S. A.: Social support and hypertension among blacks and whites in a rural, southern community. *Am. J. Epidemiol.* 124:949–956, 1986.

Suarez, B. K., Crouse, J. D., and O'Rourke, D. H.: Genetic variation in North Amerindian populations: The geography of gene frequencies. *Am. J. Phys. Anthropol.* 67:217–232, 1985a.

Suarez, B. K., O'Rourke, D. H., and Crouse, J. D.: Genetic variation in North Amerindian populations: Association with sociocultural complexity. *Am. J. Phys. Anthropol.* 67:233–239, 1985b.

Suarez, L., and Martin, J.: Primary liver cancer mortality and incidence in Texas Mexican Americans, 1969–80. *Am. J. Public Health* 77:631–633, 1987.

Sumithran, E., and Looi, L. M.: Race-related morphologic variations in hepatocellular carcinoma. *Cancer* 56:1124–1127, 1985.

Summers, K. M.: DNA polymorphisms in human populations: A review. *Ann. Hum. Biol.* 14:203–217, 1987.

Sun, S.: Epidemiology of hypertension on the Tibetan plateau. *Hum. Biol.* 58:507–515, 1986.

Susser, M.: Apartheid and the causes of death: Disentangling ideology and laws from class and race. *Am. J. Public Health* 73:581–584, 1983.

Susser, M., Watson, W., and Hopper, K.: *Medical Sociology.* New York, Oxford University Press, 1985.

Sutherland, C. M., and Mather, F. J.: Long-term survival and prognostic factors in patients with regional breast cancer (skin, muscle, and/or chest wall attachment). *Cancer* 55:1389–1397, 1985.

Svejgaard, A., Platz, P., and Ryder, L. P.: HLA and disease—1982. A survey. *Immunol. Rev.* 70:193–218, 1983.

Swart, S., Briggs, R. S., and Millac, P. A.: Tuberculous meningitis in Asian patients. *Lancet* 2:15–16, 1981.

Swift, P. G. F.: Cot death in Hong Kong. *Lancet* 1:498, 1986.

Szathmary, E. J. E.: Genetic markers in Siberian and northern North American populations. *Yearbook Phys. Anthropol.* 24:37–73, 1981.

Szathmary, E. J. E., Ritenbaugh, C., and Goodby, C. S. M.: Dietary change and plasma glucose levels in an Amerindian population undergoing cultural transition. *Soc. Sci. Med.* 24:791–804, 1987.

Szatrowski, T. P., Peterson, A. V. Jr., Shimizi, Y., et al.: Serum cholesterol, other risk factors, and cardiovascular disease in a Japanese cohort. *J. Chron. Dis.* 37:569–584, 1984.

Szczeklik, A., Dishinger, P., Kueppers, P., et al.: Blood fibrinolytic activity, social class and habitual physical activity. II. A study of black and white men in southern Georgia. *J. Chron. Dis.* 33:291–299, 1980.

Szklo, M., Gordis, L., Tonascia, J., et al.: The changing survivorship of white and black children with leukemia. *Cancer* 42:59–66, 1978.

Tait, B. D., Popert, D. N., Harrison, L., et al.: Interaction between HLA antigens and immunoglobulin (Gm) allotypes in susceptibility to Type I diabetes. *Tissue Antigens* 27:249–255, 1986.

Takahashi, E.: Secular trend of female body shape in Japan. *Hum. Biol.* 58:293–301, 1986.

Takematsu, H., Tomita, Y., Kato, T., et al.: Melanoma in Japan: Experience at Tohoku University Hospital, Sendai. In Balch, C. M., and Milton, G. W. (eds.), *Cutaneous Melanoma.* Philadelphia, Lippincott, 1984, pp. 499–505.

Tamashiro, H., Arakaki, M., Futatsuka, M., et al.: Methylmercury exposure and mortality in southern Japan: A close look at causes of death. *J. Epidemiol. Community Health* 40:181–185, 1986.

Taylor, H. R., West, S. K., Katala, S., et al.: Trachoma: Evaluation of a new grading scheme in the United Republic of Tanzania. *Bull. WHO* 65:485–488, 1987.

Taylor, W. R., Kalisa, R., Ma-Disu, M., et al.: Measles control efforts in urban Africa complicated by high incidence of measles in the first year of life. *Am. J. Epidemiol.* 127:788–794, 1988.

Teklehaimanot, A.: Chloroquine-resistant *Plasmodium falciparum* malaria in Ethiopia. *Lancet* 2:127–129, 1986.

Terasaki, P. I.: *Histocompatibility Testing 1980.* Report of the Eighth International Histocompatibility Workshop Held in Los Angeles, CA, Feb. 4–10, 1980. Los Angeles, UCLA Tissue Typing Laboratory, 1980.

Teuscher, T., Baillod, P., Rosman, J. B., et al.: Absence of diabetes in a rural West African population with a high carbohydrate/cassava diet. *Lancet* 1:765–768, 1987.

Textor, R. B.: *A Cross-Cultural Summary.* New Haven, CT, Human Relations Area File Press, 1967.

Thelle, D. S., and Forde, O. H.: The cardiovascular study in Finnmark County: Coronary risk factors and the occurrence of myocardial infarction in first degree relatives and in subjects of different ethnic origin. *Am. J. Epidemiol.* 110:708–715, 1979.

Thernstrom, S. (ed.): *Harvard Encyclopedia of American Ethnic Groups.* Cambridge, MA, Harvard University Press, 1980.

Thiele, M., Geddes, M. E., Nobmann, E., et al.: High prevalence of iron deficiency anemia among Alaskan native children. *MMWR* 37:200–202, 1988.

Thind, I. S.: Diet and cancer—an international study. *Int. J. Epidemiol.* 15:160–163, 1986.

Thind, I. S., Najem, R., Paradiso, J., and Fuerman, M.: Cancer among blacks in Newark, New Jersey, 1970–1977. A national and international comparison. *Cancer* 50:180–186, 1982.

Thom, T. J., Epstein, F. H., Feldman, J. J., and Leaverton, P. E.: Trends in total mortality and mortality from heart disease in 26 countries from 1950 to 1978. *Int. J. Epidemiol.* 14:510–520, 1985.

Thomas, J. D., Doucette, M. M., Thomas, D. C., et al.: Disease, lifestyle, and consanguinity in 58 American Gypsies. *Lancet* 1:377–379, 1987.

Thompson, M. H.: The role of diet in relation to faecal bile acid concentration and large bowel cancer. In Malt, R. A., and Williamson, B. C. N. (eds.), *Colonic Carcinogenesis.* Boston, MTP Press, 1982, pp. 31–46.

Thompson, S. E., and Washington, A. E.: Epidemiology of sexually transmitted *Chlamydia trachomatis* infections. *Epidemiol. Rev.* 5:96–123, 1983.

Thomson, G.: The human histocompatibility system: Anthropological considerations. *Am. J. Phys. Anthropol.* 62:81–89, 1983.

Thomson, N.: Aboriginal health—current status. *Aust. N.Z. J. Med.* 14:705–718, 1984.

Thylefors, B.: A simplified methodology for the assessment of blindness and its main causes. *World Health Stat. Q.* 40:129–134, 1987.

Tielsch, J. M., West, K. P. Jr., Katz, J., Chirambo, M. C., et al.: Prevalence and severity of xerophthalmia in southern Malawi. *Am. J. Epidemiol.* 124:561–568, 1986.

Tikhomirov, E.: Meningococcal meningitis: Global situation and control measures. *World Health Stat. Q.* 40:98–109, 1987.

Tills, D., Kopec, A. C., and Tills, R. E.: *The Distribution of the Human Blood Groups and Other Polymorphisms, Supplement 1.* Oxford, U.K., Oxford University Press, 1983a.

Tills, D., Warlow, A., Lord, J. M., et al.: Genetic factors in the population of Plati, Greece. *Am. J. Phys. Anthropol.* 61:145–156, 1983b.

Ting, R. Y.: Diseases of the Chinese. In Rothschild, H. (ed.), *Biocultural Aspects of Disease.* New York, Academic Press, 1981, pp. 327–355.

Titus, E. A. B., Hunt, J. A., and Hsia, Y. E.: Alpha-thalassemia variants and quadruple zeta-genes in a Laotian population. *Am. J. Hum. Genet.* 41:A317, 1987.

Tiwari, J. L., and Terasaki, P. I.: *HLA and Disease Associations.* New York, Springer-Verlag, 1985.

Tokudome, S., Kono, S., Ikeda, M., et al.: Cancer and other causes of death among leprosy patients. *JNCI* 67:285–289, 1981.

Toukanm, A. U., and Schable, C. A.: Human immunodeficiency virus (HIV) infection in Jordan: A seroprevalence study. *Int. J. Epidemiol.* 16:462–465, 1987.

Trent, R. J., Buchanan, J. G., Webb, A., et al.: Globin genes are useful markers to identify genetic similarities between Fijians and Pacific Islanders from Polynesia and Melanesia. *Am. J. Hum. Genet.* 42:601–607, 1988.

Trevino, F. M.: Standardized terminology for Hispanic populations. *Am. J. Public Health* 77:69–72, 1987.

Trevisan, M., Ostrow, D., Cooper, R. S., et al.: Sex and race differences in sodium–lithium countertransport and red cell sodium concentration. *Am. J. Epidemiol.* 120:537–541, 1984.

Tsega, E., Mengesha, B., Hansson, B. G., et al.: Hepatitis A,B, and delta infection in Ethiopia: A serologic survey with demographic data. *Am. J. Epidemiol.* 123:344–351, 1986.

Tsui, L. C., Buetow, K., and Buchwald, M.: Genetic analysis of cystic fibrosis using linked DNA markers. *Am. J. Hum. Genet.* 39:720–728, 1986.

Tsuji, S., Choudary, P. V., Martin, B. M., et al.: A mutation in the human glucocerebrosidase gene in neuropathic Gaucher's disease. *N. Engl. J. Med.* 316:570–575, 1987.

Tsukuma, H., Oshima, A., Hiyama, T., et al.: Time trends of the prevalences of hepatitis B e antigen positives among hepatitis B virus carriers in Japan. *Int. J. Epidemiol.* 16:579–583, 1987.

Tunstall-Pedoe, H.: The World Health Organization MONICA project (monitoring trends and determinants in cardiovascular disease): A major international collaboration. *J. Clin. Epidemiol.* 41:105–114, 1988.

Tuomilehto, J., Geboers, J., Joosens, J. V., et al.: Trends in stroke and stomach cancer in Austria compared to selected Eastern and Western European countries. *Cancer Detect. Prev.* 10:311–319, 1987.

Tyroler, H. A.: Race, education, and 5-year mortality in HDFP stratum I referred-care males. In Gross, F., and Strasser, T. (eds.), *Mild Hypertension: Recent Advances.* New York, Raven Press, 1983, pp. 163–176.

Tyroler, H. A., Knowles, M. G., Wing, S. B., et al.: Ischemic heart disease risk factors and twenty-year mortality in middle-age Evans County black males. *Am. Heart J.* 108:738–746, 1984.

Ubukata, T., Oshima, A., and Fujimoto, I.: Mortality among Koreans living in Osaka, Japan, 1973–1982. *Int. J. Epidemiol.* 15:218–225, 1986.

Ueshima, H., Kitada, M., Iida, M., et al.: Serum total cholesterol triglyceride level and dietary intake in Japanese students aged 15 years. *Am. J. Epidemiol.* 116:343–352, 1982.

Ueshima, H., Tatara, K., and Asakura, S.: Declining mortality from ischemic heart disease and changes in coronary risk factors in Japan, 1956–1980. *Am. J. Epidemiol.* 125:62–72, 1987.

Valenzuela, C. Y.: Pubertal origin of the larger sex dimorphism for adult stature in a Chilean population. *Am. J. Phys. Anthropol.* 60:53–60, 1983.

Van Ark, G. N., and Howells, W. W. (eds.): *Multivariate Statistical Methods in Physical Anthropology.* Hingham, MA, Kluwer Academic, 1984.

Van Griensven, G. J. P., Tielman, R. A. P., Goudsmit, J., et al.: Risk factors and prevalence of HIV antibodies in homosexual men in the Netherlands. *Am. J. Epidemiol.* 125:1048–1057, 1987.

Van Itallie, T. B.: Health implications of overweight and obesity in the United States. *Ann. Intern. Med.* 103:983–988, 1985.

Vanlandingham, M. J., Buehler, J. W., Hogue, C. J. R., et al.: Birthweight-specific infant mortality for native Americans compared with whites, six states, 1980. *Am. J. Public Health* 78:499–503, 1988.

Vega, W., Warheit, G., Buhl-Auth, J., and Meinhardt, K.: The prevalence of depressive symptoms among Mexican Americans and Anglos. *Am. J. Epidemiol.* 120:592–607, 1984.

Vega, W., Sallis, J. F., Patterson, T., et al.: Assessing knowledge of cardiovascular health-related diet and exercise behaviors in Anglo- and Mexican-Americans. *Prev. Med.* 16:696–709, 1987.

Velema, J. P., and Walker, A. M.: The age curve of nervous system tumor incidence in adults: Common shape but changing levels by sex, race and geographical location. *Int. J. Epidemiol.* 16:177–183, 1987.

Vital Statistics of the United States 1980 and 1985, Vol. II: *Mortality*. Hyattsville, MD, U.S. Department of Health and Human Services, Public Health Service, National Center for Health Statistics, 1985 and 1988.

Vitale, E., Devoto, M., Mastella, G., et al.: Homogeneity of cystic fibrosis in Italy. *Am. J. Hum. Genet.* 39:832–836, 1986.

Vittecoq, D., May, T., Roue, R. T., et al.: Acquired immunodeficiency syndrome after travelling in Africa: An epidemiological study in seventeen Caucasian patients. *Lancet* 1:612–614, 1987.

Volberding, P. A., Abrams, D. I., Conant, M., et al.: Vinblastine therapy for Kaposi's sarcoma in the acquired immunodeficiency syndrome. *Ann. Intern. Med.* 103:335–338, 1985.

Voss, R., Herz, B., and Chemke, J.: Study of DNA markers linked to the cystic fibrosis gene in 19 Israeli families. *Am. J. Hum. Genet.* 41:A109, 1987.

Wachter, W., Mvungi, M., Konig, A., et al.: Prevalence of goitre and hypothyroidism in southern Tanzania: Effect of iodised oil on thyroid hormone deficiency. *J. Epidemiol. Community Health* 40:86–90, 1986.

Wafula, E. M., and Onyango, F. E.: Acute respiratory infections in developing countries. *East Afr. Med. J.* 63:211–219, 1986.

Wahrendorf, J., Munoz, N., Bang, L. J., et al.: Blood, retinol and zinc riboflavin status in relation to precancerous lesions of the esophagus: Findings from a vitamin intervention trial in the People's Republic of China. *Cancer Res.* 48:2280–2283, 1988.

Walensky, N. A., and O'Brien, M. P.: Anatomical factors relative to the racial selectivity of femoral neck fracture. *Am. J. Phys. Anthropol.* 28:93–96, 1968.

Walker, A. R. P., and Walker, B. F.: Coronary heart disease in Indians overseas. *Lancet* 2:158, 1986.

Walker, A. R. P., Walker, B. F., and Walker, A. J.: Faecal pH, dietary fibre intake, and proneness to colon cancer in four South African populations. *Br. J. Cancer* 53:489–495, 1986.

Wallace, D. C., Garrison, K., and Knowler, W. C.: Dramatic founder effects in Amerindian mitochondrial DNAs. *Am. J. Phys. Anthropol.* 68:149–155, 1985.

Wallace, R. E., and Anderson, R. A.: Blood lipids, lipid-related measures, and the risk of atherosclerotic cardiovascular disease. *Epidemiol. Rev.* 9:95–119, 1987.

Walters, T. R., Bushmore, M., and Simon, J.: Poor prognosis in Negro children with acute lymphocytic leukemia. *Cancer* 29:210–214, 1972.

Wang, J., Palmer, R. M., and Chung, C. S.: The role of major gene in clubfoot. *Am. J. Hum. Genet.* 42:772–776, 1988.

Wang, F. W., Yu, Z. Q., Xy, J. J., et al.: HLA and hypertrophic Hashimoto's thyroiditis in Shanghai Chinese. *Tissue Antigens* 32:235–236, 1988.

Wangsuphachart, V., Thomas, D. B., Koetsawang, A., et al.: Risk factors for invasive cervical cancer and reduction of risk by 'Pap' smears in Thai women. *Int. J. Epidemiol.* 16:362–366, 1987.

Wan-Sheng, L., Gong-Shao, Y., and Zi-zhi, L.: Cigarette smoking divided by professional groups in Beijing. *Chin. Med. J.* 99:15–20, 1986.

Ward, J. I., Lum, M. K. W., Margolis, H. S., Fraser, D. W., et al.: Haemophilus influenzae disease in Alaskan Eskimos: Characteristics of a population with an unusual incidence of invasive disease. *Lancet* 1:1281–1285, 1981.

Ward, R. H., Marshall, H. W., Leppert, M., et al.: Apolipoprotein genes, lipid profiles and risk of coronary heart disease (CHD). *Am. J. Hum. Genet.* 41:A110, 1987.

Warshauer, M. E., Silverman, D. T., Schottenfeld, D., and Pollack, E. S.: Stomach and colorectal cancers in Puerto Rican-born residents of New York City. *JNCI* 76:591–595, 1986.

Wassermann, H. P.: Human pigmentation and environmental adaptation. *Arch. Environ. Health* 11:691–694, 1965.

Waterhouse, J., Muir, C., Shanmugaratnam, K., and Powell, J. P.: *Cancer Incidence in Five Continents*, Vol. IV. IARC Publication No. 42. Lyon, France, International Agency for Research on Cancer, 1982.

Watson, D. S.: A case of sorcery. *Lancet* 1:1289–1290, 1984.

Watt, G., Adapon, B., Long, G. W., et al.: Praziquantel in treatment of cerebral schistosomiasis. *Lancet* 2:529–532, 1986.

Watts, E. S.: The biological race concept and diseases of modern man. In Rothschild, H. (ed.), *Biocultural Aspects of Disease.* New York, Academic Press, 1981, pp. 3–23.

Watts, S. J.: Human behaviour and the transmission of dracunculiasis: A case study from the Ilorin area of Nigeria. *Int. J. Epidemiol.* 15:252–256, 1986.

Weatherall, D. J., and Clegg, J. B.: *The Thalassemia Syndromes.* Oxford, U.K., Blackwell Scientific, 1981.

Webb, S. G., and Thorne, A. G.: A congenital meningocoele in prehistoric Australia. *Am. J. Phys. Anthropol.* 68:525–533, 1985.

Weinberger, J. B., Blazey, D. L., Matthews, T. J., et al.: Adult T-cell leukemia/lymphoma associated with human T-lymphotropic virus type I (HTLV-I) infection—North Carolina. *MMWR* 36:804–812, 1987.

Weiner, J. S.: Nose shape and climate. *Am. J. Phys. Anthropol.* 12:1–4, 1954.

Weisburger, H., Reddy, B. S., Barnes, W. S., et al.: Bile acids, but not neutral sterols, are tumor promoters in the colon in man and in rodents. *Environ. Health Perspect.* 50:101–107, 1983.

Weiss, K. M.: Phenotypic amplification, as illustrated by cancer of the gallbladder in New World peoples. In Chakraborty, R., and Szathmary, E. J. E. (eds.), *Diseases of Complex Etiology in Small Populations.* New York, Alan R. Liss, 1985, pp. 179–198.

Weiss, K. M., Ferrell, R. E., and Hanis, C. L.: A New World syndrome of metabolic diseases with a genetic and evolutionary basis. *Yearbook Phys. Anthropol.* 27:153–178, 1984.

Weiss, K. M., Chakraborty, R., Smouse, P. E., et al.: Familial aggregation of cancer in Laredo, Texas: A generally low-risk Mexican-American population. *Genet. Epidemiol.* 3:121–143, 1986.

Weiss, K. M., Georges, E., Aguirre, A., et al.: Cleft lip/palate in Mayans of the state of Campeche, Mexico. *Hum. Biol.* 59:775–783, 1987.

Welte, J. W., and Abel, E. I.: Homicide and race in Erie County, New York. *Am. J. Epidemiol.* 124:666–670, 1986.

Westermeyer, J.: Prevention of mental disorder among Hmong refugees in the U.S.: Lessons from the period 1976–1986. *Soc. Sci. Med.* 25:941–947, 1987.

Westermeyer, J.: A matched pair study of depression among Hmong refugees with particular reference to predisposing factors and treatment outcome. *Soc. Psychiatr. Epidemiol.* 23:64–71, 1988.

Westoff, C. F.: Fertility in the United States. *Science* 234:554–559, 1986.

Wienker, C. W.: Admixture in a biologically African caste of black Americans. *Am. J. Phys. Anthropol.* 74:265–273, 1987.

Williams, R. R., and Horm, J. W.: Association of cancer sites with tobacco and alcohol consumption and socioeconomic status of patients: Interview study from the Third National Cancer Survey. *JNCI* 59:525–547, 1977.

Wilson, P. W. F., Savage, D. D., Castelli, W. P., et al.: HDL–cholesterol in a sample of black adults: The Framingham minority study. *Metabolism* 32:328–332, 1983.

Wilson, T. W.: History of salt supplies in West Africa and blood pressures today. *Lancet* 1:784–786, 1986.

Wilson, V., Byam, N., Adam, M., and McFarlane, H.: HLA antigens in diabetics of African descent in Trinidad. *West Indian Med. J.* 35:26, 1986.

Winkleby, M. A., Ragland, D. R., Syme, S. L., et al.: Heightened risk of hypertension among black males: The masking effects of covariables. *Am. J. Epidemiol.* 128:1075–1083, 1988.

Winter, W. E., MacLaren, N. K., Riley, W. J., et al.: Maturity-onset diabetes of youth in black Americans. *N. Engl. J. Med.* 316:285–291, 1987.

Winter, W. P. (ed.): *Hemoglobin Variants in Human Populations*, 2 Vols. Boca Raton, FL, CRC Press, 1986.

Wise, P. H., Kotelchuck, M., Wilson, M., et al.: Racial and socioeconomic disparities in childhood mortality in Boston. *N. Engl. J. Med.* 313:360–366, 1985.

Wissow, L. S., Gittelsohn, A. M., Szklo, M., et al.: Poverty, race and hospitalization for childhood asthma. *Am. J. Public Health* 78:777–782, 1988.

Wong, P. C. N.: Epidemiology of fractures of bones of the forearm in a mixed South East Asian community, Singapore. 1. A preliminary study. *Acta Orthop. Scand.* 36:153–167, 1965.

Wong, P. C. N.: Fracture epidemiology in a mixed southeastern Asian community (Singapore). *Clin. Orthop.* 45:55–61, 1966.

Wood, C. S.: ABO blood groups related to selection of human hosts by yellow fever vector. *Hum. Biol.* 48:337–341, 1976.

Woodfield, D. G., Simpson, L. A., Seber, G. A. F., et al.: Blood groups and other genetic markers in New Zealand Europeans and Maoris. *Ann. Hum. Biol.* 14:29–37, 1987.

Woodruff, A. W., Suni, A. E., Kaku, M., Adamson, E. A., Maughan, T. S., and Bundru, N.: Infants in Juba, southern Sudan: The first twelve months of life. *Lancet* 2:506–509, 1984.

Woodruff, A. W., Suni, A. E., Kaku, M., Adamson, E. A., et al.: Children in Juba, southern Sudan: The second and third years of life. *Lancet* 2:615–618, 1986.

Woolhandler, S., Himmelstein, D. V., Silber, R., et al.: Medical care and mortality: Racial differences in preventable deaths. *Int. J. Health Serv.* 15:1–11, 1985.

World Health Organization (WHO): *The International Pilot Study of Schizophrenia*, Vol. 1. Geneva, WHO, 1973.

World Health Organization (WHO): *International Statistical Classification of Diseases, Injuries and Causes of Death*, 9th Rev., Vol. 1. Geneva, WHO, 1977.

World Health Organization (WHO): *Apartheid and Health*. Geneva, WHO, 1983.

World Health Organization (WHO): *Targets for Health for All 2000*. Copenhagen, WHO, 1985.

World Health Organization (WHO): Major parasitic infections: A global view. *World Health Statist. Q.* 39:145–160, 1986.

World Health Organization (WHO): *World Health Statistics Annual.* Geneva, WHO, 1987.

Wright, E. J., and Whitehead, T. L.: Perceptions of body size and obesity: A selected review of the literature. *J. Community Health* 12:117–128, 1987.

Wright, W. E., Bernstein, L., Peters, J. M., et al.: Adenocarcinoma of the stomach and exposure to occupational dust. *Am. J. Epidemiol.* 128:64–73, 1988.

Wyndham, C. H.: Comparison and ranking of cancer mortality rates in the various populations of the RSA in 1970. *S. Afr. Med. J.* 67:584–587, 1985.

Xiao, X., Cao, M., Miller, T., et al.: Papillovirus DNA in cervical carcinoma specimens from central China. *Lancet* 2:902, 1988.

Xu, Z. Y., and Blot, W. J.: Geographic variation of female lung cancer in China. *Am. J. Public Health* 76:1250–1251, 1986.

Yanagawa, H., Nakamura, Y., Kawasaki, T., et al.: Nationwide epidemic of Kawasaki disease in Japan during winter of 1985–86. *Lancet* 2:1138–1139, 1986.

Yang, L., Zuo, C., Su, L. S., and Eaton, M. T.: Depression in Chinese inpatients. *Am. J. Psychiatry* 144:226–228, 1987.

Yankauer, A.: Hispanic/Latino—what's in a name? *Am. J. Public Health* 77:15–17, 1987.

Yano, K., Blackwelder, W. C., Kagan, A., et al.: Childhood cultural experiences and the incidence of coronary heart disease in Hawaii Japanese men. *Am. J. Epidemiol.* 109:440–450, 1979.

Yano, K., Reed, D. M., and McGee, D. L.: Ten-year incidence of coronary heart disease in the Honolulu heart program. *Am. J. Epidemiol.* 119:653–666, 1984.

Yano, K., MacLean, C. J., Reed, D. M., et al.: A comparison of the 12-year mortality and predictive factors of coronary heart disease among Japanese men in Japan and Hawaii. *Am. J. Epidemiol.* 127:476–487, 1988.

Yao, S., and Huang, L.: Neuroepidemiologic survey in Nanning suburbs of Guangxi Zhuang autonomous region, People's Republic of China. *Neuroepidemiology* 5:50–51, 1988.

Yates, M. D., Grange, J. M., and Collins, C. H.: The nature of mycobacterial disease in south east England, 1977–84. *J. Epidemiol. Community Health* 40:295–300, 1986.

Yeh, F. S., Mo, C. C., Luo, S., et al.: A serological case-control study of primary hepatocellular carcinoma in Guangxi, China. *Cancer Res.* 45:872–873, 1985.

Yelin, E. H., Kramer, J. S., and Epstein, W. V.: Is health care use equivalent across social groups? A diagnosis-based study. *Am. J. Public Health* 73:563–571, 1983.

Yiping, S., and Changxing, S.: HLA polymorphisms in Beijing Chinese. *Tissue Antigens* 25:115–118, 1985.

Yoshida, S., Mulder, D. W., Kurland, L. T., et al.: Follow-up study on amyotrophic lateral sclerosis in Rochester, Minn., 1925 through 1984. *Neuroepidemiology* 5:61–70, 1986.

Young, J. L. Jr., Percy, C. L., and Asire, A. J. (eds.): *Surveillance, Epidemiology and End Results: Incidence and Mortality Data, 1973–77*, NIH Publication No. 81-2330. Bethesda, MD, U.S. Department of Health and Human Services, Public Health Service, 1981.

Young, J. L. Jr., Ries, L. G., and Pollack, E. S.: Cancer patient survival among ethnic groups in the United States. *JNCI* 73:341–352, 1984.

Young, S. A., and Kaufman, M.: Promoting breastfeeding at a migrant center. *Am. J. Public Health* 78:523–525, 1988.

Young, T. K., and Frank, J. W.: Cancer surveillance in a remote Indian population in northwestern Ontario. *Am. J. Public Health* 73:515–520, 1983.

Yu, M. C., Ho, J. H. C., Lang, S. H., and Henderson, B. E.: Cantonese-style salted fish as a cause of nasopharyngeal cancer in Hong Kong. *Cancer Res.* 46:956–961, 1986.

Yuan, J. M., Yu, M. C., Ross, R. K., et al.: Risk factors for breast cancer in Chinese women in Shanghai. *Cancer Res.* 48:1949–1953, 1988.

Zagury, D., Bernard, J., Leonard, R., et al.: Long-term cultures of HTLV-III-infected T cell depletion and AIDS. *Science* 231:850–853, 1986.

Zahavi, I., Goldbourt, U., Cohen-Mandelzweig, L., et al.: Distributions of total cholesterol, triglycerides, and high-density lipoprotein cholesterol in Israeli Jewish children of different geographic–ethnic origins, ages 9–17 years. *Prev. Med.* 16:35–51, 1987.

Zemel, B. S., and Katz, S. H.: The contribution of adrenal and gonadal androgens to the growth in height of adolescent males. *Am. J. Phys. Anthropol.* 71:459–466, 1986.

Zemer, D., Pras, M., Sohar, E., et al.: Colchicine in the prevention and treatment of the amyloidosis of familial Mediterranean fever. *N. Engl. J. Med.* 314:1001–1005, 1986.

Zeng, Y. T., and Huang, S. Z.: Disorders of haemoglobin in China. *J. Med. Genet.* 24:578–583, 1987.

Zeng, Y. T., Ren, Z. R., Chen, M. J., et al.: A new unstable haemoglobin variant: Hb Shanghai [B131(H9)Gln—Pro] found in China. *Br. J. Haematol.* 67:221–223, 1987.

Zhang, J. Z., Cai, S. P., He, X., et al.: Molecular basis of β thalassemia in South China. *Hum. Hered.* 78:37–40, 1988.

Zheng, W., Blot, W. J., Liao, M. L., et al.: Lung cancer and prior tuberculosis infection in Shanghai. *Br. J. Cancer* 56:501–504, 1987.

Ziegler, R. G., Devesa, S. S., and Fraumeni, J. F. Jr.: Epidemiologic patterns of colorectal cancer. In Devita, V. T. Jr., Hellman, S., and Rosenberg, S. A. (eds.), *Important Advances in Oncology.* Philadelphia, J. B. Lippincott, 1986, pp. 209–232.

Zimmet, P., Kirk, R., Serjeantson, S., et al.: Diabetes in Pacific populations—genetic and environmental interactions. In Melish, J. S., Hanna, J., and Baba, S. (eds.), *Genetic Environmental Interactions in Diabetes Mellitus.* Amsterdam, Excerpta Medica, 1982, pp. 9–17.

Zimmet, P., Taylor, R., Ram, P., et al.: Prevalence of diabetes and impaired glucose tolerance in the biracial (Melanesian and Indian) population of Fiji: A rural–urban comparison. *Am. J. Epidemiol.* 118:673–688, 1983.

Zimmet, P., King, H., Serjeantson, S., et al.: The genetics of diabetes mellitus. *Aust. N.Z. J. Med.* 16:419–424, 1986.

Zimmet, P., Finch, C. F., Schooneveldt, M. G., et al.: Mortality from diabetes in Nauru—results of 4-year follow-up. *Diabetes Care* 11:305–310, 1988.

Zollinger, T. W., Phillips, R. L., and Kuzma, J. W.: Breast cancer survival rates among Seventh Day Adventists and non-Seventh Day Adventists. *Am. J. Epidemiol.* 119:503–509, 1984.

Zunzunegui, M. V., King, M. C., Coria, C. F., and Charlet, J.: Male influences on cervical cancer risk. *Am. J. Epidemiol.* 123:302–307, 1986.

Zurayk, H., Halabi, S., and Deeb, M.: Measures of social class based on education for use in health studies in developing countries. *J. Epidemiol. Community Health* 41:173–179, 1987.

Index

Italic *f* following a page number denotes a figure.